MANUAL OF
EMERGENCY
MEDICINE

MANUAL OF EMERGENCY MEDICINE

MICHAEL JAY BRESLER, MD, FACEP
Clinical Professor
Division of Emergency Medicine
Stanford University School of Medicine
Stanford, California
Chief, Department of Emergency Medicine
Mills-Peninsula Hospitals
Burlingame, California

GEORGE L. STERNBACH, MD, FACEP
Clinical Professor
Division of Emergency Medicine
Stanford University Medical Center
Stanford, California
Emergency Physician
Seton Medical Center
Daly City, California

SIXTH EDITION

with 57 illustrations

a mosby handbook

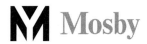

Mosby

An Affiliate of Elsevier Science

St. Louis   London   Philadelphia   Sydney   Toronto

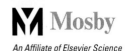

Mosby

An Affiliate of Elsevier Science

Publisher: Anne S. Patterson
Editor: Kathryn H. Falk
Developmental Editor: Carolyn M. Kruse
Project Manager: Carol Sullivan Weis
Production Editor: Rick Dudley
Series Design: Renée Duenow
Design Manager: Jen Marmarinos
Manufacturing Manager: Dave Graybill

SIXTH EDITION
Copyright © 1998 by Mosby, Inc.

Previous editions copyrighted 1963, 1968, 1973, 1983, 1989

Note: The authors and publisher of this book have made every effort to ensure that the recommended drug dosage schedules presented are accurate and in accord with sound medical practice. Because new research and experience may lead to changes in drug therapy, however, the reader is advised to verify drug dosage schedules in the manufacturer's product information insert prior to administration of the drug. This is particularly important for new or infrequently used drugs. It remains the responsibility of the physician to ascertain the suitability of the drugs and dosage regimens.

Printed in the United States of America

Mosby, Inc.
11830 Westline Industrial Drive
St. Louis, Missouri 63146

ISBN 0-8151-1142-8

02   03   04   05   /   9   8   7   6   5   4

To Benjamin, Aaron, and Adrienne
and
To Joshua and Rebecca

For their daily reminder of what life is really about

Preface

This book can be used either as a quick bedside guide for the evaluation and treatment of nearly any patient who presents to an emergency department or as a brief textbook of emergency medicine. It is equally useful for the emergency medicine specialist, as well as for the primary care physician confronted with medical or surgical emergencies. House officers, residents in training, and medical students will find it invaluable, whether they are specializing in emergency medicine or just rotating through the ED as part of their education. Emergency nurses and paramedics will also find the book useful for background, as well as for diagnostic and treatment regimens.

The sixth edition represents an extensive revision of the book. We have totally rewritten many chapters and updated all the rest. The rewritten chapters include Shock; Overview of Major Trauma; Abdominal Trauma; Cardiac Emergencies; Respiratory Emergencies; Abdominal Emergencies; Pediatric Emergencies; and Altered Level of Consciousness, Metabolic Encephalopathy, and Neurologic Emergencies. We have updated the discussion of immunosuppressed patients, including those with HIV, and have added a new chapter on the ED evaluation of the patient with a history of organ transplantation.

We have included the latest diagnostic and therapeutic modalities, even "stopping the presses" to add drugs just approved by the FDA after the manuscript had been delivered to the publisher.

We have tried to cover all the important aspects of Emergency Medicine, giving equal emphasis to both traumatic and nontraumatic emergencies, to both critical and urgent and not-so-urgent disorders—essentially to the broad spectrum of problems for which emergency patients seek our help.

A particularly unique aspect of this book is the inclusion of clinical pathways formulated by the American College of Emergency Physicians (ACEP). Although such pathways are admittedly controversial, they are here to stay; and all physicians will have to become familiar with the concept, as well as the reality, of diagnostic and treatment protocols. It is our opinion that if they are well written, clinical pathways can help all of us provide the best possible care for our patients. It is also our opinion that such pathways are best written by those who will use them in the real world. It is for this reason that we have included the Quick Reference Forms written by ACEP to summarize their Clinical Policies.

While the sixth edition is in many ways an entirely new book, we would like to give credit to the initial author of the first three editions, John Schneewind, M.D., who had the vision to create a clinical manual for the treatment of medical and surgical emergencies before the field of Emergency Medicine even existed. We would also like to thank our former colleague Michael Eliastam, M.D., with whom we co-authored the fourth and fifth editions. The book still bears the strong influence of both of these physicians.

We hope this book will be your friend, a companion to help keep both you and your patients secure when the library is closed, when the consultants are asleep—when it is just you in the "pit" at 3AM. We are both veteran emergency physicians, each with more than two decades' experience teaching Emergency Medicine in major academic centers, as well as practicing our specialty in the community hospital setting. We know what it is like to be alone with a difficult patient and no one else to turn to for assistance.

We hope this book will provide that assistance.

Michael Jay Bresler, MD, FACEP
George L. Sternbach, MD, FACEP

Contents

Part One: Overview, *1*
1. Shock, *3*
2. Electrolyte and Acid-Base Disorders, *10*

Part Two: Traumatic Emergencies, *27*
3. Overview of Major Trauma, *29*
4. Thoracic Trauma, *32*
5. Abdominal Trauma, *46*
6. Genitourinary Tract Trauma, *49*
7. Neurologic Trauma, *53*
8. Orthopedic Trauma, *60*
9. Hand Injuries, *70*
10. Facial Injuries, *81*
11. Ophthalmologic Injuries, *88*
12. Anesthesia, Analgesia, and Sedation, *92*
13. Laceration Repair, *106*
14. Soft Tissue Infections, *113*

Part Three: Nontraumatic Emergencies, *122*
15. Cardiac Emergencies, *124*
16. Vascular Emergencies (Traumatic and Nontraumatic), *155*
17. Respiratory Emergencies, *163*
18. Abdominal Emergencies, *185*
19. Genitourinary Tract Emergencies, *197*
20. Gynecologic and Obstetric Emergencies, *203*
21. Altered Level of Consciousness, Metabolic Encephalopathy, and Neurologic Emergencies, *211*
22. Head and Neck Emergencies, *233*
23. Ophthalmologic Emergencies, *242*
24. AIDS and Oncologic and Hematologic Emergencies, *246*
25. Emergencies in the Patient With Prior Organ Transplant, *266*
26. Dermatologic Emergencies, *271*
27. Environmental Emergencies, *281*
28. Poisoning, Overdose, and Envenomation, *291*
29. Psychiatric Emergencies, *329*
30. Pediatric Emergencies, *347*

Appendix A: Symptom-Oriented Clinical Pathways *363*
American College of Emergency Physicians
Quick Reference Forms for Clinical Policies
Acute Blunt Trauma *365*
Penetrating Extremity Trauma *375*
Chest Pain *379*
Abdominal Pain *389*
Vaginal Bleeding *393*
Headache *400*
Seizure *410*
Toxic Ingestion or Dermal or Inhalation Exposure *417*
Fever in Children Under the Age of 2 Years *422*

Appendix B: Suggested Readings *429*

MANUAL OF
EMERGENCY
MEDICINE

PART I

Overview

1

Shock

I. GENERAL CONSIDERATIONS.

A. Shock is defined as inadequate tissue perfusion to meet the metabolic needs of the cells, usually as a result of low blood pressure.

B. Shock is caused by impairment of one or more of the three components of normal blood pressure:
   1. Low *blood* volume.
   2. *Cardiac* dysfunction.
   3. Alteration of *vessel* lumen diameter.

C. Arterial blood pressure (BP) is proportional to both cardiac output (CO) and peripheral arterial vascular resistance (PVR). In fact, it equals the product of the two.

$$BP = CO \times PVR$$

Since CO = stroke volume (SV) × heart rate (HR), we can define BP:

$$BP = SV \times HR \times PVR$$

D. Shock is caused by the lowering of SV, HR, and/or PVR.

E. The only way that the body can compensate for shock—or that the physician can reverse shock—is to elevate SV, HR, and/or PVR.

II. MECHANISMS OF SHOCK.

A. **Categories of shock.** There are four general categories of shock (Table 1-1):
   1. *Hypovolemic* shock is caused by low blood volume (decreased SV) resulting from hemorrhage or dehydration.
   2. *Cardiogenic* shock is caused by decreased cardiac contractility (decreased SV), usually resulting from massive myocardial infarction (MI). Rhythm disturbance can also cause shock. By decreasing HR, bradycardia directly decreases CO and potentially BP. Although tachycardia is by definition increased HR, this effect may be outweighed by a lowering of SV sufficient to decrease CO and thus cause hypotension. (Tachycardia may leave insufficient time for diastolic filling or myocardial perfusion.) Thus dysrhythmias can cause shock, but the term

TABLE 1-1
Categories of Shock

Type of shock	Mechanism	Etiology
Hypovolemic	Hemorrhage	Internal or external bleeding
	Dehydration	
	Gastrointestinal	Vomiting, diarrhea
	Evaporation	Burns
	Third spacing	Burns, pancreatitis
Cardiogenic	Pump failure	Massive myocardial infarction
Distributive	Loss of vascular tone	Spinal cord trauma
		Sepsis
		Anaphylaxis
		Drug overdose
Obstructive	Obstructed flow through	Pericardial tamponade
	central circulation	Tension pneumothorax
		Pulmonary embolus
		Aortic dissection

      cardiogenic usually implies pump failure resulting from massive MI.

  3. *Distributive* shock is caused by loss of normal arterial tone (decreased PVR) such that blood cannot be distributed throughout the body (e.g., sepsis, anaphylaxis, spinal cord transection, drug overdose, endocrine deficiency).

  4. *Obstructive* shock is caused by obstruction of central circulation (decreased SV; e.g., massive pulmonary embolus, pericardial tamponade, tension pneumothorax, or thoracic aortic dissection, which decreases the effective "SV" distal to the dissection).

B. Compensation. The body compensates by activating the sympathetic branch of the autonomic nervous system, as well as by metabolic mechanisms.

  1. α-adrenergic → vasoconstriction.

    a. Arterial vasoconstriction raises PVR directly. Differential arterial vasoconstriction shunts blood from areas of decreased need (e.g., skin, gut, kidneys) to the crucial organs (e.g., heart, lung, brain).

    b. Venous vasoconstriction decreases circulation time and shunts blood to the arterial circulation. It also increases cardiac preload, thereby increasing contractility (SV) in accordance with the Frank-Starling principle.

  2. β₁-adrenergic → cardiac.

    a. Increased contractility (SV).

    b. Increased HR.

  3. Metabolic activity.

    a. Sodium and water retention by the kidneys (SV).

    b. Mobilization of extravascular fluid into the vessels (SV).

    c. Thirst (SV).

HYPOKALEMIC SHOCK

    d. Over time, increased blood cell production by the bone marrow.

III. CLINICAL FINDINGS.

A. Subjective symptoms are fairly nonspecific: anxiety, restlessness, feeling of impending doom, nausea, weakness, and thirst.

B. Objective findings on examination reflect decreased organ perfusion and compensatory mechanisms.

1. *Tachycardia. Except in patients taking β-blocking medication, and in spinal cord transection above T10, which interrupts sympathetic innervation of the heart.*

2. *Cool, pale, clammy skin with delayed capillary refill. Except in distributive shock, where the primary mechanism is inability to maintain even normal vascular tone. In dark-complected patients, skin color can be evaluated at the nailbeds, palm, or oral mucosa.*

3. *Narrow pulse pressure. This occurs before blood pressure falls and is thus a subtle but crucial sign of impending shock.* Pulse pressure narrows early in *nondistributive* forms of shock as compensatory α-adrenergic vasoconstriction elevates diastolic pressure.

4. *Decreased BP.* Systolic pressure can be maintained at normal levels until 15% to 25% of blood volume is lost, and thus a pulse pressure below 40 mm Hg can be a tip-off of impending hypotension.

5. *Altered mental status, tachypnea, dilated pupils.*

6. *Decreased urine output.*

C. Clinical pearls.

1. Massive hypovolemia can be masked by good compensation, particularly in young people, resulting in temporarily adequate systolic blood pressure. Tachycardia, pulse pressure below 40 mm Hg, and delayed capillary refill may be early warning signs.

2. Failed compensation in the elderly patients, and taking β-blockers, can result in normal pulse rate despite shock.

3. Distributive shock causes warm, perfused skin—unless accompanied by hypovolemia (e.g., spinal cord transection with occult intraabdominal hemorrhage).

4. Spinal cord transection above T10 is often accompanied by bradycardia because normal sympathetic tone to the heart is impaired. Thus paradoxical bradycardia in the presence of hypotension may be a tip-off of cord transection in a comatose patient whose motor function cannot adequately be assessed.

5. Brain injury does not cause shock. Shock accompanying head injury is due to another cause such as occult hemorrhage, massive scalp hemorrhage, or cord transection.

6. Infants can bleed sufficiently into their heads to develop hypovolemic shock because the head is large relative to the rest of their body and because open sutures allow expansion.

7. Hypovolemic shock causes flat neck veins. Shock accompanied by distended neck veins is probably obstructive shock. Evaluate for tension pneumothorax (diminished breath

sounds, tracheal or mediastinal shift) or pericardial tamponade (normal breath sounds).

8. Septic and anaphylactic shock are caused primarily by vasodilation, resulting in distributive shock. However, both may also cause intravascular hypovolemia resulting from increased capillary permeability, as well as impaired cardiac contractility resulting from presumed cardiotoxic substances.

9. Distributive shock typically causes warm, perfused skin, whereas the other types of shock cause cool, pale, often clammy skin. However, impairment of microcirculation in shock can result in a mottled skin appearance. Septic shock is particularly likely to cause this phenomenon.

IV. TREATMENT.

A. General measures.

1. As discussed in Chapter 3, a rapid initial assessment is followed by a more detailed physical examination.

2. Airway, breathing, circulation, and spine are assessed and stabilized as necessary. Oxygen is applied to all patients in shock, and large-bore intravenous lines (IV) are established (except in cardiogenic shock, where major volume expansion may be deleterious).

3. A urinary catheter is inserted and urine output maintained above 50 ml/hr in the adult, 1 ml/kg/hr in children, and 2 ml/kg/hr in infants under 1 year of age.

B. Treatment modalities (Table 1-2).

1. Volume expansion *(hypovolemic and distributive shock) (sometimes used very carefully in cardiogenic shock to increase preload; particularly helpful in right ventricular MI).*

   TRENDELENBURG

   a. Leg elevation.
   b. IV crystalloid, colloid, and blood products.
   c. Medical (or military) antishock trousers (MAST), also known as pneumatic antishock garment (PASG).

2. α-adrenergic vasoconstrictors *(distributive shock).*
   a. Dopamine greater than 10 μg/kg/min, or:
   b. Neosynephrine, norepinephrine, or metaraminol.

3. β₁-adrenergic inotropes *(cardiogenic shock).*
   a. Dopamine 2 to 10 μg/kg/min, or:
   b. Dobutamine 2.5 to 10 μg/kg/min.

4. Specific measures.
   a. Control hemorrhage *(hypovolemic shock).*
   b. Splint fractures *(hypovolemic shock).*
   c. Decompress pneumothorax and pericardial tamponade *(obstructive shock).*   ↑ FOR ACUTE ONSET CVA
   d. Heparin, tissue plasminogen activator (t-PA), and catheter or surgical removal of pulmonary embolus *(obstructive shock).*
   e. Antiallergic measures: diphenhydramine 50 mg IV; epinephrine 0.3 mg subcutaneously (SC) or slow IV *(anaphylactic distributive shock).*
   f. Antibiotics *(septic distributive shock).*

TABLE 1-2
Summary of Shock Treatment Modalities

Type of shock	Volume expansion	α-Adrenergic vasoconstrictors	β₁-Adrenergic inotropes	Other specific measures
Hypovolemic	Yes	No	No	Control hemorrhage Splint fractures
Cardiogenic	No (unless dehydrated or right ventricular MI)	No	Yes	Aortic balloon pump
Distributive	Yes	Yes	No	Antibiotics Antihistamines
Obstructive	Yes	No	No	Decompress: Tamponade Tension pneumothorax

C. Hemorrhagic hypovolemic shock.

1. This is the most common form of shock in the emergency department (ED). Restoring intravascular volume is crucial (as is controlling hemorrhage). IV crystalloid based on sodium is the immediate treatment: 1 to 2 L of normal saline or Ringer's solution for adults or 20 ml/kg for children.

2. Large-bore (14- or 16-gauge), short peripheral IV catheters are most easily used. Even wider catheters (8 French) may be inserted through either peripheral cutdown or centrally via Seldinger wire technique.

3. Colloid agents such as albumin or dextran are usually reserved for a later phase of treatment when the dangers of continued bleeding and capillary leak syndrome diminish. Colloid other than blood is generally not used in the ED.

4. If there is no response to the initial 1 to 2 L of crystalloid, or if massive hemorrhage is obvious, blood replacement is indicated. Packed red cells with normal saline are readily available and are most commonly used. Whole blood is also acceptable.

5. Crossmatched blood (whether packed cells or whole blood) is optimal. However, full crossmatching may take up to an hour, which may be too long in critically bleeding patients. Type-specific blood is generally available within 10 minutes and is fairly safe. If the patient is too unstable to wait even for type-specific blood, type O can be used, preferably O negative, especially for women of childbearing age.

6. If significant amounts of fluid are rapidly administered, prewarming the fluid will help avoid iatrogenic hypothermia. Heating lamps should also be used to help prevent radiant heat loss from the undressed patient's skin.

7. Autotransfusion of noncontaminated blood (e.g., from hemothorax) may be lifesaving. Commercial devices are available.

8. Dilutional coagulopathy may develop in patients receiving massive transfusions because banked blood is devoid of viable platelets and clotting factors V and VIII. Although this is rarely a problem during the ED phase of care, baseline coagulation studies should be obtained to guide later replacement therapy if required.

9. The MAST (PASG) device may be of help, but it is controversial; many authorities do not recommend its use. It reduces blood flow to the legs and possibly the abdomen, thus "shunting" blood to the central circulation. It does not take the place of fluid resuscitation and is contraindicated in pulmonary edema and uncontrolled hemorrhage outside the inflation area. Inflation of the abdominal compartment is contraindicated in pregnancy and diaphragmatic rupture. The device must be deflated slowly beginning with the abdominal compartment, pausing with every 5–mm Hg drop in blood pressure to replace blood volume with IV fluids.

10. Fluid overload should be avoided to prevent adult respiratory distress syndrome in any critically injured patient and cerebral edema in the head injury victim. Some authorities believe that even moderately excessive fluid replacement may interfere with hemostasis at the bleeding sites, the increased hydrostatic pressure "washing out" the clot and causing increased hemorrhage. Care thus should be taken not to raise the blood pressure beyond normal limits with fluid rescuscitation if hemostasis has not yet been achieved.

2

Electrolyte and Acid-Base Disorders

I. ACID-BASE BALANCE.

A. General considerations.
Changes in the acid-base balance are identified by the evaluation of arterial blood gases (ABGs). Nomograms or simple formulas (examples occur throughout the chapter) can be used to define acid-base abnormalities, which may be either acidosis or alkalosis. Both can be produced by respiratory or metabolic causes, and mixed abnormalities may coexist because one may compensate for the effect of the other. The four states are metabolic acidosis, metabolic alkalosis, respiratory acidosis, and respiratory alkalosis. The bicarbonate (HCO_3) level is reported with both the blood gas values and the laboratory electrolyte results. If there is a possibility of a complex abnormality, the electrolyte HCO_3- is more accurate because it is directly measured, whereas the HCO_3- reported with the blood gas evaluation is derived indirectly from pH and PCO_2 levels.

B. Respiratory acidosis.

1. *Mechanism of production.* Hypoventilation resulting from the following:
   a. Retention of CO_2 resulting from primary pulmonary disease (e.g., chronic obstructive pulmonary disease [COPD] or asthma).
   b. Centrally acting drugs interfering with ventilation and producing CO_2 retention.
   c. Neuromuscular diseases, thoracic or spinal trauma, massive obesity, and airway obstruction interfering with ventilation, which leads to CO_2 retention.

2. *Clinical presentation.*
   a. The signs and symptoms of the condition that causes the hypoventilation.
   b. Possible altered level of consciousness resulting from severe CO_2 retention.

c. ABGs.
  (1) $PaCO_2$ elevated above the normal range of 38 to 42 mm Hg; calculate the expected pH for the patient's $PaCO_2$. For every 10 mm Hg above a $PaCO_2$ of 40, the pH usually falls 0.08. For example, for $PaCO_2 = 50$, the calculated or expected pH = 7.32.
  (2) If the patient's pH is significantly below the calculated or expected pH, metabolic acidosis is present in addition to respiratory acidosis or alkalosis.
  (3) If the patient's pH is significantly above the expected value, metabolic alkalosis is present in addition to the respiratory abnormality.
  (4) The PO_2 value should be compared with the expected value for the patient's age:

$$\text{Age-adjusted } PO_2 = 104 - 0.4 \times \text{age}$$

  Because of the shape of the oxyhemoglobin dissociation curve, a PaO_2 above 60 mm Hg is acceptable because it represents 90% saturation. Even small decreases below 60 mm Hg represent significant falls in the saturation level, portending potential tissue hypoxia.

d. Serum electrolytes. The serum bicarbonate level will be normal in the acute setting and elevated in the chronic or compensated state because of reabsorption of bicarbonate by the kidney. Look for anion gap, and consider osmolal gap as well, if clinically appropriate (see Section I, C, 2, b, 3).

3. *Treatment.*
  a. Treat the underlying cause of the hypoventilation.
  b. Improve ventilation by airway suction, bag-valve mask ventilation, and if necessary, nasal or endotracheal intubation.
  c. Rarely is $NaHCO_3$ administration indicated for pure respiratory acidosis. Correction of hypoventilation is the correct initial treatment. Recheck ABG concentrations as necessary to evaluate any improvement in the ventilation.

C. Metabolic acidosis.

1. *Mechanisms of production.*
  a. Diseases such as diabetic ketoacidosis, alcoholic ketoacidosis, and uremia result in an excess of acidic ions that cannot be excreted rapidly enough to prevent acidosis.
  b. Ingestion of acidic compounds such as methanol, aspirin, ethylene glycol, and paraldehyde produces severe metabolic acidosis.
  c. Anaerobic metabolism after cellular hypoxia produces lactic acidosis. This may occur in persons with sepsis, shock, convulsions, ketoacidosis, and uremia.

2. *Clinical presentations and diagnosis.*
  a. The signs and symptoms of the underlying condition that causes the acidosis may be present.

b. ABGs.
  (1) $PaCO_2$ should be evaluated (see Section I, B, 2) for evidence of hypoventilation (i.e., $PaCO_2$ higher than 40 mm Hg). The expected pH should be calculated.
  (2) The patient's pH should be compared with the expected pH calculated from the $PaCO_2$. If the patient's pH is less than the expected pH, metabolic acidosis is present. A pH below 7.1 can have serious effects on cardiac and neurologic function.
  (3) Check serum osmolality, electrolytes, and renal function tests.
      (a) Serum osmolality is calculated and compared with the measured level from the laboratory. A significant osmolal gap indicates the presence of additional solutes in the serum.
      (b) Electrolytes are evaluated to assess the anion gap.

$$Na - (Cl + HCO_3) = \text{anion gap}$$

      An anion gap greater than 15 indicates an excess of lactate or similar acidic ions producing metabolic acidosis.
      (c) An elevated blood urea nitrogen (BUN) level indicates renal failure or prerenal or postrenal azotemia.
  (4) Toxicology screen. If an overdose is suspected, a blood, urine, and gastric aspirate examination may identify the ingestion of drugs producing metabolic acidosis.

3. Treatment.

a. Treat the underlying cause.
b. $NaHCO_3$ administration should be considered if the pH is below 7.1 and HCO_3 is below 10.

Dosage = (desired HCO_3 − observed HCO_3)
      $\times (0.4) \times$ weight in kg = mEq HCO_3 needed

However, only one third to one half of this dose should be administered before ABGs and serum electrolytes are rechecked.
c. For patients with values for pH above 7.1 and $NaHCO_3$ above 10, only aggressive treatment of the underlying condition is indicated initially.

D. Respiratory alkalosis.

1. Mechanisms of production.

a. Hyperventilation resulting from psychogenic anxiety is the most common form of respiratory alkalosis seen in the ED. However, the "hyperventilation syndrome" should be diagnosed only after excluding the more dangerous causes, particularly hypoxia.

b. Hypoxia resulting from congestive heart failure or pulmonary disorders such as pulmonary embolus or pneumonia are also common causes of hyperventilation.

c. Compensatory hyperventilation may follow metabolic acidosis because of stimulation of the medullary respiratory center by the acidic ions.

d. The central action of certain drugs and brain stem disorders or trauma also may produce hyperventilation.

2. Clinical presentation.

a. A common presentation of psychogenic hyperventilation is paresthesias of the extremities and the circumoral area, dizziness, chest discomfort, and rarely carpal pedal spasm.

b. ABGs.
The Pa_{CO_2} is decreased below normal, and the calculated or expected pH is elevated. If the patient's actual pH is significantly below the calculated or expected pH, metabolic acidosis is also present.

3. Treatment.

a. If hypoxia is present, correct it immediately.

b. Look for and treat any underlying cause such as pulmonary embolus, bronchospasm, pulmonary edema, pneumonia, or metabolic acidosis (e.g., diabetic ketoacidosis).

c. For psychogenic hyperventilation only, a mild tranquilizer may be used, such as diazepam, 5 to 10 mg orally, along with reassurance and counseling. Breathing into a paper bag is sometimes used to raise the P_{CO_2} level, but this can actually cause hypoxia.

E. Metabolic alkalosis.

1. Mechanisms of production.

a. Loss of acid through vomiting or excessive gastric suction.

b. Chronic or excessive diuretic administration, producing hyperchloremia and leading to alkalosis.

c. Severe K^+ depletion resulting in the movement of H^+ into the cells, thus producing alkalosis.

2. Clinical presentation.

a. Signs and symptoms of the underlying condition.

b. ABGs. Blood pH and HCO_3 levels elevated above normal.

c. Serum electrolytes. Serum K^+ is decreased, Cl^- is decreased, and HCO_3 is increased.

3. Treatment.

a. Replace K^+ if needed as described in Section V, D, 3.

b. Cl^- replacement is calculated by first determining the bicarbonate excess.

$$NaHCO_3 \text{ excess} = (\text{desired } HCO_3 - \text{observed } HCO_3)$$
$$\times 0.4 \times \text{weight in kg} = Cl^- \text{ deficiency}$$

c. Replace the Cl^- lost when using NaCl and KCl, depending on the K^+ level (see Section V, D, 3).

II. HYPERNATREMIA.
A. Mechanisms of production.
1. Significant hypernatremia occurs when thirst cannot compensate for a hypertonic state. This occurs most frequently with severe vomiting or diarrhea, obtundation, or lack of water intake, or in infants who are unable to make their needs known.
2. *Water loss in excess of sodium loss (both are lost).* This is the most common mechanism of hypernatremia. Causes include gastroenteritis, sweating, and osmotic diuresis (e.g., caused by hyperglycemia, iatrogenic mannitol, or the urea load of infant formulas).
3. *Pure water loss without sodium loss.* This is much less common. Causes include diabetes insipidus (hypothalamic or nephrogenic) and excessive sweating from hypermetabolic states (e.g., hyperpyrexia or hyperthyroidism).
4. *Excess intake of sodium.* This occurs mostly by accident or iatrogenically. Among the causes are excessive administration of sodium bicarbonate during cardiac resuscitation, inadvertent use of IV hypertonic saline solutions, accidental substitution of salt for sugar in the preparation of infant formulas, and drinking of seawater after shipwrecks.
B. Causes (NOTE: Table 2-1 compares the causes listed below with the mechanisms described above).
1. Gastrointestinal water loss.
2. Sweat loss.
3. Osmotic diuresis.
4. Diabetes insipidus.
5. Hypermetabolic states.
6. Accidental or iatrogenic.
C. Clinical presentation.
1. Nearly all the symptoms of hypernatremia are due to cellular dehydration caused by a fluid shift from the isotonic in-

TABLE 2-1
Etiology of Hypernatremia

Cause	H_2O loss > Na loss	Pure H_2O loss	Increased NA intake
Gastrointestinal loss	X		
Sweat loss	X	X	
Osmotic diuresis	X		
Diabetes insipidus		X	
Hypermetabolic states		X	
Accidental or iatrogenic	X		X

tracellular compartment into the hypertonic extracellular compartment.

2. If there is a net loss of total body sodium and water, the volume of the extracellular (and therefore intravascular) compartment will decrease. This may lead to significant or even lethal hypotension.

3. Neurologic symptoms predominate in persons with hypernatremia: thirst, lethargy, coma, muscle irritability, and seizures. Severe cerebral dehydration may lead to hemorrhage as the brain shrinks away from its vascular attachments.

D. Treatment.

1. Replacement of water is central to correction of hypernatremia. Oral intake may suffice. IV 5% dextrose in water may also be used.

2. If a significant amount of sodium has been lost, IV normal saline will replace both water and sodium, and it is hypotonic relative to the patient's hypertonic serum.

3. Rapid correction of hypernatremia may lead to significant rebound cerebral edema. Correction should therefore be limited to half the fluid loss over the first 24 hours.

Fluid loss = normal total-body water − current total-body water

Normal total-body water (L) = 0.6 × normal body weight (kg)

Current total-body water = normal total-body water $\times \dfrac{\text{normal serum Na}^+}{\text{current serum Na}^+}$

III. HYPONATREMIA.

A. Mechanisms of production.

1. Water retention greater than sodium retention (but both are retained).

a. The total-body water content is increased, total-body sodium content is increased, and urinary sodium levels are usually less than 10 mEq/L.

b. The patient usually is clinically *edematous.*

c. Disorders include congestive heart failure, nephrosis, and cirrhosis.

2. Sodium loss greater than water loss (but both are lost).

a. The total-body water content is decreased, total-body sodium content is decreased, and urinary sodium levels are usually less than 10 mEq/L if sodium and water loss are nonrenal. Urinary sodium is usually more than 10 mEq/L if sodium and water loss are renal.

b. The patient is in a net state of *dehydration.*

c. Disorders include the following:

(1) Nonrenal loss: vomiting, diarrhea, excessive sweating, extensive burns, pancreatitis, massive trauma.

(2) Renal loss: diuretics, adrenal mineralocorticoid insufficiency, salt-wasting nephropathy, renal tubular acidosis.

3. *Water retention without sodium retention* (some sodium may be lost through compensatory mechanisms, but the principal abnormality is water retention rather than sodium loss).

a. The total-body water content is increased, total-body sodium content may be somewhat decreased, and urinary sodium levels are usually more than 20 mEq/L.

b. The patient does not usually demonstrate edema or dehydration.

c. Disorders include the syndrome of inappropriate antidiuretic hormone (SIADH), hypothyroidism, adrenocorticosteroid insufficiency, and water intoxication.

4. *Additional osmotically active solutes in the serum.* (The elevated osmotic pressure of the serum attracts water from the cells into the intravascular space, thereby diluting the serum sodium, resulting in hyponatremia.)

a. The additional osmotic agents are most often glucose in hyperglycemia and mannitol administered iatrogenically.

b. Total-body water and sodium concentrations are usually decreased because of osmotic diuresis.

c. In profound hyperglycemia, the measured serum sodium concentration is decreased because of laboratory testing artifact. True sodium concentration can be calculated by adding 2 mEq/L to the measured sodium concentration for each 100 mg/L increase in the serum glucose concentration above 200 mg/L.

B. Causes (NOTE: Table 2-2 compares the causes listed below with the mechanisms described above).

1. *Protein loss.* Nephrosis, cirrhosis.
2. *Congestive heart failure.*
3. *Dehydration.* Vomiting, diarrhea, sweating, burns, pancreatitis, massive trauma.
4. *Renal.* Nephrosis, salt-wasting nephritis, renal tubular acidosis.
5. *Adrenal.* Mineralocorticoid insufficiency, corticosteroid insufficiency.
6. *Diuretics.*
7. *SIADH.*
8. *Water intoxication.*
9. *Hypertonic states not resulting from sodium.* Hyperglycemia, mannitol administration.

C. Clinical presentation.

1. Symptoms and signs of the underlying process.
2. Symptoms resulting from hyponatremia are largely dependent on the rate of development. A sudden decrease in the serum sodium concentration from 140 to 120 mEq/L may cause severe symptoms, whereas a gradual decline to 120 mEq/L may be asymptomatic.

TABLE 2-2
Etiology of Hyponatremia

Cause	H_2O retention > Na retention	Na loss > H_2O loss	Pure H_2O retention	Increased osmoles
Protein loss (nephrosis, cirrhosis)	X			
Congestive heart failure	X			
Dehydration (vomiting, diarrhea, sweating, burns, pancreatitis, massive trauma)		X		
Renal				
Nephrosis	X			
Salt-wasting nephritis		X		
Renal tubular acidosis		X		
Adrenal				
Mineralocorticoid insufficiency		X		
Corticosteroid insufficiency			X	
Diuretics		X		
SIADH			X	
H_2O intoxication			X	
Hypertonic states not resulting from Na (hyperglycemia, excess mannitol administration)				X

   3. Symptoms generally occur at a serum sodium level below 120 mEq/L.
     a. Gastrointestinal: anorexia, nausea, vomiting.
     b. Neurologic: lethargy, confusion, coma, seizures.
D. Treatment.
   1. Water restriction is usually the principal treatment, particularly when water retention is the primary abnormality (see Sections III, A, 1 and 3).
   2. Administration of *isotonic* saline is often appropriate treatment for states in which sodium loss exceeds water loss (see Section III, A, 2).
   3. Correction of the underlying problem is essential.
   4. The antidiuretic hormone (ADH) inhibitor demeclocycline (300 to 600 mg given orally twice a day) may be useful for treating SIADH.

5. If potentially life-threatening symptoms occur (usually with a serum sodium level below 110 mEq/L), IV administration of hypertonic saline may be indicated.
   a. Three percent saline is given intravenously in small quantities sufficient to correct the serum sodium level no more than halfway to normal over a period of 8 hours (see Section II, D).

   $$Na^+ \text{ replacement (mEq)} = (\text{desired serum } Na^+ \\ - \text{current serum } Na^+) \times \text{current total-body water}$$

   b. Hypertonic saline should be given only when *absolutely* necessary. This will usually be limited to states of acute symptomatic water intoxication.
6. Another modality involves the use of a diuretic (furosemide or mannitol) to induce water diuresis, followed by replacement (if appropriate) of sodium and potassium lost in the urine. This regimen is potentially quite dangerous if there is already a net total deficit of sodium or potassium. It should be used only for severe hyponatremia concurrently with treatment of the underlying abnormality. (Diuretics may, of course, be required for the treatment of specific disorders such as congestive heart failure.)

E. Falsely low serum sodium measurements—pseudohyponatremia.
1. The nonaqueous phase of serum is expanded in hyperlipidemias and hyperproteinemias such as macroglobulinemia and multiple myeloma.
2. Since sodium is confined to the aqueous phase but is measured per total volume of serum (aqueous plus nonaqueous), such states will lower the measured sodium concentration. The actual aqueous sodium concentration, however, is unchanged.
3. Because the symptoms of hyponatremia depend on the aqueous-phase sodium concentration, such states cause no symptoms and require no treatment.

IV. HYPERKALEMIA.
A. Mechanisms of production.
1. *Increase in potassium load.* This is an uncommon cause of hyperkalemia in the patient with normal renal function. However, the patient who receives medications containing potassium is at risk for developing hyperkalemia if renal function deteriorates. Potassium overload may also be the result of the release of potassium from injured tissue (e.g., crush injury).
2. *Alteration of the distribution of potassium in the body.* Since most of the body's potassium is intracellular, the redistribution of potassium to the extracellular fluid may result in hyperkalemia. This is most commonly due to acidosis.

   3. Decrease in the renal excretion of potassium. This may be due to acute renal failure or the use of potassium-sparing diuretics. Patients with chronic renal failure usually maintain normal potassium excretion.

B. Causes.

   1. Acute renal failure.
   2. Acute acidosis (e.g., diabetic ketoacidosis).
   3. Adrenal insufficiency.
   4. Extensive transfusion with old banked blood.
   5. Cellular injury.
      a. Burns.
      b. Crushing injury.
      c. Rhabdomyolysis.
      d. Chemotherapy.
   6. Potassium-sparing diuretics (e.g., triamterene, spironolactone).

C. Clinical presentation.

   1. *Neuromuscular.* Interference with resting neuromuscular membrane potential results in paresthesias, muscular cramping, weakness, or paralysis.
   2. *Gastrointestinal.* Nausea, vomiting, anorexia, and abdominal pain.
   3. *Cardiac.* Hyperkalemia affects the cardiac membrane potential, which results in conduction disturbances and dysrhythmias. Peaking of the T waves and shortening of the Q-T interval are early findings. These are followed by flattening or disappearance of the P wave and prolongation of the QRS complex. Ventricular fibrillation or asystole is the ultimate result of uncorrected hyperkalemia.

D. Treatment.

   1. The presence of neuromuscular symptoms, electrocardiographic abnormalities, and a serum potassium level greater than 6.5 mEq/L are indications for treatment.
   2. In the face of paralysis or severe cardiac conduction disturbance, the effects of hyperkalemia may rapidly be reversed by restoring normal membrane excitability. This is done by administering 10% calcium gluconate, 10 to 30 ml intravenously over a period of 3 to 4 minutes. The calcium has a transient effect, does not actually lower serum potassium levels, and should be followed by additional treatment measures.
   3. Promoting the movement of potassium into cells results in a lowering of the serum potassium level. The IV administration of 50 ml of 50% dextrose and 10 units of regular insulin may be expected to lower the serum potassium concentration by 1 to 2 mEq/L within 30 minutes. In the acidotic patient, the administration of IV sodium bicarbonate will accomplish the same purpose.
   4. Removal of potassium from the body is a slower therapeutic process than the temporizing measures described above. It

may be accomplished by enhancing renal or gastrointestinal tract excretion. Diuresis with a thiazide diuretic or furosemide will increase urinary potassium excretion but is not appropriate for all clinical settings, for example, hypovolemia or renal failure. Polystyrene sulfonate (Kayexalate) exchange resin causes potassium to transfer into the gastrointestinal tract by colonic cation exchange. The oral dose is 20 g with 100 ml of 20% sorbitol solution. Retention enemas of 50 to 100 g of polystyrene sulfonate with 50 to 100 ml of 70% sorbitol may be repeated every 4 hours as needed.

- **E. Falsely elevated serum potassium level measurements.**
  1. Hemolysis during sample collection results in falsely high levels.
  2. Exercise of the extremity before sampling may result in muscular potassium being released into the serum.
  3. Leukocytosis and thrombocytosis may also result in a falsely elevated potassium level.

V. HYPOKALEMIA.
- **A. Mechanisms of production.**
  1. *Increased potassium excretion.* This is the most frequent cause of hypokalemia. Increased excretion may be renal (e.g., diuretics) or gastrointestinal (e.g., vomiting or diarrhea).
  2. *Inadequate potassium intake.* This is an unusual cause of hypokalemia except in persons with a remarkably deficient diet.
  3. *Alteration of the distribution of potassium in the body.* This is the mechanism of production of hypokalemia in alkalosis and other less common conditions.
- **B. Causes.**
  1. Excessive potassium loss.
     - a. Gastrointestinal.
       - (1) Protracted vomiting.
       - (2) Diarrhea, laxative abuse.
       - (3) Nasogastric suction.
     - b. Renal.
       - (1) Diuretics.
       - (2) Osmotic diuretics.
       - (3) Aldosteronism.
       - (4) Potassium-wasting nephritis.
  2. Inadequate dietary intake.
     - a. Starvation.
     - b. Unusual diet.
     - c. Alcoholism.
  3. Other causes.
     - a. Hypokalemic periodic paralysis.
     - b. Alkalosis.
     - c. Cushing's syndrome.

C. Clinical presentation.
   1. Symptoms of hypokalemia tend to be vague and mild if the level of serum potassium is above 3.0 mEq/L. Severe complications usually occur at serum levels less than 2.0 mEq/L.
   2. *Mental status.* Patients with hypokalemia may be depressed, confused, or agitated.
   3. *Neuromuscular.* Fatigue, muscular weakness, or frank paralysis may develop because of interference with the neuromuscular transmembrane resting potential. Apnea secondary to respiratory muscle failure may occur at serum potassium levels of 1.0 to 1.5 mEq/L.
   4. *Cardiac.* Dysrhythmias may be caused by hypokalemia. These include atrial, nodal, and ventricular premature beats or tachycardia. Hypokalemia is especially likely to lead to serious dysrhythmia in patients taking digitalis. Electrocardiographic changes of hypokalemia include T wave flattening or inversion, Q-T interval prolongation, and prominent U waves.

D. Treatment.
   1. Whenever a condition is reversible, treatment should be directed toward this.
   2. If hypokalemia is minor, dietary potassium intake may be supplemented by the addition of bananas or orange juice. Potassium chloride elixir, a 10% solution containing 20 mEq/15 ml, may be administered as a supplement. Potassium pills are more expensive but also more palatable. Forty to 60 mEq/day is adequate replacement therapy for most patients who have hypokalemia resulting from diuretic use.
   3. For severe hypokalemia—serum potassium level less than 2 mEq/L—IV replacement is necessary. The rate of infusion should depend on the severity of symptoms. The administration of 5 to 20 mEq/hr is adequate for most cases. Potassium may be administered as rapidly as 50 mEq/hr in extreme emergencies. During IV potassium replacement, the electrocardiogram should be monitored for the reversion of inverted T waves to normal. Since hyperkalemia is generally far more hazardous than hypokalemia, all patients receiving rapid potassium replacement should be monitored with extreme caution.

VI. HYPERCALCEMIA.
   (NOTE: Laboratory determinations of serum calcium levels measure total calcium, but clinical symptoms are based on only the ionized portion.)
   A. Mechanisms of production.
      1. *Increased gastrointestinal absorption.* This may be due to the increased intake of dietary calcium, as in the milk-alkali syndrome, or to enhanced intestinal absorption.

     2. *Mobilization of calcium from bone.* This may be caused by increased bone resorption or osteolysis.

     3. *Reduced renal excretion of calcium.*

B. Causes.

  1. Hyperparathyroidism.

  2. Malignant disease, most commonly cancer of the lung, breast, and kidney.

  3. Granulomatous illness.

    a. Sarcoidosis.

    b. Tuberculosis.

    c. Histoplasmosis.

    d. Coccidioidomycosis.

  4. Vitamin D intoxication.

  5. Immobilization.

  6. Milk-alkali syndrome.

  7. Hyperthyroidism.

  8. Addison's disease.

  9. Use of thiazide diuretics.

C. Clinical presentation.

  1. *Gastrointestinal tract.* Anorexia, nausea, vomiting, constipation, and abdominal pain are manifestations of hypercalcemia.

  2. *Urinary tract.* Hypercalcemia may cause polyuria, polydipsia, and stone formation in the urinary tract.

  3. *Neurologic.* Fatigue, muscular weakness, and diminished deep-tendon reflexes are the result of hypercalcemia. Severe hypercalcemia is accompanied by alterations in mental status: apathy, depression, psychotic behavior, disorientation, stupor, or coma.

  4. *Electrocardiographic.* Hypercalcemia causes shortening of the Q-T interval.

D. Treatment.

  1. Infusion of normal saline to overcome dehydration and lower the calcium concentration is the simplest way to treat hypercalcemia. Urinary calcium excretion is enhanced by increased sodium excretion. The infusion of IV normal saline and the administration of 40 to 80 mg of IV furosemide may therefore be used to lower the serum calcium concentration. Care should be taken to prevent circulatory overload. Thiazide diuretics, which may cause hypercalcemia, should be avoided.

  2. Mithramycin lowers the calcium concentration by inhibiting bone resorption. A single dose of 25 μg/kg in 5% dextrose in water (D_5W) given in an IV infusion over a period of 3 to 4 hours results in a lowered calcium concentration in 12 to 24 hours. Repeated administration may cause thrombocytopenia and serious renal or hepatic toxicity.

  3. Glucocorticoids reduce the level of serum calcium over the course of several days. Hydrocortisone, 250 mg intravenously every 6 hours, or the equivalent may be given.

  4. Ethylenediaminetetraacetic acid (EDTA) increases the urinary excretion of calcium and forms complexes with calcium in the blood. It is the most effective way to reduce the

calcium concentration. From 15 to 50 mg/kg should be given over the course of 4 hours. Since there is a significant risk of acute renal failure with EDTA, its use should be restricted to life-threatening emergencies.

5. Administration of inorganic phosphate is also a rapid means of reducing the calcium concentration. IV infusion of elemental phosphorus, 20 to 30 mg/kg over a period of 12 to 16 hours, will lower the calcium concentration rapidly. However, soft-tissue calcification, renal necrosis, and cardiac arrest may result from the use of elemental phosphate.

E. Falsely elevated serum calcium level measurements.

1. The level of serum calcium may be falsely elevated if there is venous stasis resulting from the prolonged application of a tourniquet.

2. Since almost half the serum calcium is protein bound, a decrease in the levels of plasma albumin and globulin should result in a decrease in the upper limit for the normal calcium level. As a consequence, a patient with a low plasma protein level may display signs of hypercalcemia even though the measured serum calcium level is in the normal range.

3. By contrast, alkalosis results in increased binding of calcium to protein. The alkalotic patient may display signs of hypocalcemia even though the total serum calcium concentration is in the normal range.

VII. HYPOCALCEMIA. (N O T E: Laboratory determinations of serum calcium levels measure total calcium, but clinical symptoms are based on only the ionized portion.)

A. Mechanisms of production.

1. *Hypoalbuminemia.* From 40% to 45% of the total serum calcium is protein bound. When the serum protein level decreases, homeostasis of the ionized portion of serum calcium is maintained, with an amount equivalent to that formerly bound to protein now absorbed into bone. Thus the total serum calcium level falls in hypoalbuminemia, but the ionized portion remains normal, and there are no symptoms.

2. *Decreased mobilization of calcium from bone.* This involves the parathyroid hormone (PTH) system, as well as magnesium interaction with this system.

3. *Decreased levels of vitamin D or its metabolites.* This may involve dietary insufficiency, malabsorption, metabolic abnormalities, or excessive excretion.

4. *Conversion of ionized to nonionized calcium.*

B. Causes.

1. Hypoalbuminemia.

2. Disorders of the PTH system.
   a. Decreased PTH production.
   b. Decreased end-organ sensitivity to PTH (pseudohypoparathyroidism).
   c. Decreased level of serum magnesium.

3. Disorders of vitamin D.
   a. Decreased dietary intake of vitamin D.
   b. Decreased gastrointestinal tract absorption of vitamin D.
   c. Decreased conversion of vitamin D to active metabolite.
   d. Increased conversion of vitamin D to inactive metabolite.
   e. Increased excretion of active metabolite.
4. Precipitation of ionized calcium resulting from hyperphosphatemia or pancreatitis.
5. Alkalosis.
6. Increased incorporation of calcium into new bone formation resulting from osteoblastic metastases.

C. Clinical presentation.

1. Neurologic. The initial symptoms are circumoral or peripheral paresthesias, muscle cramping, carpopedal spasm, and confusion. Symptoms may progress in severe hypocalcemia to frank tetany or convulsions. A significant decrease of the serum ionized calcium level is reflected by Chvostek's sign (facial muscle spasm induced by tapping over the facial nerve) and Trousseau's sign (carpal spasm induced by inflation of an arm tourniquet).

2. Electrocardiographic. Prolonged Q-T intervals may be seen.

D. Treatment.

1. In persons with chronic hypocalcemia, the dietary intake of calcium and vitamin D is increased.
2. Emergent treatment is necessary if the clinical signs of hypocalcemia are present. Unless these are due to a transient abnormality such as the respiratory alkalosis of hyperventilation, IV calcium should be given; 100 to 300 mg is administered over a span of several minutes as 10 to 30 ml of a 10% solution of calcium gluconate. A slow IV infusion can be then titrated to serum levels.
3. If the level of serum magnesium is also low (<0.8 mEq/L), 1 to 2 g of magnesium sulfate (8 to 10 mEq of elemental magnesium) is given intravenously as a 10% solution over a period of 15 minutes.

VIII. HYPERMAGNESEMIA.

A. Mechanisms of production.

1. Much less common than hypomagnesemia.
2. Usually caused by increased ingestion of magnesium, coupled with diminished elimination.

B. Causes.

1. Severe renal failure.
2. Excess ingestion of magnesium-containing medications, usually in patients with renal failure.

C. Clinical presentation.

1. Usually asymptomatic unless serum level is greater than 5 mEq/L.

   2. Hypotension.
   3. Cardiac rhythm disturbances: bradycardia, heart block, atrial fibrillation.
   4. CNS depression: decreased level of consciousness.
   5. Respiratory depression.
D. **Treatment.**
   1. Calcium chloride 5 ml of a 10% solution intravenously over 30 seconds.
   2. Normal saline solution intravenously in patients with normal renal function. Monitor for overhydration.
   3. Dialysis in patients with severe hypermagnesemia:
      a. Serum level greater than 8 mEq/L.
      b. Severely symptomatic.
      c. Severe renal impairment.

IX. HYPOMAGNESEMIA.
A. Mechanisms of production.
   1. Severe malnutrition.
   2. Magnesium loss resulting from diuresis, especially caused by alcoholism.
   3. Magnesium malabsorption.
B. Causes.
   1. Alcoholism (the most common cause).
   2. Malabsorption syndromes with steatorrhea.
   3. Renal disorders, for example, chronic renal failure, renal tubular acidosis, nephrotic syndrome.
C. Clinical presentation.
   1. Central nervous system (CNS) hyperexcitability:
      a. Mental status alteration: irritability, combative behavior, disorientation, confusion.
      b. Ataxia, nystagmus, athetosis.
      c. Grand mal seizures.
   2. Respiratory muscle weakness.
   3. Anorexia, nausea, vomiting.
D. Treatment.
   1. Mild (serum magnesium > 1 mEq/L and patient is asymptomatic): augment magnesium intake with dietary supplement.
   2. Severe (serum magnesium < 1 mEq/L or patient is severely symptomatic): IV magnesium sulfate, 2 g over 5 to 15 minutes, followed by 5 g over the next 6 hours. If the serum level is less than 1 mEq/L but symptoms are mild, 6 g may be given over 3 hours.

PART II

Traumatic Emergencies

3

Overview of Major Trauma

Severly traumatized patients should be evaluated and managed in a systematic fashion, with emphasis placed on establishing priorities of care based on the nature and severity of injury. Initial assessment consists of a very rapid primary survey of airway, breathing, and circulation (ABC)–together with stabilization of vital functions–followed by a thorough secondary survey, which includes complete physical examination and diagnostic studies as indicated.

I. AIRWAY.

Airway management is of the highest priority. Patency of the upper airway should be ensured, with consideration given to the possibility of injury to the cervical spine.

A. In the unconscious patient, positioning maneuvers such as the chin lift and jaw thrust may produce airway patency. However, the neck should not be hyperextended in an effort to clear the airway.

B. Suctioning of the airway may clear it of particulate matter.

C. Insertion of a nasopharyngeal or oropharyngeal airway may help maintain airway patency in an unconscious or stuporous patient.

II. BREATHING AND VENTILATION.

Oxygenation and air exchange must be ensured.

A. All major trauma victims should have high-flow oxygen applied unless there is a specific contraindication.

B. Ventilatory support with bag-valve-mask apparatus should be initiated if respiratory effort is inadequate.

C. Endotracheal intubation should be performed as soon as possible when indicated. The cervical spine should be stabilized manually and/or by rigid collar if there is any possibility of neck injury. Oral or nasotracheal intubation may be achieved with the help of Magill forceps or fiberoptic bronchoscope, if neck stabilization renders routine intubation difficult. Rapid-sequence intubation with pharmacologic paralysis may be necessary (see Chapter 12). When intubation is not successful or is precluded by major facial fractures, a surgical airway can be achieved by cricothyrotomy (see Chapter 4).

D. The chest should be evaluated by inspection, palpation, percussion, and auscultation for signs of rib fracture, pneumothorax (simple, tension, or open), hemothorax, pulmonary contusion, or flail chest.

III. CIRCULATION.

A rough estimate of the adequacy of perfusion can be obtained by assessing skin color and temperature, capillary refill, pulse rate, and level of consciousness.

A. Pressure is applied to all visible significant external hemorrhage sites.

B. If there is any question of significant trauma, two large-bore IV lines are inserted, and normal saline or lactated Ringer's solution is infused, the rate of infusion to depend on the patient's clinical status (see Chapter 1). Pneumatic antishock trousers are controversial but are sometimes useful.

IV. NEUROLOGIC STATUS.

Once airway, breathing, and ventilation have been secured, together with spinal immobilization as indicated, a rapid neurologic assessment is performed. Mental status and gross motor function are documented.

V. SECONDARY SURVEY.

The entire body is then examined. The patient should be undressed and at some point the back examined, usually by "logrolling" the patient without flexing the spine:

A. Head, including cranium, face, eyes, ears, nose, and mouth.

B. Neck, including spine, trachea, and neck veins.

C. Chest, including ribs, sternum, and clavicle.

D. Abdomen.

E. Pelvic bones.

F. Perineum, rectum, and genitalia.

G. Extremities.

H. Neurologic system.

I. Back, including entire spine, posterior chest, flanks, and buttocks.

VI. MONITORING.

Frequent and repeated evaluation of the major trauma patient is crucial. If there is any change in the patient's status, the vital signs, abdomen, and chest should be reevaluated.

Monitoring of vital signs is of course crucial, and the following procedures may also be indicated:

A. Foley catheterization and maintenance of urinary output of at least 50 ml/hr in adults, 1 ml/kg/hr in children, and 2 ml/kg/hr in infants below 1 year of age. A urinary catheter should not be inserted if there is suspicion of a urethral injury on the basis of blood at the urethral meatus, displacement of the prostate, or other findings. A retrograde urethrogram is indicated in this instance.

B. Nasogastric tube insertion to prevent gastric distention and detect gastrointestinal bleeding or diaphragmatic herniation. The orogastric route should be used if there is midfacial injury that may produce a cribriform plate fracture.

C. Central venous pressure monitoring to guide volume resuscitation and to detect the presence of obstruction of the central circulation resulting from pericardial tamponade or tension pneumothorax.

4

Thoracic Trauma

Chest Injuries

I. GENERAL CONSIDERATIONS.

A. Patients with injuries to the chest are frequently in critical condition and require rapid diagnosis and adequate treatment. Emergency thoracotomy is needed in only about 10% of the cases of major thoracic trauma. The other 90% need resuscitation procedures that are available in a well-equipped ED followed by appropriate inpatient care.

B. The ABCs should be evaluated immediately after the patient arrives in the ED: the airway must be secured and breathing and circulation supported, if needed.

C. Airway.

1. If the airway is not patent, it must be made so immediately. Obstruction is often caused by the patient's tongue, and a jaw thrust extending the mandible forward is often sufficient to clear the airway. Adjuncts such as an oral or a nasal airway may also help. Foreign bodies, including displaced dentures, must be removed.

2. Endotracheal (ET) intubation may be required if the airway cannot be secured by the aforementioned measures or if the patient is not ventilating adequately.

   a. Orotracheal intubation can be performed if cervical spine trauma is ruled out clinically or radiographically. If the possibility of spinal injury exists and intubation must be instituted, the head should be stabilized and held in a neutral position by an assistant and the procedure carried out without motion of the cervical spine.

   b. Cricothyrotomy may be necessary if intubation is unsuccessful, if there is a strong possibility of cervical spine injury, or in cases of massive facial trauma.

      (1) Cricothyrotomy is preferred over formal tracheostomy in the ED because it is easier to perform rapidly.

      (2) Cricothyrotomy is performed in the following manner:

         (a) The cricothyroid membrane is located at the transverse slit lying caudal to the thyroid cartilage and cephalad to the cricoid cartilage.

    (b) The thyroid cartilage is stabilized with one hand while a 1- to 2-cm transverse incision is made with the other hand. The incision is carried through the skin and cricothyroid membrane.

    (c) The incision is then spread and a tube inserted. Either a tracheostomy device or a small endotracheal tube (e.g., number 4) cut short can be used.

    (d) A large-bore needle or commercially available cricothyrotomy device may be inserted temporarily as an easier and more rapid alternative to a formal surgical cricothyrotomy. However, such smaller airways should be replaced as soon as possible with a larger tube inserted through an incision.

D. Breathing. Even if the airway is clear, the patient's breathing may not be adequate. Observe the chest and auscultate the lungs. If needed, assist ventilation with a bag-valve device connected to a mask or ET tube.

E. Circulation. Perfusion must be maintained by control of bleeding, infusion of fluid and blood through large-bore IV lines as indicated, decompression of tension pneumothorax or pericardial tamponade, or open thoracotomy with aortic compression and internal cardiac massage (see the following items).

F. The initial evaluation may reveal serous underlying pathology such as the following:

    1. Pneumothorax. Dyspnea with decreased breath sounds and tympany on one side, perhaps with subcutaneous emphysema.

    2. Tension pneumothorax. The aforementioned signs plus the eventual development of tracheal deviation, distended neck veins, cyanosis, and shock.

    3. Open pneumothorax (sucking chest wound). An obvious penetrating wound with air flow through the chest wall defect.

    4. Flail chest. A segment of the chest wall moving paradoxically, that is, inward during inspiration and outward during expiration.

    5. Pericardial tamponade. Hypotension that may be accompanied by distended neck veins but symmetric breath sounds.

II. DIAGNOSIS AND TREATMENT OF THORACIC TRAUMA.

Trauma to the chest can be either blunt or penetrating and may result in injuries that range from trivial to lethal.

A. Rib fracture.

    1. General.

        a. A simple rib fracture is painful but rarely serious. However, pain may curtail respiration and prevent adequate coughing, particularly in the elderly, thereby leading to atelectasis and pneumonia.

b. Multiple rib fractures may cause a flail chest (see Section II, B).

c. Fractures of the first or second rib are associated with a significant incidence of major vessel injury. Consideration should be given to aortography.

d. Fractures of the lower ribs may be associated with splenic, hepatic, or renal injury.

2. Diagnosis.

a. The patient with a simple rib fracture has tenderness on palpation and complains of pain aggravated by coughing, deep breathing, or motion.

b. A chest radiograph, including rib detail, confirms the diagnosis and helps rule out the presence of underlying pneumothorax or hemothorax.

c. Much of the anterior chest wall may consist of noncalcified cartilage, which is not radiopaque. A fractured rib cartilage thus does not appear on radiography but clinically resembles a rib fracture.

3. Treatment.

a. Pain is usually relieved with an oral analgesic such as hydrocodone or codeine combined with aspirin or acetaminophen every 4 hours.

b. Intercostal nerve block can be used to manage severe pain from rib fracture.

 (1) Bupivacaine (Marcaine), 0.5% 2 to 5 ml, is infiltrated around the intercostal nerve of the fractured rib, as well as the ribs above and below the injury.

 (2) The site of injection is beneath the lower edge of the rib, between the fracture and the spinous process. Care must be taken to avoid the intercostal vessels and the lung parenchyma.

c. Tight binding is not recommended because it may restrict breathing. An easily removable rib belt fastened with Velcro can provide comfort, but the patient must be reminded of the importance of periodic sighing or deep breathing to prevent hypoaeration, retention of secretions, and pneumonia.

d. Factors that might warrant hospital admission are age, underlying cardiorespiratory disease, significant associated injuries, multiple fractures, abnormal blood gas values, or complications such as pneumothorax.

B. Flail chest.

1. General.

a. When several ribs or the sternum are fractured on both sides of the point of impact, an unstable or flail chest may result (Fig. 4–1).

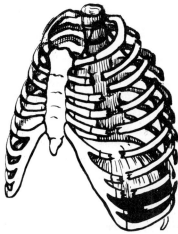

FIG. 4-1 Flail chest. — *USUALLY occurring on one SIDE*

b. The unsupported chest wall segment moves in a paradoxical manner, moving inward with negative intrathoracic pressure during inspiration and moving outward during expiration.

c. This paradoxical motion results in decreased tidal volume, which leads to a functional right-to-left shunt and hypoxia. The main contributing factor to hypoxia in these injuries, however, is coexisting pulmonary contusion. The more severe and extensive the contusion, the more severe are the gas exchange abnormalities (see Section E).

Bruising of the lungs

2. **Diagnosis.** The paradoxical motion of the flail segment can be discerned by direct observation or palpation.

3. **Treatment.**

a. The flail segment must be stabilized. In the field, paramedics may place the patient in a supine or decubitus position so that the flail segment lies against the gurney.

b. In the ED, internal stabilization is the best approach for significant cases of flail chest, especially if blood gas analysis reveals inadequate ventilation or oxygenation. Internal stabilization consists of ET intubation and positive-pressure ventilation.

c. Associated injuries such as pneumothorax and hemothorax are treated with tube thoracostomy. Because positive-pressure ventilation can induce pneumothorax in an in-

BUM

jured lung, chest tubes are often inserted in these patients
when mechanical ventilation is instituted (see Section C).

d. Intercostal nerve block is particularly helpful for severe
pain.

C. Pneumothorax.

1. General.

a. Traumatic pneumothorax may follow blunt or penetrating
injuries and can be associated with hemothorax. Air may
enter the pleural space from either the trachea, bronchi, or
lungs, if these are damaged, or from the surrounding at-
mosphere if the chest wall is penetrated.

b. It is important to ascertain the relative amount of air in the
pleural space and to determine whether it is under tension.

c. Pneumothoraxes may be classified as simple, tension, or
open. The last two categories in particular may be rapidly
fatal.

2. Simple pneumothorax.

a. The parietal and visceral pleura are normally held in contact by the combined actions of negative intrapleural pressure and the capillary attraction provided by a small
amount of pleural fluid.

b. When air enters the pleural space, both of these factors are
negated.

c. The lung on the affected side begins to collapse, and oxygenation becomes impaired (Fig. 4–2).

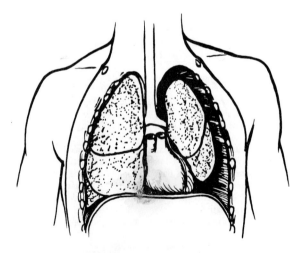

FIG. 4-2 Simple pneumothorax.

3. *Tension pneumothorax.*
   a. If more air enters the pleural space during inspiration than escapes during expiration, a ball-valve effect is created.
   b. Intrapleural pressure increases even after the lung completely collapses.
   c. Eventually this pressure becomes so high that the mediastinum is pushed to the opposite side, thus leading to compression of the opposite lung as well (Fig. 4–3).
   d. Extreme hypoxia can result.
   e. As intrapleural pressure increases and both lungs are compressed, blood flow through the central circulation declines significantly, thereby resulting in arterial hypotension and shock.
   f. Tension pneumothorax is an extreme emergency. It can be lethal within minutes if not immediately corrected (see Section C).

4. *Open pneumothorax (sucking chest wound).*
   a. Even with penetrating trauma to the chest wall, most air enters the pleural space from the damaged lung rather than through the chest wall defect.
   b. If the chest wall defect is sufficiently large, however, air may enter and leave the pleural space with each breath, thus leading to collapse of the underlying lung.
   c. An open pneumothorax can be rapidly fatal unless corrected immediately (see Section C).

PENETRATING TRAUMA

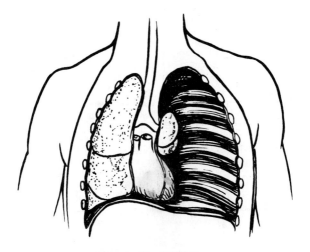

FIG. 4-3 Tension pneumothorax.

5. *Diagnosis.*
  a. Symptoms: dyspnea and pleuritic chest pain.
  b. Physical examination.
    (1) Simple pneumothorax.
      (a) Diminished breath sounds are auscultated over the affected side of the chest.
      (b) Tympany to percussion may be elicited.
      (c) Subcutaneous emphysema may be present.
      (d) These signs may not be apparent if the pneumothorax is small.
    (2) Tension pneumothorax.
      (a) Neck vein distention—often difficult to appreciate, especially if there is significant concomitant blood loss.
      (b) Tracheal deviation to the side opposite the pneumothorax, as detected by palpation of the neck.
      (c) Cardiac displacement to the opposite side as detected by percussion and auscultation of the chest.
      (d) Shock. *Shock with distended neck veins strongly suggests tension pneumothorax if breath sounds are diminished or asymmetric, or pericardial tamponade if breath sounds are normal* (see Section J). Shock resulting from blood loss should cause collapse of the neck veins.
    (3) Open pneumothorax.
      (a) Air bubbles may be seen to move through blood overlying the wound.
      (b) A characteristic hissing sound may be heard as air traverses the chest wall defect.
  c. Chest radiograph.
    (1) Separation of the visceral from the parietal pleural surface is the hallmark of pneumothorax.
      (a) A distinct lung margin is seen medial to the parietal pleura.
      (b) Pulmonary vascular markings are absent in the region between the two pleural surfaces.
    (2) An expiratory view may help reveal a subtle pneumothorax because the lung is smaller with more concentrated markings on expiration while the amount of pleural air remains constant.
    (3) An upright film is strongly recommended if there is no spinal fracture and the patient is hemodynamically stable. Small and moderate-sized pneumothoraxes may not be readily apparent on supine films because the air is layered above the entire lung surface in the supine position.

(4) The following clues to pneumothorax may be detected on a supine film:
  (a) Lucency of one lung field compared with the other.
  (b) Pneumomediastinum.
  (c) Pneumopericardium.
  (d) Subcutaneous emphysema.

6. *Treatment.*

a. Observation may be sufficient treatment for small (<10%) spontaneous pneumothoraxes with no significant symptoms.

b. Insertion of a unidirectional valve device through the chest wall may be used without suction to drain small pneumothoraxes.

c. Tube thoracostomy with continuous suction is advisable for all but the most minor traumatic pneumothoraxes, as well as for spontaneous pneumothoraxes of moderate to large size.

d. Technique of tube thoracostomy:
  (1) The second intercostal space, midclavicular line, can be used in a spontaneous pneumothorax.
  (2) The fourth to sixth intercostal spaces, midaxillary line, should be used in trauma for better drainage of a possible hemothorax. This location is also effective for spontaneous pneumothorax.
  (3) Percuss during full expiration to be sure the site does not overlie the liver or spleen.
  (4) After preparing the skin, infiltrate thoroughly with lidocaine (Xylocaine) down to the periosteum and the pleural surface.
  (5) Make a small incision down to the rib.
  (6) Using a small hemostat, dissect bluntly up over the superior margin of the rib, thereby avoiding the neurovascular bundle running along the bottom rib margin.
  (7) Enter the pleural space and spread the hemostat to enlarge the pleural opening.
  (8) Insert a gloved finger into the pleural space to make sure that the pleural space has been entered and that no adhesions will interfere with placement of the tube.
  (9) Attach a clamp to the tube and insert. Be sure that all side holes in the tube are inside the pleural space.
  (10) Connect the tube to a water seal and continuous suction at −20 cm water.
  (11) Secure the tube to the chest wall with a horizontal mattress suture and apply an airtight petrolatum dressing.

(12) Use of a trocar is controversial but is definitely dangerous if the pneumothorax is small.

(13) For patients with trauma, use a large-bore tube (36 French). A spontaneous pneumothorax can be treated with a smaller tube (10 to 12 French).

e. Tension pneumothorax.

(1) Air under tension must be released rapidly.

(2) A large-bore needle (preferably mounted on a saline-filled syringe barrel) should be used to relieve the tension.

(3) This is performed through the second intercostal space in the midclavicular line.

(4) A chest tube is then inserted as described above.

f. Open pneumothorax.

(1) The sucking wound must be closed immediately. The examiner's gloved hand can be used initially, with a petrolatum gauze dressing applied as soon as possible.

(2) If occlusion of the sucking wound is not followed immediately by tube thoracostomy—especially if intubation and assisted ventilation are required—a tension pneumothorax may sometimes develop. If this occurs, remove the occlusive dressing to allow the air to decompress through the chest wall defect.

(3) Tube drainage of the thorax should begin as soon as possible through a separate incision.

(4) The patient may require definitive operative repair of the chest wall.

D. Hemothorax.

1. General.

a. Hemothorax is an accumulation of blood in the pleural cavity. It occurs frequently in the setting of major chest trauma and is often accompanied by a pneumothorax.

b. Hemothorax may be caused by injury to the chest wall vasculature, the great vessels, or the intrathoracic organs such as the lung, heart, or esophagus.

c. Large hemothoraxes may lead to the following:

(1) Hypovolemic shock.

(2) Hypoxia resulting from interference with lung expansion.

2. Diagnosis.

a. Symptoms.

(1) Pleuritic chest pain.

(2) Dyspnea.

b. Physical examination.

(1) Diminished breath sounds.

(2) Dullness to percussion unless there is a significant accompanying pneumothorax.

     c. Chest radiograph.
       (1) Fluid is apparent below the base of the lung on an upright film.
       (2) Hemothorax may be subtle on a supine film and cause only a hazy dullness on the affected side.

3. Treatment.
     a. A very small hemothorax can be managed by observation.
     b. Any significant hemothorax should be drained via a thoracostomy tube connected to a water seal. The blood is removed and the lung reexpanded. Drainage through the chest tube should reflect the rate of hemorrhage.
     c. Restoration of blood volume with IV fluid or blood should begin immediately.
     d. Thoracotomy in the operating room should be strongly considered if there is initial thoracostomy tube drainage of blood greater than 20 ml/kg, if there is persistent bleeding at a rate greater than 7 ml/kg/hr, or if the patient remains hypotensive despite adequate resuscitation and other sites of hemorrhage have been excluded.

E. Pulmonary contusion (see also Chapter 17).
   1. Lung contusion may develop immediately after trauma or within the first 72 hours and is characterized by dyspnea, decreasing arterial PO_2, rales, and infiltrates seen on chest radiograph.
   2. Severe lung contusion may be associated with voluminous tracheobronchial secretions, hemoptysis, and pulmonary edema.
   3. The treatment of a significant contusion is ET intubation to permit suctioning and to apply mechanical ventilation with continuous positive end-expiratory pressure (PEEP).
   4. Lung contusion may lead to adult respiratory distress syndrome (see Chapter 17).

F. Tracheal or bronchial rupture.
   1. Pneumomediastinum or pneumothorax usually occurs.
   2. Tension pneumothorax may develop.
   3. If the patient requires mechanical ventilation, tension pneumomediastinum may arise and cause tracheal compression.
   4. Rupture of the airway can result in inadequate air delivery to the lungs.
   5. Subcutaneous emphysema, especially in the neck, may indicate a serious airway injury.
   6. Bronchoscopy will establish a diagnosis.
   7. Tracheostomy may be used to control respiration, to remove secretions, and to prevent further leakage of air from the high intratracheal pressures that occur with coughing or Valsalva's maneuver.
   8. One or more chest tubes should be inserted if a pneumothorax is present.

9. Operative repair of the tracheal or bronchial laceration is indicated as soon as possible after the patient's condition is stabilized.

G. Diaphragmatic rupture.

1. Rupture of the diaphragm may be seen after blunt trauma to either the chest or the abdomen. Evidence of rupture may be present immediately or may be delayed many months.
2. The tear is usually on the left. If the defect is large, the abdominal contents may herniate into the chest.
3. Changes in respiratory physiology are much like those seen with a pneumothorax.
4. With acute herniation, the first complaints are dyspnea and left-sided chest pain, which may be referred to the shoulder.
5. The diagnosis is made with a radiograph, which may reveal loops of bowel in the thorax. However, initial radiographic findings may be subtle, revealing only basilar atelectasis or haziness of the diaphragmatic margin.
6. Treatment: operative reduction of the herniation and repair of the ruptured diaphragm are performed as soon as possible.

H. Injuries to the aorta and great vessels.

1. Penetrating injuries to the thoracic aorta may result in cardiac tamponade or hemothorax, depending on whether the site of the vessel injury is intrapericardial or extrapericardial.
2. Rapid deceleration is the most common mechanism of non-penetrating aortic trauma and leads to extrapericardial dissection or rupture.
3. Such injuries are usually fatal immediately, but a small number of victims may survive long enough to reach the hospital.
4. Fluid resuscitation should be used to maintain blood pressure.
5. Aortography or chest computed tomography (CT) should be performed if the chest radiograph reveals a widened mediastinum or if there is a strong clinical suspicion of major vessel injury. Fracture of the first or second rib may be accompanied by great vessel injury.
6. Treatment is surgical.

I. Myocardial contusion.

1. Blunt trauma to the chest may cause contusion of the myocardium. The resulting injury can resemble myocardial infarction, although the damage may heal completely and the clinical course is usually more benign.
2. Enzyme changes and electrocardiographic (ECG) abnormalities may occur over the same time course as in nontraumatic infarction. Thus a contusion may not be apparent at the time of presentation.
3. ECG changes may include sinus tachycardia, right bundle-branch block, various conduction disturbances, and other dysrhythmias. These findings usually occur early. Their ab-

sence after several hours greatly reduces the likelihood of myocardial contusion.

4. Because the clinical course includes the risk of serious dysrhythmias and other complications, the patient suspected of
having sustained a myocardial contusion should be admitted
to the hospital for cardiac monitoring.

J. Cardiac tamponade.

1. Cardiac tamponade occurs from an accumulation of blood in
the pericardial sac resulting from either blunt or penetrating
trauma.

2. Diastolic filling and stroke volume decline.

3. In persons with thoracic trauma, falling blood pressure and distended neck veins (in the absence of other signs of tension
pneumothorax) strongly indicate acute pericardial tamponade.

4. Severe shock out of proportion to the amount of blood lost
strongly suggests tamponade.

5. Other findings in tamponade may include narrowed pulse
pressure, muffled heart sounds, and pulsus paradoxus (blood
pressure fall of more than 10 mm Hg during inspiration).
However, these signs may not be present, and their absence
does not rule out acute cardiac tamponade.

6. Treatment.

   a. If a pulse is palpable, needle aspiration is the initial treatment and often is lifesaving (Fig. 4–4). (If there is no pulse,
   see Section K on emergency thoracotomy.)

      (1) Aspiration is performed with a 16- or 18-gauge, short-
      bevel spinal needle attached to a three-way stopcock
      and a 50-ml syringe.

      (2) The needle is inserted slightly to the left of the
      xiphoid process and is directed cephalad and to the
      left until blood can be aspirated. The depth of inser-
      tion usually is 3 to 4 cm. Unless there is great ur-
      gency, this should be done with ECG monitoring.
      An alligator clamp is used as an ECG lead and at-
      tached to the needle, which is then advanced until a
      current of injury appears on the monitor. The needle,
      which is now touching the epicardial surface, is then
      slightly withdrawn back into the pericardial space,
      and fluid is aspirated.

      (3) A central venous catheter can be threaded through
      the needle and left in place to allow periodic aspira-
      tion to prevent the reaccumulation of fluid.

   b. Needle aspiration of an acute traumatic pericardial tamponade may be difficult and is often only a temporizing
   procedure. Traumatic pericardial fluid is primarily blood
   (hemopericardium), and clots are not easily aspirated
   through a needle. Immediate thoracotomy in the ED is
   sometimes necessary to sustain life until definitive surgery
   can be done in the operating room (see Section K).

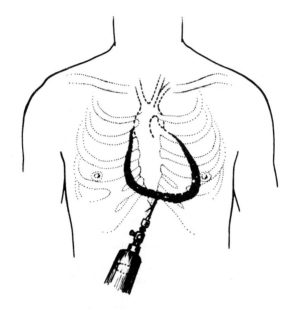

FIG. 4-4 Needle aspiration of pericardial fluid.

    c. Thoracotomy in the operating room is the definitive treatment for all patients with penetrating wounds of the heart and acute hemopericardium and tamponade.

K. Open thoracotomy in the ED.

    1. Indications.

        a. Trauma.

            (1) Hemorrhage from any source with unobtainable carotid and femoral pulse.

            (2) Chest injury with an unobtainable pulse.

        b. Refractory ventricular fibrillation with a basically healthy heart.

            (1) Electrocution.

            (2) Hypothermia.

    2. Procedure.

        a. An incision is made in the left fourth intercostal space from a point 2 to 3 cm lateral to the sternum (to avoid the internal thoracic vessels) to the midaxillary line.

        b. Rib-spreading retractors are used to expose the heart.

        c. For exsanguinating hemorrhage, the aorta is compressed just above the diaphragm with a vascular clamp or the physician's finger. Blood is thus shunted to the vital organs.

d. If there is any possibility of hemopericardium, the pericardium is opened. The coronary arteries should be visible through the pericardium in the absence of pericardial hemorrhage. If the coronary arteries are obscured by fat, or if the pericardium appears opaque because of subpericardial blood, open the pericardium by the following method:
   (1) The phrenic nerve is first identified.
   (2) A longitudinal incision in the pericardium is made parallel to the phrenic nerve.
   (3) The pericardial sac is evacuated of clots, and the heart is delivered outside the pericardium.
   (4) Cardiac wounds can be controlled temporarily with finger pressure. Only a minority require suturing in the ED.
e. In persons with refractory ventricular fibrillation, internal paddles can be applied directly to the heart. Moist saline gauze pads should be used to separate the paddles from the pericardial surface. From 30 to 50 J is appropriate.
   (1) In electrocution, this may be sufficient.
   (2) In hypothermia, warming the heart in warm saline may allow successful defibrillation.
f. Throughout the procedure, internal cardiac massage is performed as indicated.
g. The patient is taken to the operating room as soon as possible for definitive treatment.

5

Abdominal Trauma

I. GENERAL CONSIDERATIONS.

A. Trauma to the abdomen may be blunt or penetrating. Either type may lead to hemorrhage from either solid organ or direct vascular damage, or to peritonitis caused by spillage of contents from a ruptured viscus.

B. Serious injuries may occur without a visible mark or contusion on the abdominal wall. A seemingly trivial injury may rupture the bowel or spleen. Clinical evidence of injury may not appear until several hours after the injury. Thus the possibility of inapparent but significant injury must be kept in mind constantly and the patient examined at frequent intervals.

II. INITIAL EVALUATION AND STABILIZATION.

A. An accurate history may be extremely helpful for assessing the possibility of major injury.

B. An initial assessment is conducted as discussed in Chapter 3. The ABCs of airway, breathing, and circulation are secured, along with spinal immobilization as indicated.

C. The abdomen is visualized, auscultated, percussed, and palpated.

D. The back should also be evaluated, with the patient "logrolled" to prevent spinal motion if appropriate.

E. Rectal and vaginal examinations should be conducted in patients with potentially serious truncal injury.

F. For major trauma cases, several large-bore IV lines, a nasogastric tube, and a urinary (Foley) catheter are inserted as discussed in Chapters 1 and 3.

III. DIAGNOSTIC STUDIES.

A. Blood is drawn for complete blood count (CBC), type and cross, and other relevant studies such as renal function, electrolytes, and coagulation. Urine is analyzed for blood.

B. Whereas supine, upright, and decubitus radiographs of the abdomen may be of help in detecting free air in the stable patient, plain radiographs are generally of very limited value in assessing the traumatized abdomen. Peritoneal lavage, CT, and possibly ultrasonography are the appropriate modalities.

C. Unstable patients may have to be rushed immediately to the operating room, but if sufficiently stable, they can undergo *diagnostic peritoneal lavage* (DPL) in the ED. This procedure can be performed rapidly and is highly sensitive for detecting blood.

1. The bladder and stomach are decompressed with a urinary catheter and nasogastric tube, respectively.

2. After antiseptic preparation, lidocaine (Xylocaine) with epinephrine (to limit local bleeding) is injected in the midline, one third of the distance from the umbilicus toward the pubis.

3. A small vertical incision is made sufficiently deep to visualize the fascia, which is then grasped and elevated with clamps. A small cut is made in the fascia and its adherent, underlying peritoneum.

4. A peritoneal dialysis catheter is then inserted through the cut and advanced into the pelvis.

5. A syringe is attached and aspirated. Return of frank blood indicates hemoperitoneum.

6. If blood is not aspirated, 10 ml/kg (maximum 1 L) of (preferably warmed) normal saline or Ringer's lactate solution is instilled and allowed to remain for 5 to 10 minutes if the patient is sufficiently stable. Sensitivity is increased by gentle agitation of the abdomen, or by logrolling the patient onto each side for several minutes if the clinical condition permits. This allows the fluid to mix with blood that might be localized.

7. The IV bag is then vented and placed on the floor, allowing the fluid to drain from the abdomen.

8. A positive tap is defined as greater than 100,000 red blood cells (RBCs)/mm^3 or greater than 500 white blood cells (WBCs)/mm^3. The presence of stool, bile, or significant amylase is also indicative of intraabdominal injury.

9. Relative contraindications to DPL include prior abdominal surgery, coagulopathy, and pregnancy.

10. Varying amounts of the instilled fluid remain in the abdomen after DPL. Subsequent CT may not be able to distinguish this fluid from blood, thus rendering CT after DPL much less useful.

D. If the patient is sufficiently stable to go to the radiology department, *CT* of the abdomen and pelvis is very useful for detecting the presence of intraperitoneal blood, although it is not quite as sensitive as DPL. However, CT can also detect intraperitoneal air, locate the exact site(s) of damage, and evaluate the retroperitoneal space—none of which can be done with DPL. Intestinal trauma may escape detection by CT, however.

E. *Ultrasonography* has been increasingly utilized to detect abdominal injuries. It is fast and can be done at the bedside in the ED, but it is highly operator dependent.

IV. SPECIAL CONSIDERATIONS.

A. Blunt vs. penetrating trauma.

1. Either mechanism may lead to fatal injuries. The stable blunt trauma patient whose DPL or CT does not reveal evidence of major injury can be observed closely, thus often avoiding laparotomy.

2. Knife wound patients may also be treated expectantly in some cases if they remain stable. However, victims of gunshot wounds that have penetrated the peritoneal cavity must be explored surgically.

3. Early surgical consultation is important for any seriously injured patient. As with any trauma victim, the most crucial factor is frequently repeated clinical evaluation.

B. Thoracic trauma. (See Chapter 4 for full discussion of chest injuries.)

1. Depending on the phase of respiration, the diaphragm may be found anywhere from the fourth intercostal space (nipple level) to the lower costal margins just above the sacral crest. Thus injuries to the abdomen may also involve the chest, and vice versa.

2. Any penetrating injury between the nipple line and the umbilicus must be evaluated carefully to rule out thoracic injuries, as well as abdominal injuries.

C. Pelvic trauma. (See Chapter 6 for full discussion of genitourinary tract trauma.)

1. Pelvic injuries can be devastating because of their tendency to cause major hemorrhage and the difficulty of achieving hemostasis.

2. Shock should be treated as in Chapter 1. The PASG, or MAST, may provide temporary control of bleeding caused by major pelvic fractures. However, the best treatment of unstable pelvic ring fractures is the application of an external pelvic fixation device.

D. Retroperitoneal trauma.

1. Hemorrhage into the retroperitoneal space may be quite severe yet may not cause much abdominal tenderness on palpation. It is not detected by DPL. CT evaluation of the retroperitoneal space, however, is quite sensitive.

2. If possible, retroperitoneal hemorrhage is treated conservatively, allowing the increasing pressure of the confined hematoma to tamponade the bleeding.

6

Genitourinary Tract Trauma

I. RENAL INJURIES.

A. The kidney is injured less frequently than the liver or spleen because of its retroperitoneal position and protection by heavy musculature and the rib cage. Moreover, the fatty capsule may help tamponade renal hemorrhage. However, because the renal parenchyma is soft and highly vascular, it cannot easily withstand severe blunt or penetrating trauma.

B. Renal injuries may involve simple contusion, minor laceration without urinary extravasation, major lacerations or fractures, and pedicle injuries.

C. Blunt trauma to the abdomen produces renal injury by transmitting the impact in all directions or by impinging the kidney against a solid structure such as the vertebral column.

D. Penetrating renal trauma is often associated with other visceral injuries.

E. The findings with renal trauma may include flank pain, hematuria, shock, a flank mass, and abdominal guarding or rigidity.

F. Shock should be treated immediately because it is potentially lethal (see Chapter 1). Early treatment is also important because a patient in shock may not excrete contrast medium, and the resulting nonvisualization of the kidney may be mistaken for a seriously damaged kidney.

G. Diagnosis.

1. Urinalysis typically reveals hematuria. Whereas microscopic hematuria (<100 RBCs/HPF) can be treated by observation and repeat urinalysis, gross hematuria warrants further evaluation by CT or possibly intravenous pyelography (IVP).

2. CT with IV contrast material is the preferred modality for evaluating the genitourinary system in any multiple-trauma victim.

3. IVP has a limited role in trauma. IVP may be used as a screening procedure for isolated flank trauma. However, if such pa-

tients are strongly suspected to have sustained renal injury, initial CT scanning is advisable.

   a. A negative IVP rules out significant renal damage.

   b. A "one-shot" IVP just before laparotomy may be useful in patients too unstable to await CT scanning. Contrast material is injected and a single radiograph can then determine the existence of two functioning kidneys or the presence of gross renal trauma.

H. Treatment.

   1. In less serious injuries, conservative measures are recommended.

     a. Carefully monitor vital organs and observe the size of any flank mass.

     b. Record urinary output and the amount of hematuria.

     c. Stabilize the blood pressure and pulse with IV fluids and blood.

     d. Repeat CT as necessary.

   2. Surgery is indicated when the vital signs cannot be maintained with adequate fluid and blood replacement, or when there is an expanding flank mass, falling central venous pressure (CVP), continued inadequate urine output, or continued gross hematuria.

II. URETERAL INJURIES.

A. Because of its well-protected position, the ureter is rarely injured by blunt trauma. Penetrating injury is more common.

B. Findings may include an increasing mass in the flank or free urine within the peritoneal cavity. CT or IV urography may reveal the site of the rupture or extravasation or may show dilation of the collecting system proximal to the site of injury.

III. BLADDER INJURIES.

A. The most common bladder injuries are due to either direct trauma or associated pelvic fractures. A distended bladder may suffer extensive injury from minimal trauma, whereas an empty, collapsed bladder may escape injury.

B. Rupture of the bladder may be into the intraperitoneal space or more commonly the extraperitoneal space, depending on the section of bladder wall damaged.

C. The patient has tenderness in the suprapubic region and often hematuria or the inability to urinate.

D. An IVP or CT usually reveals extravasated contrast material; however, false-negative results do occur even with large tears. If there is still a strong clinical suspicion, a stress cystogram should be obtained.

E. Large intraperitoneal ruptures often require surgery. Extraperitoneal ruptures can frequently be managed conservatively with an indwelling catheter and anticholinergic medication.

IV. URETHRAL INJURIES.

A. Posterior urethral injuries (membranous and prostatic urethra) are classic accompaniments of pelvic fractures. Anterior urethral injuries follow direct trauma such as straddle injuries.

B. Depending on the site of the injury, urethral damage may allow urinary extravasation superior to the urogenital diaphragm into the pelvis, or below the urogenital diaphragm into the superficial perineal space, scrotum, or lower anterior abdominal wall.

C. Rectal examination may reveal a boggy fullness with loss of the prostatic outline.

D. Blood at the urethral meatus, or obvious penile or vulval trauma, suggests urethral damage. A retrograde urethrogram should be performed before urethral catheterization to avoid further injury.

E. If the urethrogram demonstrates extravasation of contrast, a suprapubic bladder catheter can be inserted and urologic consultation obtained.

V. PENILE TRAUMA.

A. Contusions of the penis are characterized by edema or, in more serious injuries, by ecchymosis that may spread to the scrotum and even to the anterior abdominal wall. The treatment is rest, ice packs, and an indwelling urethral catheter if there is interference with urination.

B. Fracture of the penis results from severe trauma to the erect organ, with resulting rupture of the corpora cavernosa. Bleeding into the subcutaneous tissues is extensive, with severe swelling and pain along the penile shaft.

C. Wounds of the penis are rare, and usually due to a gunshot, bite, or stabbing. Occasionally, avulsion occurs when clothing is caught in machinery.

D. Although simple lacerations may be sutured in the ED (see Chapter 13), any significant injury requires accurate surgical repair, usually in the operating room.

VI. INJURY TO THE SCROTUM AND ITS CONTENTS.

A. The scrotum is commonly damaged by kicks, blows, straddle injuries, gunshot wounds, or machinery accidents. Because of the mobility of scrotal skin over its contents, and because of cremasteric muscle contraction, the testes are somewhat protected. However, when injured, severe testicular swelling resulting from traumatic orchitis, hydrocele, or hematocele may occur. If the testes prolapse through an injury in the scrotal sac, they must be reinserted and the defect repaired operatively.

B. Closed injuries to the scrotum and its contents are generally treated conservatively. Scrotal support is indicated, and ice packs and analgesics are also used. After 48 hours, warm, moist packs may be helpful. Occasionally, evacuation of the hematocele may be necessary.

C. Lacerations of the scrotum are treated by thorough cleansing, debridement, and suturing, together with adequate drainage if needed (see Chapter 13). Scrotal skin has a good blood supply and usually heals very well.

D. If a testis has sustained a major injury, or if physical examination suggests extravasation of testicular tissue into the scrotal sac, urologic consultation is indicated to assess the need for immediate operative repair.

7

Neurologic Trauma

I. HEAD INJURIES.

A. Be sure the airway is clear and ensure that ventilation is adequate. If intubation is needed, use the orotracheal route with manual in-line traction. If facial injuries make intubation hazardous, consider immediate cricothyroidotomy (see Chapter 4).

B. Stop active bleeding with pressure unless a spurting vessel can be seen and clamped. Do not clamp facial vessels, however, because of their proximity to nerves.

C. Investigate other parts of the body for life-threatening injuries.

D. Keep the neck immobilized until cervical injury is ruled out on clinical or, when indicated, radiologic grounds.

E. Perform a neurologic examination, and record the results.

1. Evaluate the state of consciousness.
   a. Is the patient awake?
   b. If drowsy, can the patient be readily awakened?
   c. Are questions answered appropriately and commands obeyed?
   d. Is the patient oriented to person, time, place, and situation?
   e. Can the patient give a detailed history of the traumatic event, or is there retrograde amnesia?

2. Examine the eyes for pupillary size and reaction to light.
   a. Unilateral enlargement of a pupil may indicate increasing intracranial pressure, especially when the patient is unresponsive.
   b. Whenever pupillary inequality is visible on the initial examination, it should carefully be evaluated. Even in the alert patient, it may indicate early herniation.
   c. Nonreactive midsize or small pupils may indicate a midbrain or pontine lesion.
   d. The finding of normal fundi does not preclude intracranial trauma.

3. Eye movement.
   a. If the patient is unconscious and cervical injury has been ruled out, gentle rotation of the head from side to side permits determination of whether the eyeballs stay with

the head (doll's eyes absent) or move to the opposite side (doll's eyes present); movement indicates preservation of the oculocephalic (proprioceptive head turning) reflex. If cervical injury has not been ruled out, keep the neck immobilized. Consider caloric testing if it is important to rule out brain stem injury when CT is not available.

b. Nystagmus may reflect cerebellar or vestibular disturbance or recent indulgence in alcohol or other drugs such as phencyclidine hydrochloride (PCP).

4. Evaluate motor function in the face and extremities.
   a. Does the patient follow command?
   b. If not, is there purposeful movement or response to painful stimulus?
   c. Is the movement restricted to arm flexion (decorticate posturing) or arm and leg extension (decerebrate posturing)?

5. Reflexes.
   a. Deep tendon reflexes should be elicited.
   b. Babinski's reflex and similar abnormal reflexes indicate impairment of CNS pathways.

6. Bleeding from the ear and nose.
   a. Investigate to see whether the blood is from an adjacent laceration.
   b. Admixture of blood with cerebrospinal fluid, or leakage of clear fluid alone, indicates a basilar skull fracture.
   c. Blood arising in the ear (e.g., bulging or discolored eardrum) also indicates a basilar skull fracture.

F. Closed head injuries.
   1. Cervical spine x-rays should be considered in patients with head injury accompanied by unconsciousness, especially if there is any alteration of mental status remaining by the time of examination. Care must be taken to consider injuries to the spine before twisting or turning the patient's neck. For every patient, the C7 and T1 bodies must be visualized on the radiograph. Downward traction on the arms and/or swimmer's views may be required. (See Section II.)
   2. CT scanning of the head should be considered for head injury patients who do not improve promptly and for all patients who show signs of neurologic deterioration.
   3. X-ray films of the head are generally not indicated but may be helpful in identifying skull fractures in children whose neurologic status does not warrant CT scanning.
   4. Epidural hematomas must be evacuated in the operating room. The prognosis is often good if treated emergently because the underlying brain is often not seriously injured. Delay in evacuation, however, is likely to result in major brain damage or death from herniation caused by the expanding hematoma.
   5. Subdural hematomas must also be evacuated, but the location of the bleeding often implies a more forceful blow to

the head, resulting in direct brain trauma in addition to the hemorrhage. The prognosis is generally not as good as that of emergently treated epidural hematoma.

6. Frequent monitoring of vital signs and neurologic status is important to detect deterioration and the need for repeat CT scanning and appropriate treatment.

7. Convulsions may be controlled with diazepam (Valium), 10 to 15 mg IV, 5 mg/min, followed by phenytoin (Dilantin) loading. Alternative drugs are available (see Chapter 21).

8. Significant elevation of intracranial pressure, especially if there are signs of brain stem herniation such as a dilating pupil, should be treated with endotracheal intubation and controlled hyperventilation to a $PaCO_2$ of 25 to 30 mm Hg.

9. In the rapidly deteriorating patient, mannitol, 1 to 1.5 g/kg IV, should be given to reduce intracranial pressure.

10. The use of steroids to reduce cerebral edema resulting from trauma is controversial. If used, dexamethasone (Decadron), 20 mg, should be administered IV, followed by 10 mg every 4 hours for 24 hours.

G. Penetrating head injuries.

1. Penetrating wounds of the cranial cavity require debridement and closure, generally in the operating room. If a knife or foreign object protrudes from the head, it should be removed in the operating room.

2. Soft-tissue scalp wounds can be sutured as described in Chapter 13. Simple outer table skull fractures may sometimes be debrided in the ED, but any significant open skull fracture, especially if the inner table is violated or if there is any depression, should be treated in the operating room by a neurosurgeon.

II. SPINE AND CORD INJURIES.

A. Any patient who has fallen or has been involved in an accident may have an injury to the spine and its contents. A high degree of suspicion is particularly warranted for any unconscious patient. Movements should be gentle and guarded. If there is any suspicion of spinal trauma, a rigid cervical collar should be applied and the patient placed on a spine board.

B. Examination.

1. The spine should be palpated from head to sacrum for obvious protrusion, malalignment, and areas of tenderness.

2. If the patient needs to be turned, the head and body should be moved en bloc ("log-rolled") to avoid twisting the neck and spine until the examiner is sure there is no injury.

3. If the patient is conscious, neurologic examination can rapidly detect spinal cord damage.

   a. Voluntary movement of various parts of the extremities is requested.

   b. Sensation and deep tendon reflexes are tested.

c. In questionable cases, testing of other reflexes may be helpful, such as plantar, abdominal, and cremasteric responses in men.
4. In the unconscious patient, several findings may indicate cord injury.
   a. Deep tendon reflexes and response to painful stimulus may be absent with either cord or brain injury.
   b. The absence of rectal tone may indicate severe cord damage.
   c. Priapism is a strong indicator of cord injury.
   d. Hypotension without tachycardia suggests spinal shock

TABLE 7-1
Motor Levels

Action	Muscles	Spinal cord levels
Shrugging shoulders	Trapezius	Accessory nerve, C2, C3
Flexion of forearm at elbow	Biceps	C5, C6
Extension of arm at elbow	Triceps	C6, C7
Abduction and adduction of fingers	Interosseous and lumbricals	C8, T1
Flexion of thigh on abdomen	Iliopsoas	L1, L2, L3
Extension of lower leg at knee	Quadriceps	L2, L3, L4
Dorsiflexion of foot and great toe	Anterior tibial and peroneal muscles	L4, L5
Plantar flexion of foot	Gastrocnemius	L5, S1

TABLE 7-2
Sensory Levels

Areas of body	Spinal cord levels	Vertebral body levels
Neck to clavicle	C2-C4	C2-C4
Outer deltoid	C5	C5
Thumb	C6	C6
Index finger	C7	C7
Little finger	C8	T1
Nipple	T3	T2
Umbilicus	T10	T8
Inguinal area (groin)	L1	T10
Thigh above knee	L3	T11
Lateral part of calf	L4	T11-T12
Foot dorsum	L5	T12
Lateral part of foot and small toe	S1	L1
Buttock	S3-S5	L1-L2

resulting from loss of both normal vascular tone and reflex tachycardia (see Chapter 1).

   e. Diaphragmatic breathing without intercostal motion may indicate a high cervical cord lesion.

5. The level of spinal cord injury can be determined by the neurologic findings in most cases (Tables 7-1 and 7-2 and Fig. 7-1).

   a. In the cervical area, the vertebral bodies correspond to the spinal cord segments. In the thoracic region, the bodies are 1 to 2 segments higher than the cord levels. The lumbar and sacral areas of the cord are compressed from the level of T10 to the interspace between L1 and L2, where the cord normally ends. Pinprick sensation can be

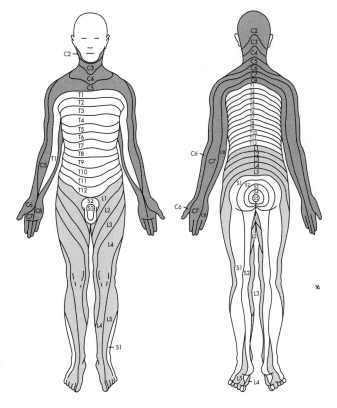

FIG. 7-1 Sensory dermatome.
(From Hockberger RS: Spinal injury. In Rund D et al: *Essentials of emergency medicine*, ed 2, St Louis, 1996, Mosby.)

checked on both sides of the body and also on the back and front for discrepancies and better localization.

b. Retention of superficial and deep pain discrimination indicates an incomplete lesion and lateral-column preservation. Sacral sparing (retained anal sensation and sphincter function) also indicates an incomplete lesion and is often a good prognostic sign.

6. Spinal injuries may be stable or unstable (Table 7-3).

a. The most common serious injuries to the spine that are compatible with life are those at C5 to C6 and those at T12 to L1.

b. Lesions at or above C4 usually involve phrenic centers and apnea. Those at C5 to C6 cause sensory loss below the clavicles and on the surface of the arm and the ulnar side of the hand.

TABLE 7-3
Classification of Spinal Injuries

Mechanisms of spinal injury	Stability
Flexion	
Wedge fracture	Stable
Clay shoveler's fracture	Stable
Subluxation	Potentially unstable
Bilateral facet dislocation	Always unstable
Flexion teardrop fracture	Extremely unstable
Atlantooccipital dislocation	Unstable
Anterior atlantoaxial dislocation with or without fracture	Unstable
Odontoid fracture with lateral displacement fracture	Unstable
Fracture of transverse process	Stable
Rotation	
Unilateral facet dislocation	Stable
Rotary atlantoaxial dislocation	Unstable
Extension	
Posterior neural arch fracture (C1)	Unstable
Hangman's fracture (C2)	Unstable
Extension teardrop fracture	Usually stable in flexion, unstable in extension
Posterior atlantoaxial dislocation with or without fracture	Unstable
Vertical compression	
Bursting fracture of vertebral body	Stable
Jefferson's fracture (C1)	Extremely unstable
Isolated fractures of articular pillar and vertebral body	Stable

      c. Lesions at L1 involve the conus medullaris and produce saddle anesthesia and sphincter tone loss.

  7. Radiographs of the relevant portions of the spine should be obtained, with care to avoid movement. If a fracture is found, x-rays should generally be taken of the entire spine.

      a. The area at C6 to T1, especially in large men, may be difficult to visualize unless the arms are pulled down while the film is taken. Swimmer's views may be required. Oblique views, again without moving the patient, may be needed.

      b. CT scanning of the spine may be very helpful in questionable cases and also to delineate the extent of injury found on plain films.

C. Treatment.

  1. Ensure that the airway is patent and ventilation is adequate. High cord lesions may produce apnea. If endotracheal intubation is needed, use the orotracheal route with manual in-line traction.

  2. If radiographs show a fracture or dislocation, or if there is clinical evidence of cord injury, spinal immobilization should be maintained.

  3. Administration of corticosteroids within 8 hours of injury is recommended for patients with spinal cord injury: methylprednisolone, 30 mg/kg IV, followed by an infusion of 5.4 mg/kg/hr for the following 23 hours.

  4. Neurosurgical and/or orthopedic consultation is recommended for any patient with a spine fracture or cord injury.

  5. Patients with unstable fractures, fracture-dislocations, or neurologic deficit should be considered for early transfer to a regional spinal cord center if one is available. Early telephone consultation should address patient management before and during transfer.

8

Orthopedic Trauma

I. GENERAL CONSIDERATIONS.
A. Priorities.
1. Priorities for treatment must be established for any patient with multiple injuries. An adequate airway must be established and maintained and hemorrhage controlled. Injuries to the chest, abdomen, or great vessels require priority treatment because they may be critical.
2. A check of neurologic function and of the circulation and pulses distal to a fracture is essential, as is complete documentation of such assessment.
B. Radiographs. Adequate roentgenograms of the area of injury are imperative.
1. Standard radiographic (usually posteroanterior, lateral, and oblique) views must be obtained as indicated.
2. Additional special views may be needed such as mortise or oblique views in ankle injuries.
3. For extremity injuries in children and adolescents, the opposite side is available for comparison if there are any questions in interpreting the film.
4. Films should include the joints proximal and distal to the area traumatized.
5. Always obtain postreduction radiographs after manipulation.
C. Casts.
1. Application of a plaster splint to immobilize a fracture until swelling subsides may be indicated in the acute setting. If major swelling is not anticipated, a cylindric cast may be applied.
2. If the cast must later be split and spread, the padding must be divided down to the skin; otherwise, underlying strands of sheet wadding may remain to impair circulation.
3. Be certain that the patient understands to return immediately if the extremity becomes cold or numb or if there is increased pain.

II. THE UPPER EXTREMITY.
A. Clavicle.
1. Complications such as nonunion of the clavicle are uncommon.

2. A sling may relieve much of the pain of undisplaced fractures. An active person will be most comfortable in a clavicular figure-eight brace.

B. Scapula.

1. Fractures may be caused by direct trauma or avulsion of muscle origins or insertions.
2. The patient should be examined for associated injuries such as rib fractures or pneumothorax.
3. For simple fractures and most avulsions, using a shoulder immobilizer during the time of acute pain is sufficient.

C. Dislocation of the shoulder.

1. Dislocation is anterior in 90% of cases and is apparent clinically. The lateral aspect of the shoulder is flat instead of rounded, and a deep depression is palpable between the head of the humerus and the acromion laterally.
2. Examination for associated brachial plexus injury is mandatory. The radial pulse should also be palpated and its presence noted in the record.
   a. Injury to the axillary nerve is common. Hypesthesia over the deltoid prominence indicates some compromise of sensory branches.
3. Evaluate adequate roentgenograms to discover any associated fractures before attempting reduction.
4. Reduction.
   a. A number of reduction techniques may be used, including the following:
      (1) Passive traction.
         (a) The patient is given an appropriate dose of IV analgesia or sedation (see Chapter 12). Alternatively, 20 ml of 1% lidocaine can be injected into the joint inferior and lateral to the acromion, aspirating as much blood as possible before injecting. Wait 15 minutes for maximum analgesia.
         (b) The patient then lies face down on the examining table with a shoulder over the edge and the affected extremity dependent.
         (c) From 10 to 15 lb of weight is tied to the wrist with gauze bandages.
         (d) The dislocation may be reduced after 10 to 15 minutes of this traction.
      (2) Method of Hippocrates.
         (a) Administer analgesia and sedation as above.
         (b) Exert slow, gentle longitudinal traction on the extremity, with countertraction exerted on the axilla.
         (c) Then, slowly and without force, bring the extremity to the midline while maintaining traction.
      (3) Scapular rotation.
         (a) Have the patient lie prone on the examination table with the arm hanging over the edge, or have

the patient sitting upright and have an assistant apply traction to the arm.
   (b) Push the tip of the scapula medially and the superior aspect of the scapula laterally.
5. After the dislocation is reduced, immobilize the extremity by applying a shoulder immobilizer.
   a. A bias-cut stockinette is good for this dressing.
6. Always obtain postreduction films.
7. Refer the patient for orthopedic follow-up care.

D. Acromioclavicular separation.
   1. The patient complains of pain localized just medial to the acromioclavicular joint. The mechanism of injury is a fall on the point of the shoulder.
   2. The injury may involve torn acromioclavicular ligaments only or, in more severe injuries, a tear of the coracoclavicular ligaments. In the second instance, the upwardly displaced distal end of the clavicle is much more prominent.
   3. Examination reveals local tenderness and pain at the acromioclavicular joint on downward traction of the forearm with the elbow flexed at 90 degrees. Roentgenograms of the acromioclavicular joint with the patient holding 10 lb of weight in his or her hand should readily demonstrate disruption of the joint.
   4. Either injury may be treated conservatively.
      a. Circumferential strapping extending around the flexed elbow up over the angle of the shoulder and the clavicle may be used to hold the separation reduced.
      b. Alternatively, a commercially produced acromioclavicular splint or shoulder immobilizer may be applied.
   5. For complete separation, reduction and internal fixation may be indicated.

E. Humerus.
   1. Fracture of the surgical neck.
      a. This fracture is common in elderly patients after falls onto the shoulder.
      b. Manipulation usually will not appreciably improve the position, especially with marked comminution. A shoulder immobilizer and administration of analgesics is appropriate initial therapy in most cases.
      c. Function is the most important factor. Arrange for close orthopedic follow-up.
      d. If the fracture is associated with a brachial plexus injury or dislocation of the head, open reduction and exploration may be indicated.
   2. Shaft fractures.
      a. In the elderly, it is often elected to apply a posterior plaster splint and ensure orthopedic follow-up.
      b. In young patients, nonunion or malunion is fairly common. A hanging arm cast or sling and swath dressing should be applied.

  c. Radial nerve injury is common; it may appear some hours after the initial injury from motion at the fracture site.

  d. Open surgical management usually is not indicated.

 3. Supracondylar fracture.

  a. This fracture requires immediate attention.

  b. The possibility of Volkmann's ischemic contracture after this injury makes it extremely dangerous. Examine the patient for increasing pain, pallor, absent pulse, paresthesias, and paralysis, the classic findings in ischemic injury.

F. Elbow.

 1. Central subluxation of the head of the radius, also known as *nursemaids' elbow.*

  a. This is a very common injury, and its history is important; typically, a sudden, longitudinal traction has been exerted on the upper extremity of a young child, usually under the age of 3.

  b. There is pain when passive flexion or extension of the elbow is attempted.

  c. The forearm is held in pronation; attempts at passive supination aggravate the pain.

  d. Obtain radiographs of the elbow before manipulation if the diagnosis is in doubt.

  e. With the examiner's thumb on the radial head, quick supination of the forearm by using very little force is all that is needed to thrust the radial head back through the annular ligament and relieve the painful disability completely.

  f. Ideally, a sling with a posterior plaster splint may be applied to hold the forearm in supination after the reduction. Young children, however, rarely tolerate the application of a sling or splint and usually do well without them.

 2. Dislocation of the elbow.

  a. The mechanism of injury is usually a fall. The elbow is markedly deformed, with disruption of the relationships of the bony prominences of the elbow.

  b. Obtain radiographs before attempting manipulation.

  c. Always check for associated neurovascular injuries, especially brachial artery and ulnar or median nerve damage.

  d. Reduction is by the application of longitudinal traction on the forearm with countertraction on the arm. Reduction may be difficult to achieve, and general anesthesia may be required.

  e. After reduction, immobilize the arm in a posterior plaster splint with the elbow flexed beyond a right angle. Check the distal pulses, and observe the circulation of the hand.

 3. Radial head fractures.

  a. Most will do well with immobilization in a posterior plaster splint until the acute pain subsides.

  b. Selected cases may need surgical treatment.

 4. Olecranon fractures.

  a. If the fracture is undisplaced, the extremity may be immobilized with the elbow in 90 degrees of flexion.

b. Even the slightest displacement is unacceptable, and open reduction with internal fixation is indicated.

5. "Tennis elbow."

   a. The patient often gives a history of repetitive use of the extremity.

   b. Pain is localized over and distal to the lateral epicondyle of the humerus near the origin of the extensor muscles.

   c. The pain may radiate down the forearm and is aggravated by pronation of the forearm, flexion of the wrist, and strong grip.

   d. Roentgenograms are normal.

   e. Local injection of corticosteroids and application of a sling for several days usually relieve the pain.

   f. Analgesics should be prescribed for several days, and the extremity should not be used. Oral antiinflammatory drugs may be helpful.

   g. Pain often returns after subsequent use, and the extremity may require prolonged rest.

G. Forearm.

1. Radius-ulna shaft fractures.

   a. If pronation and supination are to be preserved in the forearm, close to an anatomic reduction of both fractures is necessary.

   b. In children, with their great potential for growth and remodeling, some degree of displacement may be acceptable.

2. Distal radius (Colles') fractures.

   a. This is a common injury, especially in older patients after a fall onto the outstretched hand. A deformity involving the dorsum of the distal forearm is often visible. There may be an associated ulnar styloid fracture.

   b. Anesthesia for reduction may be achieved by hematoma block or Bier block.

   c. For reduction, apply longitudinal traction with countertraction to the elbow. Increase the deformity by forcible dorsiflexion of the wrist. In this position of hyperextension, the distal fragment can be pushed toward the palm to the proper relationship with the proximal radius. The wrist is then flexed, and the distal radial fragment is molded toward the palm and the ulna to correct angulation and radial displacement.

   d. A well-molded short-arm cast or sugar-tong splint is usually adequate to relieve discomfort in an older patient, but a long-arm cast may be desirable for the comminuted fracture. The cast should be split to prevent the development of ischemia resulting from swelling.

   e. It no longer is accepted practice to place the hand in extreme palmar flexion and ulnar deviation; this may help maintain a reduction, but it leaves the wrist stiff, a poor position in the older patient.

H. Wrist and hand.
  1. Navicular fractures.
      a. The mechanism of injury is usually a fall onto the outstretched hand. The patient complains of pain in the wrist, especially over the region of the anatomic snuff box. There is pain on extension and ulnar deviation of the wrist.
      b. Initial roentgenograms of the wrist may fail to demonstrate the fracture, but special navicular views are often more sensitive.
      c. In confirmed navicular fractures or those suspected on clinical grounds, apply a short-arm cast incorporating the thumb to the interphalangeal joint in a position of abduction and opposition.
      d. If initial films are normal, repeat radiographs out of plaster in 7 to 10 days. Callus and resorption of bone at the fracture site may then be apparent.
  2. Metacarpal fractures.
      a. Fractures occur at the neck of the second to fifth metacarpals from direct trauma, as in a blow with the fist.
      b. The most common fractures are of the fourth and fifth metacarpals (boxer's fracture). There is palmar angulation of the metacarpal head.
      c. Local infiltration of the fracture hematoma with 1% lidocaine usually provides sufficient anesthesia for reduction.
      d. Flex the metacarpophalangeal and proximal interphalangeal joints to 90 degrees, and exert strong pressure over the proximal interphalangeal joint dorsally along the axis of the proximal phalanx. This may correct the angulation in a recent injury.
      e. Immobilize the hand with the metacarpophalangeal and proximal interphalangeal joints of the injured finger in the functional position in a short-arm cast.
      f. A good functional result can be obtained with less than anatomic reduction. Up to 40 degrees of volar angulation is acceptable.

III. THE LOWER EXTREMITY.
A. The Hip.
  1. Fractures.
      a. These may occur with relatively minor trauma in the elderly.
      b. Classically, the shortened lower extremity lies in external rotation (greater in intertrochanteric than in neck fractures).
      c. Movement or rotation at the hip causes groin or knee pain.
      d. There is pain on pressure over the greater trochanter.
      e. Such fractures are best treated by open reduction and internal fixation.

2. Dislocation.
   a. This injury is the result of severe violence. Automobile accidents are the most common cause. On physical examination, the hip is flexed and adducted; the leg is shortened and internally rotated. Sciatic nerve injury is sometimes associated.
   b. Early reduction is imperative and lessens such complications as late aseptic necrosis of the femoral head and pressure injury of the sciatic nerve. Reduction is frequently difficult, and general anesthesia may be required.
   c. Evaluate for associated fractures to the femoral shaft and pelvis.
3. Trochanteric bursitis.
   a. This may be confused with hip joint disease or with a herniated intervertebral disk.
   b. Either the subcutaneous or, more commonly, the deep trochanteric bursa may be involved. The bursitis is usually aseptic.
   c. Direct pressure over the bursa duplicates the pain.
   d. The patient may be treated with nonsteroidal antiinflammatory medications. The condition also responds to local corticosteroid injection.

B. Femoral shaft.

1. Diaphyseal fractures.
   a. There may be appreciable blood loss into the thigh. Signs of hemorrhage can be easily missed if the patient is not carefully monitored.
   b. Initial management includes immediate immobilization in a traction splint, evaluation of the extent of volume loss, and administration of IV fluids and blood, as indicated.
   c. Surgical repair is required.
2. Supracondylar fractures: Popliteal artery injury may be a complication. A careful evaluation of distal circulation is imperative. Early consultation with orthopedic and vascular surgeons and arteriography should be obtained in any case in which circulatory impairment is suspected.

C. The knee.

1. Patellar fractures.
   a. Undisplaced longitudinal fractures may be immobilized with the knee in extension in a cylinder cast or knee immobilizer.
   b. If the fragments are separated as they frequently are in horizontal fractures, surgical reduction is required.
2. Patellar dislocations.
   a. Most frequently, these occur laterally. Adolescent girls and young women are most often affected.
   b. Reduction is achieved by applying pressure medially over the lateral side of the patella while slowly extending the knee.
   c. Recurrences may require surgical stabilization.

ACL
MCL INJURIES

3. Nonbony injury.
    a. A common injury is a torn medial meniscus, sometimes associated with anterior cruciate and medial collateral ligament tears. A typical history is the sudden onset of pain after internal rotation of the femur on the fixed tibia and foot.
    b. If the development of swelling was slow (over a period of hours), a serous effusion is likely; anticipate a cartilage injury only.
    c. If swelling was rapid in onset, anticipate ligament tears or a fracture with a hemarthrosis. However, complete ligament tears may not result in significant effusion.
    d. Arthrocentesis should be performed if a large effusion is present.
        (1) Always aspirate the knee under strict aseptic conditions.
        (2) Note whether the aspirated fluid is serous or bloody.
        (3) Let the tube into which the joint fluid is injected stand. If globules of fat (marrow) rise to the surface, anticipate an osteochondral fracture, which may not be apparent on roentgenograms.
    e. Examination.
        (1) With the knee flexed at 30 degrees, check for abnormal mobility with medial or lateral pressure applied to the lower part of the leg. If a medial or lateral collateral ligament is torn, excessive motion will be felt, and a fingertip on the joint line will feel the joint rock open on the injured side.
        (2) Test for excess anteroposterior motion of the head of the tibia with the knee flexed to 90 degrees. Excessive anterior motion of the tibia is possible with a torn anterior cruciate ligament, and excessive posterior motion is possible with the less common tear of the posterior cruciate ligament.
        (3) Many tests demonstrate torn cartilages, but none is exceptionally reliable. The leg may be held in full internal or external rotation with the knee acutely flexed.
            (a) A snap or click is sometimes felt or heard as the knee is then brought into full extension while the leg is rotated. There are many variations and eponyms for such tests.
            (b) Abnormal laxity, "pops," "clicks," or other findings may be bilateral and unrelated to the injury.
4. Radiographs: Obtain adequate roentgenograms of the knee; these should include "tunnel" or intercondylar notch views and "skyline" or tangential views of the patella if indicated.
5. Management.
    a. Early surgical repair is usually advised for torn collateral ligaments or a torn meniscus.

    b. If adequate examination is prohibited by excessive pain or swelling, the patient must have follow-up arrangements made for reexamination in several days.

D. Tibial shaft fracture.

1. Most can be treated satisfactorily by closed reduction. These fractures should be reduced under general anesthesia if the position is not satisfactory. Associated vascular injury probably occurs more often than is suspected clinically.

2. Proximal shaft fractures are through cancellous bone and usually heal with no difficulty. Fractures through the distal third are in an area of poor blood supply; delayed union is common, and nonunion is by no means rare. Prolonged immobilization may be necessary in this case, sometimes for 6 to 9 months.

E. The ankle.

1. Sprain.

    a. The anterior talofibular ligament is the most commonly injured, and there is point tenderness anterior to the lateral malleolus.

    b. For the uncomplicated sprain, elastic bandages and taping or prefabricated splints are used in treatment along with ice, elevation, and crutches.

2. Fractures.

    a. Films must include anteroposterior, lateral, and mortise (oblique) views. The "joint line" around the talus should be the same width on both sides and top.

    b. Early reduction before significant swelling occurs is important. Some cases require open reduction.

F. The foot.

1. Calcaneal fractures.

    a. Check for associated compression fractures of the spine because the mechanism of injury is usually a fall from a height.

    b. The best results seem to follow elevation of the extremity after the application of pressure dressings. Early motion of the foot and ankle without bearing weight for 4 to 8 weeks usually gives a good functional result.

2. Fracture of the base of the fifth metatarsal (ballet fracture).

    a. The peroneus brevis muscle inserts at the base of the fifth metatarsal. The mechanism of injury of the fracture is the avulsion of the base of the metatarsal by a sharp, sudden inversion.

    b. It is a common injury often confused with a sprained ankle. The tenderness and swelling are anterior around the fifth metatarsal base, not around the anterior tip of the lateral malleolus.

    c. These patients are often reasonably comfortable in shoes with a hard sole to limit motion. If they experience great pain during walking, they may need a short-leg walking cast.

3. Phalangeal fractures.
    a. Firm, well-fitting shoes relieve much of the pain during walking.
    b. Taping adjacent toes together helps relieve pain but may lead to skin maceration unless there is adequate padding between the toes.

IV. PELVIS.

A. Pelvic fractures are potentially the most dangerous of bony injuries, being capable of producing exsanguinating hemorrhage.
    1. The source of bleeding is usually the vascular plexus lining the pelvic walls, but there may also be injury to iliac, iliolumbar, or femoral vessels.
    2. When signs of hypovolemic shock are present, fluid resuscitation is indicated, and early transfusion of blood may be required.
    3. Application of the pneumatic antishock garment may be of particular benefit in pelvic fractures.
    4. Operative reduction of unstable fractures will also diminish bleeding.
B. Fractures with which hemorrhage is most often associated are those of the sacrum or ilium, bilateral pubic rami, separation of the symphysis pubis, and dislocations of the sacroiliac joint.
C. Urinary tract injury accompanies approximately 10% of pelvic fractures.
    1. Hematuria is usually present.
    2. Urethral injuries in male patients usually occur at the level of the prostatic apex.
        a. Gross blood may be seen at the urethral meatus.
        b. Pubic fractures may be palpable on rectal examination, and the prostate may be displaced superiorly and surrounded by a boggy hematoma.
        c. Insertion of a urethral catheter in trauma patients with meatal bleeding is contraindicated. The diagnosis should be verified by retrograde urethrography and a suprapubic cystostomy catheter inserted.

V. THE SPINE.

For a discussion of spinal injury, refer to Chapter 7.

9

Hand Injuries

Note: See Chapter 8 for a discussion of hand fractures, Chapter 14 for a discussion of antibiotic prophylaxis and treatment of infection, and Chapter 12 for discussion of regional anesthesia.

I. GENERAL PRINCIPLES.

A. Evaluation of the patient as a whole must precede diagnosis and treatment of the specific hand injury.

1. Inquiry must be made as to whether the patient has a chronic systemic disease that may retard wound healing such as diabetes, circulatory insufficiency, or neoplasm.

2. It should also be learned whether the patient is receiving steroid therapy and what the status of his or her tetanus immunization is.

3. Treatment priorities must be established for the patient with multiple injuries. Life-threatening conditions must be dealt with at once.

B. An accurate history of the specific hand injury must be obtained. Important considerations are the time elapsed since injury, how and where the injury was sustained, right or left hand dominance, and the occupation of the patient.

C. Old scars and previous injuries should be well documented. Sensory, motor, and vascular status must be evaluated. A diagram is useful for describing all lacerations, scars, and deficits.

D. Radiographs may be helpful in delineating hand injuries that involve bone or foreign bodies.

II. FUNCTIONAL ANATOMY OF THE HAND.

An accurate diagnosis of injuries and infections requires precise knowledge of the anatomy.

A. **Palmar surface of the wrist** (Fig. 9-1).

1. The palmar surface of the wrist contains three easily palpable tendons: palmaris longus in the middle with flexor carpi radialis and flexor carpi ulnaris to either side. (Palmaris longus is absent unilaterally in approximately 15% of patients and absent bilaterally in 7%.)

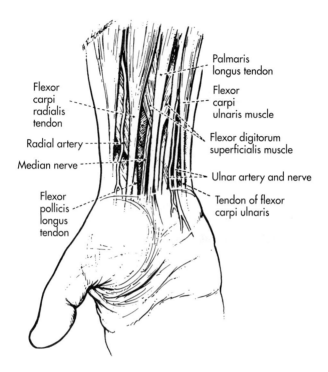

FIG. 9-1 Palmar aspect of a wrist.

2. The median nerve lies just deep to palmaris longus on its radial side. The ulnar nerve and artery lie deep to flexor carpi ulnaris on its radial side. The radial artery lies just radial to flexor carpi radialis.

B. Palm of the hand (Fig. 9-2).

1. The transverse carpal ligament forms the roof of the carpal tunnel. This space contains nine tendons and one nerve: the superficialis and profundus tendons to the fingers, the flexor policis longus tendon, and the median nerve.

2. The ulnar artery and nerve occupy a separate compartment formed by the volar carpal ligament.

3. The motor branch of the median nerve leaves the main trunk at the distal edge of the transverse carpal ligament to innervate the thenar muscles and the radial lumbricals.

C. Dorsum of the hand and wrist (Fig. 9-3).

1. The extensor tendons of the fingers insert at the base of the middle phalanges.

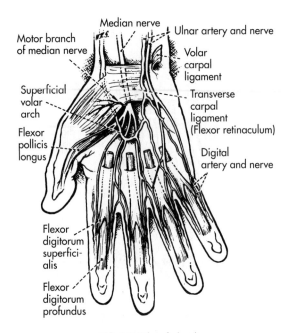

Median nerve

Motor branch
of median nerve

Ulnar artery and nerve

Volar
carpal
ligament

Superficial
volar
arch

Transverse
carpal
ligament
(Flexor retinaculum)

Flexor
pollicis
longus

Digital
artery and nerve

Flexor
digitorum
superfici-
alis

Flexor
digitorum
profundus

FIG. 9-2 Palm of a hand.

2. There are two tendons to the index finger and (with consid-
erable anatomic variation) two tendons to the fifth finger.

D. Radial aspect of the wrist (Fig 9-4).

1. This region is injured frequently. The long and short extensor tendons and their insertions and the abductor pollicis
longus tendon of the thumb are shown in Fig. 9-4.

2. Of greater practical importance is the sensory (superficial)
branch of the radial nerve, which is frequently overlooked in
lacerations of this region.

3. If this structure is not repaired, the proximal end can form a
neuroma that may become tender and painful.

4. The extensor carpi radialis longus and brevis are shown in
Fig. 9-4. The brevis is ulnar to the longus and is the prime
wrist extensor.

III. DIAGNOSIS.

Before injection of a local anesthetic, it is crucial to evaluate the
vascular status, sensation, and motor function of the hand.

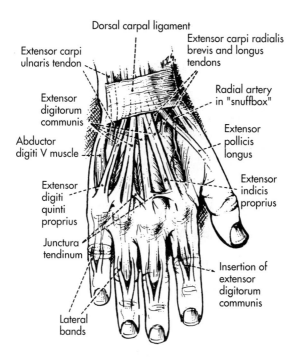

FIG. 9-3 Dorsum of a hand.
BACK OF HAND

A. Vascular status.

1. A cold, pulseless hand indicates severe arterial damage. Circulation must be restored promptly in the operating room.

2. Significant bleeding can ordinarily be controlled with a compression bandage. If bleeding persists, a padded blood pressure cuff applied to the arm and inflated to above systolic blood pressure will stop the bleeding. The cuff must be deflated every 45 minutes to allow full tissue perfusion.

3. Performance of Allen's test will help delineate vascular status in persons with wrist and forearm injuries.
   a. The hand is elevated, and both the radial and the ulnar arteries are occluded at the wrist by digital pressure.
   b. The patient is asked to open and close the fist repeatedly until venous drainage leaves the hand pale.
   c. Pressure over one artery is then released.
   d. The hand should return to pink within 15 to 30 seconds.

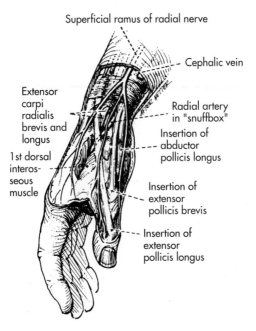

Superficial ramus of radial nerve

Cephalic vein

Extensor carpi radialis brevis and longus

Radial artery in "snuffbox"

Insertion of abductor pollicis longus

1st dorsal interosseous muscle

Insertion of extensor pollicis brevis

Insertion of extensor pollicis longus

FIG. 9-4 Superficial ramus of radial nerve.

    e. The entire procedure is then repeated and the other artery is tested.

B. Sensation (Fig. 9-5).

  1. The median nerve carries sensory fibers from the palmar surface of the thumb, index finger, middle finger, and radial half of the ring finger, as well as the portion of the palm proximal to these fingers. It also provides sensation to the distal dorsal aspects of these fingers.

  2. The radial nerve accounts for sensation over the radial aspect of the same fingers and the dorsal hand proximal to them.

  3. The ulnar nerve provides sensation to the ulnar aspect of the ring finger and the entire little finger, as well as to both the palmar and dorsal aspects of the hand proximal to its finger distribution.

  4. Anesthesia of the palm or dorsal aspect of the hand is usually accompanied by a loss of sensation to one or more fingers and implies a major nerve injury.

  5. Anesthesia of one half of a single finger indicates laceration of a digital sensory nerve.

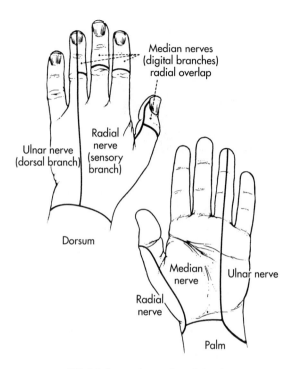

FIG. 9-5 Sensory innervation of a hand.

6. Hypesthesia of a given anatomic area is often transient and suggests that the nerve is merely contused rather than transected.

C. Motor function.

1. Partial tendon transections may leave the patient with sufficient strength to perform a requested maneuver against gravity. However, if the maneuver is performed against resistance, subtle injuries may be detected.

2. Depending on the injury, motor function evaluation should include the following:

   a. Flexion of the fingers at the proximal interphalangeal joints (flexor digitorum superficialis).

   b. Flexion of the fingers at the distal interphalangeal joints (flexor digitorum profundus).

   c. Extension of the fingers.

   d. Opposition of the thumb and little finger.

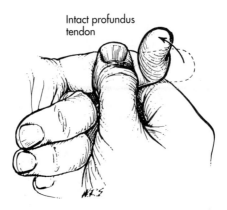

Intact profundus tendon

FIG. 9-6 Test for flexor digitorum profundus function.

    e. Abduction of the fingers.

    f. Extension and flexion of the wrist.

3. An inability to flex the distal phalanx with immobilization of the middle phalanx indicates division of the flexor digitorum profundus (Fig. 9-6).

4. Holding all fingers in extension except the one injured tests the function of the flexor digitorum superficialis (Fig. 9-7).

5. A laceration over the dorsal surface and the inability to extend the finger fully suggest severance of the following:

    a. The common extensor tendon.

    b. The extensor indicis.

    c. The extensor digiti minimi.

6. Lacerations near the distal interphalangeal joint and droop of the distal phalanx (mallet-finger deformity) indicate injury of the extensor complex in this region.

7. An inability to fully extend the distal phalanx of the thumb suggests division of the extensor pollicis longus tendon.

8. Injuries over the first metacarpal and the radial aspect of the wrist with the inability to extend and abduct the thumb suggest injuries to the short extensor and long abductor tendons. The long extensor also may be divided.

9. Even small lacerations of the thenar area may divide the motor branch of the median nerve, which innervates the thenar muscles. With such injury, the patient will be unable to strongly oppose the thumb to the base of the little finger or to abduct the thumb normally.

10. Damage to the motor branch of the ulnar nerve in the palm will make abduction or adduction of the extended fin-

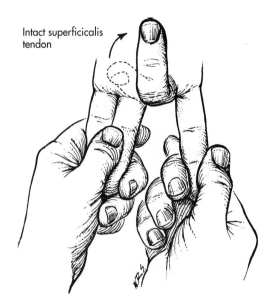

Intact superficicalis tendon

FIG. 9-7 Test for flexor digitorum superficialis function.

gers impossible because of the loss of interosseous muscle function.

a. The best test is to have the patient put the hand palm down on a table and attempt to deviate the index finger radially.

b. One may observe and palpate the first dorsal interosseous muscle located on the dorsal radial aspect of the second metacarpal bone and assay the extent of movement and muscle tone.

IV. TREATMENT.

See Chapter 12 for a discussion of nerve blocks for hand anesthesia.

A. General principles.

1. If at all possible, hand lacerations should be sutured within 6 hours of the injury to avoid infection.

2. Single-layer repair is usually sufficient unless a muscle, tendon, or nerve is involved. Multiple-layer closure on the hand increases the risk of adhesions involving deeper structures.

3. Interrupted stitches should be used. The interrupted vertical mattress technique is often helpful on the dorsum of the hand, an area especially liable to inversion of scar tissue.

4. Inspection of the wound in a bloodless field is important.
   a. A well-padded arm tourniquet can be used. The arm is elevated, and a layer of cast padding is applied. A blood pressure cuff or a commercial pneumatic tourniquet is placed over the padding and inflated to approximately 50 mm higher than systolic pressure. The rubber tubing of the cuff may require clamping to prevent air leakage. The arm will become painful, and the tourniquet should be released as soon as possible, certainly within 45 minutes.
   b. Finger tourniquets can be used. A small rubber catheter or drain can be applied to the base of the finger and secured with a hemostat, which is obviously visible (Fig. 9-8). The tourniquet time should be minimized. The laceration can often be repaired after the tourniquet is released so long as adequate inspection was achieved in a bloodless field.
5. Immobilization of the hand is essential to the healing process. If skin overlying joints is involved, those joints

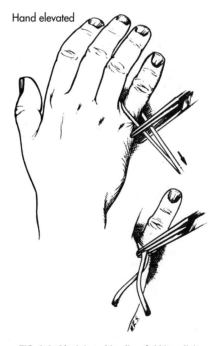

Hand elevated

FIG. 9-8 Obtaining a bloodless field in a digit.

should be splinted. In any major hand injury, the entire hand and wrist should be immobilized in a position of function.
6. Elevation of the hand with any significant injury should be encouraged, with a sling used as needed.
7. Hand sutures may generally be removed in 7 to 10 days.

B. Nerve injuries.

1. Small areas of numbness over the distal finger may be caused by nerve contusion or by the transection of sensory fibers that are too small to repair. Many of these deficits resolve spontaneously.
2. Any motor loss or significant sensory loss should be evaluated by a hand surgeon. The skin can be closed primarily and the deficit evaluated in several days if the surgeon is unavailable at the time of the injury.

C. Vascular injuries.

1. Isolated bleeding digital arterial vessels can usually be controlled with pressure alone. They should not be ligated, if possible, because of their proximity to nerves.
2. There is usually sufficient collateral circulation so that the loss of a digital artery is of little consequence. However, obvious vascular compromise with decreased capillary perfusion should be evaluated immediately by a hand surgeon.

D. Tendon injuries.

1. Flexor tendons are generally repaired by a hand surgeon in the operating room. They require extended follow-up and have a high incidence of complications.
2. Simple extensor tendon transections can be repaired in the emergency department, depending on the practice in the community and the training of the emergency physician. Nonabsorbable suture material should be used and the hand immobilized. The details of tendon repair are beyond the scope of this book.

E. Open fractures.

1. Meticulous debridement and irrigation will help prevent infection.
2. Many fractures will heal well with skin closure and immobilization, particularly digital tuft fractures. However, open reduction of fragments, including wiring, will often be necessary.
3. Antibiotics are suggested, such as cephazolin, 0.5 to 1 g intramuscularly, followed by cephalexin or dicloxacillin, 250 to 500 mg four times daily for 5 days.

F. Avulsions and amputations.

1. Avulsion of the soft-tissue volar pad over the distal phalanx will usually respond well to split-thickness skin grafting.
2. Avulsion of the soft tissue over the fingertip often will heal satisfactorily with no repair.
3. Exposed bone must be covered with soft tissue. A full-thickness skin graft, pedicle flap, or rongeuring of the bone tip with primary skin closure may be necessary.

G. Grease and paint gun injuries.

1. These may appear to be minimal puncture wounds soon after injury. However, they cause one of the most serious hand injuries. The insoluble organic compound injected into the fingertip may enter the tendon sheath and be conveyed proximally well into the hand. Delayed inflammatory reaction and swelling are extremely intense, and such injuries often lead to amputation if untreated.

2. All patients with this type of trauma should be referred immediately to a hand surgeon. Many will require decompression and debridement in the operating room.

10

Facial Injuries

I. INTRODUCTION.

A. For cases involving multiple-system injury, the entire patient must be evaluated to establish the proper priority of management (see Chapter 3).

B. If the airway is compromised by facial injury, it must be secured immediately.

C. Definitive repair of facial lacerations can be delayed several hours if necessary (see Chapter 13).

D. Reduction of facial fractures may be postponed for several days to a week until the patient's general condition has stabilized and soft-tissue swelling has subsided, at which time surgery will be easier to perform and bone position easier to maintain.

II. FACIAL BONE FRACTURES.

A. Clinical signs of facial bone fracture include point tenderness and swelling over the fracture site, bony asymmetry, and mobility of the fractured portion. Several specific findings should be ruled out by examination:

1. Malocclusion is one of the most accurate signs of a mandibular or maxillary fracture.

2. Numbness of the cheek or gum, or deficit of ocular motion, may reflect orbital fracture with entrapment of nerve or muscle.

B. Clinical findings should be confirmed with facial radiographs. Lateral and stereoscopic Waters' views are the most useful. Other views should be ordered as indicated. CT may be useful in defining injuries unclear on plain radiographs.

C. **Orbital fractures** may involve only the malar bone of the inferior orbital rim, the thin floor of the orbit, or both (Fig. 10-1). Findings may include the following:

1. Palpable irregularity and depression of the inferior orbital rim. This may be absent in isolated orbital floor fractures.

2. Depression of the level of the globe.

3. The subjective complaint of diplopia and the finding of extraocular muscle entrapment, particularly of the inferior rectus on upward gaze.

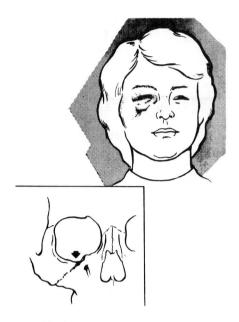

FIG. 10-1 Depressed fracture of the right malar bone.

4. Numbness in the distribution of the infraorbital nerve—the medial portion of the cheek and the upper lip and gums.
5. Radiographs may reveal a fracture line, clouding of the maxillary antrum because of blood, air in the orbit, or the herniation of soft tissue into the maxillary sinus.
6. Nerve or muscle dysfunction may be due to swelling or contusion and resolve in several days. However, entrapment caused by bone displacement, and any significant bony deformity, require surgical correction.
7. Prophylactic antibiotics such as amoxicillin or a cephalosporin are sometimes used for fractures extending into the paranasal sinuses.

D. **Zygomatic arch fractures** cause local tenderness and swelling, often with visible or palpable depression over the arch (Fig. 10-2). This fracture is most frequently caused by a direct blow.
1. Trismus and pain may occur on opening the mouth, when depressed bony fragments impinge on the underlying mandibular coronoid process and the temporalis muscle.
2. Special underpenetrated radiographs of the zygomatic arches confirm the diagnosis.
3. Depressed zygomatic fractures require surgical reduction.

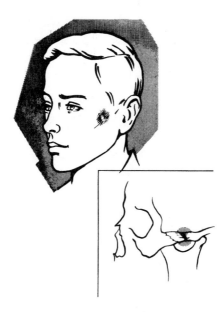

FIG. 10-2 Depressed fracture of the zygomatic arch.

E. **Mandibular fractures** cause tenderness along the mandible in one or more areas, pain on opening and closing of the mouth, and often malocclusion and irregularity of the lower teeth. Mobility of the fractured portion may occur, and occasionally so will compounding of the fracture into the oral cavity.

  1. Standard radiographs may be difficult to interpret, but special panorex views usually define the injury clearly.

  2. The condyle is the weakest portion of the mandible (Fig. 10-3). Fractures may be associated with bleeding from the external auditory canal if the walls of the canal are disrupted. An open bite suggests the presence of a mandibular dislocation or bilateral condylar fractures. Temporomandibular joint views may be required to disclose the abnormality.

  3. Fractures of the symphysis are the least common mandibular fractures. If there is injury to or edema around the mental foramen, there may be anesthesia of the chin and lower lip.

  4. Simple mandibular fractures can be treated by interdental wiring or elastic traction, but complicated fractures of the mandible require open reduction.

F. **Maxillary fractures** fall into several well-defined categories.

  1. Le Fort I. This is a transverse fracture across the maxilla (Fig. 10-4).

  2. Le Fort II. This fracture runs through the nasal bones and the frontal maxillary processes (Fig. 10-4).

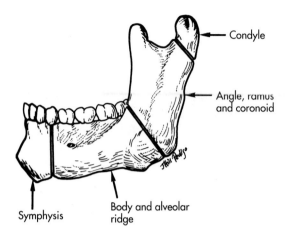

FIG. 10-3 Areas of the mandible.

3. *Le Fort III.* In this fracture, the maxilla, nasal bones, and zygoma are separated from their cranial attachments, that is, there is craniofacial dysjunction (Fig. 10-4). This type of fracture is usually associated with additional facial fractures.

4. These midface fractures may result in vertical elongation of the midface, malocclusion, and abnormal movement of the maxillary portion of the face. The latter may be demonstrated by grasping the upper teeth and palate and displacing this unit anteriorly.

5. Midface fractures usually require open reduction.

G. **Nasal fractures** may be nondisplaced, depressed, or laterally displaced. Visualization and palpation will often reveal the deformity if present.

1. Inspection of the nostrils usually reveals blood and sometimes septal hematoma or septal cartilage dislocation into either nasal airway.

2. Radiographs of the nasal bones confirm the diagnosis but are of little aid to therapy if there is no displacement on examination because nondisplaced nasal fractures without airway obstruction require no treatment. However, social or legal considerations may dictate radiologic documentation.

3. Septal hematoma should always be ruled out by inspection or palpation.

   a. If untreated, infection and necrosis of the septal cartilage can develop.

   b. Treatment consists of local lidocaine injection followed by incision over the inferior portion of the hematoma. A

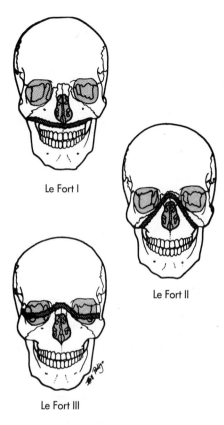

Le Fort I

Le Fort II

Le Fort III

FIG. 10-4 Le Fort types of maxillary fracture.

small drain can then be inserted and the anterior nose packed with petrolatum gauze.

4. Clear drainage from the nose may indicate a leak of cerebral spinal fluid from a basilar skull fracture.

5. When swelling is minimal, displaced fractures can be reduced during the first few hours. However, significant swelling can preclude adequate visual evaluation of reduction efforts. In this case, manipulation should be deferred for approximately 1 week until the swelling is reduced.

III. LARYNGEAL TRAUMA.

A. Laryngeal trauma may be caused by a blow to the anterior neck from a baseball bat, golf ball, or fist, or from the entanglement of a scarf or necktie in machinery. Among the most common causes are bicycle and automobile accidents.

B. Symptoms and diagnosis.

1. Rapid diagnosis and treatment are imperative to prevent airway compromise.
2. Hoarseness, dysphonia, or aphonia after trauma is suggestive of nerve or cartilage injury involving the larynx.
3. The airway should be evaluated immediately. Respiratory symptoms may range from relatively trivial to rapidly progressing stridor, dyspnea, and total airway obstruction.
4. Gentle palpation of the neck in persons with suspected laryngeal trauma may disclose subcutaneous emphysema, pain on palpation, deformity and discoloration or fixation of the thyroid or cricoid cartilages, or fracture of the hyoid bone. The thyroid cartilage may be flattened, or one ala may overlap the other anteriorly.
5. Indirect laryngoscopy may reveal hematoma, edema, vocal cord laceration, deformity of the laryngeal configuration, or impaired mobility of the vocal cords.
6. Lateral and anteroposterior neck radiographs for soft-tissue detail may reveal air in the soft-tissue spaces or disruption of airway anatomy. CT examination may be of further assistance in identifying the nature and extent of injury.
7. Fiberoptic or direct laryngoscopy is indicated for suspected laryngeal fractures.

C. Treatment.

1. The essence of therapy for laryngeal trauma is maintenance and preservation of the airway. Cricothyrotomy or tracheostomy may be required. Rapid evaluation is important in preventing airway obstruction.
2. The treatment of minimal soft-tissue injury consists of voice rest, humidification, and surveillance. If the airway becomes compromised, however, early surgical establishment of a stable airway is indicated.

IV. TRAUMATIC PERFORATION OF THE EARDRUM.

A. Tympanic membrane (TM) perforation may be caused directly by a foreign body such as a cotton-tipped applicator used to clean the ear, or indirectly from barotrauma from water skiing, diving, or a slap to the ear. Perforation resulting from otitis media can also occur.

B. **Symptoms.** Pain, bleeding, hearing loss, fullness, and tinnitus are common. Vertigo can also occur.

C. **Evaluation.** The injury is apparent on otoscopic examination. Document hearing loss before initiating treatment by testing ability to hear whispered words at 2 to 3 feet or to hear fingers lightly rubbed together close to the ear.

D. Treatment.
1. The TM perforation will usually heal spontaneously, but immediate otolaryngologic consultation should be obtained if there is significant vertigo, copious bleeding, clear fluid drainage, or major TM damage.
2. Systemic antibiotics are generally unnecessary in uncontaminated injuries such as those caused by a cotton-tipped applicator. However, many authorities recommend topical instillation of a balanced-pH otic antibiotic such as polymyxin B sulfate, bacitracin Zinc, neomycin (Neosporin)-glucocorticoid, particularly in contaminated perforations such as diving injuries.
3. The patient should be advised to keep water and other material out of the ear canal. Cotton lubricated with petroleum jelly may be loosely fitted to the bowl of the auricle during showering.

V. DENTAL TRAUMA.
A. Tooth avulsion.
1. An avulsed deciduous tooth should not be replaced because this may lead to problems with the eventual permanent tooth.
2. Avulsed permanent teeth should be replaced as rapidly as possible, preferably within the first 30 minutes.
   a. Care should be taken not to disturb the root or any soft tissue still adherent to the tooth. The tooth should not be wiped or rubbed.
   b. If necessary, any adherent clot or debris can be gently rinsed away from the socket.
   c. While the tooth may be stored temporarily in saline, it should be replaced into its socket as soon as possible.
B. Tooth displacement. A displaced tooth that is still in the socket and not grossly unstable should not be manipulated in the ED because this may lead to disruption of the blood and nerve supply and eventual death of the tooth. Many displaced teeth eventually return to normal alignment because of gradual pressure from the lip and tongue. Obviously, dental consultation is indicated.
C. Tooth fracture.
1. Immediate dental consultation is indicated for a broken tooth if the nerve is exposed, as may be suggested by bleeding from the broken tooth surface or exposure of the pink-colored pulp.
2. Temporarily covering the exposed surface with wax may provide significant analgesia.
3. If both a broken tooth and an oral laceration are present, the wound should be thoroughly explored for the missing tooth fragment.
4. The alveolar ridge should be examined to rule out a fracture.

11

Ophthalmologic Injuries

I. GENERAL CONSIDERATIONS.

A. In the patient with multiple trauma, the priorities of trauma care should be observed (see Chapter 3). Eye injury should be addressed only after life-threatening trauma is assessed and the patient stabilized.

B. In all patients with eye injury except those for whom intervention must be initiated without delay (e.g., caustic burns), visual acuity should be tested before diagnostic or therapeutic manipulation. Each eye should be tested separately and the results noted in the medical record. If the patient wears glasses, the acuity may be recorded with the glasses in place and the notation "corrected" made.

C. The standard Snellen's eye chart should be used whenever possible, and the smallest line discernible by the patient recorded. A pinhole can be used for patients who did not bring their corrective lenses. If the patient is unable to read even the largest figures on the chart, he or she should be asked to count the number of fingers the examiner holds, to detect finger movement, and to perceive light, in that order.

D. Examination of the eye should be complete in each instance, and should include a funduscopic examination. Examination with the slit lamp (if available) should be used in appropriate cases.

II. CHEMICAL EXPOSURE OF THE CONJUNCTIVA AND CORNEA.

A. The offending agents are mostly detergents, window-cleaning or other cleaning solutions, and strong acids and bases such as battery acid or lye. The most serious injury results from strong alkaline solutions.

B. The severely burned conjunctiva looks white and opaque and breaks down to shreds within a few hours; the cornea turns dull white. The moderately damaged conjunctiva appears edematous and hyperemic.

C. Irrespective of the nature of the offending agent, initial treatment consists of copious irrigation with water in the most readily available form. Tap water at room temperature is an excellent irrigating fluid. Tap water used in a washbowl or sink in which the injured person can immerse the top of his head, including the burned eye, should be recommended over the telephone to any person who reports a chemical injury to the eye. While the eye is under water, the eyelids should be moved vigorously so the water can penetrate into the recesses of the conjunctival sac.

D. In the ED, the condition must be recognized promptly and treatment instituted immediately. Sterile saline or lactated Ringer's solutions are preferable as irrigating solutions, but tap water is preferable when other fluid is not readily available. The following points should be remembered:

1. A few drops of a topical anesthetic (tetracaine, proparacaine, or a similar agent) instilled into the conjunctival sac facilitates the treatment for both patient and physician.

2. IV saline solution may be instilled through IV tubing. Alternatively, a commercial irrigation lens, such as a Morgan or Mediflow lens, may be applied if there is no gross deformity of the cornea. The stream of fluid going in should be strong, that is, on the order of several milliliters per second.

3. Spasm of the lid muscles elicited by the chemical exposure must be overcome by gentle pull on the eyelids (if necessary, with lid retractors).

4. The recesses (fornices) of the conjunctival sac, particularly the upper one, should be irrigated thoroughly and swept with a moistened cotton-tipped applicator to remove particulate matter.

5. If there is particulate foreign matter, irrigation should be continued until no more particles can be dissolved in the effluent. At least 1 L of solution should be used to irrigate the exposed eye. The pH of the inferior fornix tear film should be checked 30 minutes after irrigation is completed. Irrigation should be continued until this pH is 7.4.

E. After irrigation and examination, topical antibiotic preparations should be instilled into the eye every 3 to 4 hours for 1 or 2 days. In significant cases, acute ophthalmologic consultation may be required.

III. FOREIGN BODIES OF THE EYE.

A. Large splinters of glass, plastic, or metal can cut into the eye in such a way as to anchor but still move with the movements of the lids. The mere opening of the eye, voluntarily by the patient or manually by the examiner, can add severe trauma by pushing the foreign body deeper into the eye. Topical anesthetic such as 0.5% proparacaine or tetracaine should be instilled into the eye to aid examination. If the object has not penetrated the cornea, it may be removed as described in Section II, C.

B. Clinical findings suggestive of foreign body penetration of the cornea include a shallow anterior chamber, iris prolapse, and an irregular pupil.

C. Penetration should be suspected particularly when a metallic foreign body has been driven at high velocity such as particles propelled by a grinding wheel. If there is doubt about the presence of a foreign body, orbital radiographs may identify it. Orbital CT may also be used for this purpose, as well as to identify intraocular injuries.

D. The large majority of ocular foreign bodies, fortunately, do not carry much kinetic energy and are therefore stopped by the surface layer of the cornea or conjunctiva. Tarsal plate foreign bodies can be removed with a moistened cotton-tipped applicator after eversion of the upper lid. One or two drops of topical anesthetic may be instilled to obtain patient cooperation.

E. Foreign bodies are removed from the surface of the cornea with a cotton-tipped applicator, an ophthalmic spud, or small hypodermic syringe needle after institution of good topical anesthesia. When a slit lamp is available, it should be used.

F. Removal of a foreign body should be followed by the instillation of a topical broad-spectrum antibiotic and reexamination 24 hours later if still symptomatic. Application of a topical cycloplegic (such as 2% or 5% homatropine drops) to prevent painful ciliary muscle spasm is indicated if there is a large corneal abrasion (see the following section).

IV. CORNEAL ABRASION.

A. The cornea is covered by a squamous stratified epithelium resting on a basement membrane. Objects that brush across the cornea can rub off portions of this epithelium, thereby causing a corneal abrasion. By exposing sensory nerve endings, this elicits photophobia, lacrimation, blepharospasm, and an intense foreign-body sensation or pain.

B. The epithelial defect is often minute and demonstrable only by staining the cornea with fluorescein and examining the eye with a cobalt blue light. Only the exposed deeper layers of epithelium take the stain and fluoresce green, in sharp contrast to the undamaged, unstained surrounding surface layer of epithelium. This staining is best seen in a darkened room.

C. Corneal abrasions heal rapidly unless complicated by infection. Local anesthetics should not be prescribed topically for relief from the intense discomfort because they may inhibit the regeneration of epithelium and delay healing.

D. Treatment includes an optional eye patch and the instillation of broad-spectrum topical antibiotics (bacitracin, neomycin, sulfacetamide) every 4 to 6 hours. Oral analgesics may be prescribed and topical cycloplegics (e.g., cyclopentolate 0.5%) instilled for large abrasions.

E. The eye should be reexamined within 24 hours. In most cases, the abrasion heals completely or almost completely within that time.

V. BLUNT TRAUMA TO THE EYE.

A. For injuries of the orbital bones, see Chapter 10.

B. Blunt injuries to the eye are often inflicted by relatively large, often round objects. During the impact, the eyeball wall is stretched, and some ocular tissues (such as the choroid) tolerate this less well than others. In some of these injuries, the mechanic stress is so great that the eyeball wall ruptures. Such injuries require surgical repair.

C. In milder cases, the cornea and sclera stretch sufficiently to allow for the deformation caused by the injuring object, and intraocular hemorrhages of varying extent are the principal findings a few hours after the injury. Blood in the anterior chamber of the eye (hyphema) is frequently the result of such trauma.

   1. Treatment of hyphema includes bed rest with elevation of the head to 45 degrees, protection of the eye with a metal shield, and instillation of topical mydriatics.

   2. Although hospital admission was previously recommended for all patients with hyphema, some adults with small hyphemas are now treated as outpatients. The decision to follow this course should be made in consultation with an ophthalmologist.

VI. INJURIES TO THE EYELIDS.

A. Lacerations of the eyelids are common injuries. Before these lacerations are repaired, the following important points should be remembered:

   1. The eyes should be carefully examined for signs of injury that may be more significant than the laceration.

   2. Lacerations including those of the lid border require more than standard suturing in one or two layers if permanent notching of the border is to be avoided (see Chapter 13).

   3. Injuries of the lower lacrimal canaliculus are difficult to repair and should therefore be referred to a surgeon with special expertise.

12

Anesthesia, Analgesia, and Sedation

I. REGIONAL ANESTHESIA.

A. Local infiltration block.

1. For superficial lacerations that need approximation and debridement, this form of anesthesia is the most practical and readily available. The approach is from within the wound by injecting the local anesthetic centrifugally into the tissues.

2. Agent of choice.

   a. A 1% lidocaine (Xylocaine) solution is recommended. Lidocaine diffuses through tissues and tissue planes quickly, and a small amount of epinephrine (1:200,000) might be needed to retain the drug longer in the operative site. Epinephrine should not be used for anesthesia in the area of the end arteries, that is, fingers, toes, nose, ears, and penis.

   b. Mepivacaine (Carbocaine), 0.5%, does not diffuse as rapidly as lidocaine and may be more useful for longer procedures.

   c. If anesthetic time of several hours is anticipated, a 0.25% solution of bupivacaine (Marcaine) may be used. The maximum dose is 200 mg.

3. Procedure for infiltrating around a wound.

   a. Raise a small skin wheal by injecting anesthetic into the dermis with a ½-inch or a 25- or 27-gauge needle.

   b. After a short wait, insert the needle through the wheal and inject the anesthetic.

   c. Insert the needle to its full length at an angle to the wound, and then inject the drug as the needle is withdrawn.

   d. Repeat this step until the entire area has been injected. The discomfort produced by local infiltration can be reduced by any of the following methods:

(1) Injecting slowly.
(2) Warming the local anesthetic before use.
(3) Buffering the local anesthetic solution. One ml of 8.5% sodium bicarbonate should be added per 10 ml local anesthetic.

e. Wait several minutes until the anesthetic takes effect.
f. Observe the guidelines for the maximum dose administered. For lidocaine and mepivacaine, the recommended maximum dose is 6 to 10 mg/kg. No more than 500 mg (50 ml of 1.0%) should be administered regardless of the weight of the patient.

4. Sedating the patient may be necessary (see Section III). It may also be helpful to apply a gauze pad soaked in 4% lidocaine to the wound before local anesthetic infiltration.

B. Topical anesthesia.

1. Application of a topical anesthetic solution, such as a combination of tetracaine, adrenaline (epinephrine), and cocaine (TAC), can provide anesthesia for wound repair.
2. Because of the vasoconstricting properties of this compound, it should be avoided in the digits, ears, penis, and areas of limited vascularity. It should not be applied to mucose.

C. Regional nerve blocks.

1. Head and neck.
   a. Trigeminal nerve and its branches.
      (1) For these blocks, 2 to 4 ml of 2% lidocaine or mepivacaine with or without epinephrine is indicated.
      (2) Mandibular nerve.
         (a) *Distribution.* This block provides anesthesia to the anterior two thirds of the tongue, the temporal and mandibular regions of the face, the lower lip, and the lower teeth and gums (Fig. 12-1, *B*).
         (b) *Landmarks.* Intraoral injection of anesthetic is just medial to the mandibular ramus about 1 cm posterior to the position of the third molar. Paresthesias of the tongue or lower jaw are frequent.
      (3) Mental nerve.
         (a) *Distribution.* This block provides anesthesia to the chin, lower lip, and gums (Fig. 12-1, *A*).
         (b) *Intraoral landmarks.* Injection is at the junction of the buccal surface of the lower lip and gum at the level of the second bicuspid tooth.
         (c) *Extraoral landmarks.* Injection is percutaneous at the level of the second bicuspid, about 1 cm above the inferior mandibular border and 2.5 cm from the midline of the mandible.
      (4) Infraorbital nerve.
         (a) *Distribution.* This block provides anesthesia to the upper lip, the side of the nose, the medial portion of the cheek, and the lower eyelid (see Fig. 12-1, *A*).

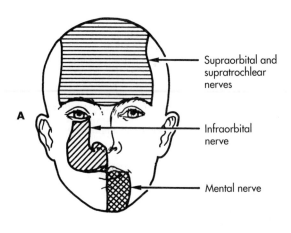

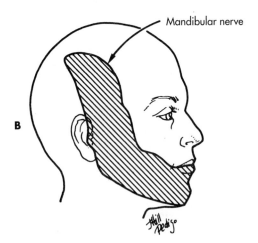

FIG. 12-1 Sensory area distribution of branches of the trigeminal nerve.

      (b) *Intraoral landmarks.* Injection is at the border of the upper gum with the buccal mucosa of the upper lip at the level of the cuspid tooth. The needle is advanced to about 1 cm inferior to the lower orbital rim.

(c) *Extraoral landmarks.* Injection is about 1 cm inferior to the infraorbital rim at its midline.

(5) Supraorbital and supratrochlear nerves.

(a) *Distribution.* The block of the branches of these nerves provides anesthesia to the forehead and the anterior half of the scalp (see Fig. 12-1, *A*).

(b) *Landmarks.* This is really a field block, and injection is across the forehead and the bridge of the nose from one lateral eyebrow border to the other, or only to the midline if only one side requires anesthesia.

(6) Superficial cervical plexus.

(a) *Distribution.* This block will provide anesthesia for skin, muscle, and subcutaneous tissues of the front of the neck and the anterior aspect of the chest almost down to the nipple line.

(b) The superficial cervical plexus is accessible at the posterior margin of the sternocleidomastoid muscle midway between the origin and the insertion. Inject 10 to 15 ml of a 1.0% or 1.5% local anesthetic.

(7) Great auricular nerve.

(a) This nerve supplies sensation to most of the ear.

(b) It may be blocked by the infiltration of 1 to 2 ml of local anesthetic at multiple sites over the mastoid process. Infiltration should be at the most inferior portion of the mastoid process, just posterior to the inferior portion of the pinna.

2. Upper extremities (see also Chapter 9).

a. Digital nerve block (Fig. 12-2).

(1) Anesthetic solution containing epinephrine should never be used for a digital block because it can cause severe vasoconstriction and necrosis.

(2) One of several techniques is presented.

(a) A solution of lidocaine hydrochloride and a No. 25 hypodermic needle are used.

(b) The needle is placed in the web space and advanced toward the palm at a 20-degree angle to the long axis of the finger being anesthetized.

(c) The needle is inserted slowly until it encounters the proximal phalanx. It is then withdrawn slightly, and the plunger is pulled back to be sure the needle point is not in a vessel.

(d) Either 2 or 3 ml of solution is then injected to produce a "ballooning" of the web space. The procedure is repeated through a separate needle puncture on the other side of the digit.

(e) Solution is placed in a position corresponding to web space injection for the radial digital nerve of

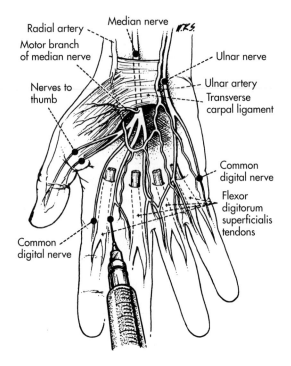

FIG. 12-2 Sites for nerve blocks.

the index finger and the ulnar digital nerve of the fifth finger.

(f) The digital nerves of the thumb flank the flexor pollicis longus tendon. From 2 to 3 ml of solution is injected on each side of the tendon at the base of the thumb on the palmar surface.

(g) If an injury affects the dorsum of the finger, particularly distal to the distal interphalangeal joint, it is advisable to supplement the digital block with a field block on the dorsum. Then 2 ml of solution is injected transversely across the dorsum at the base of the finger.

b. Median nerve block (Fig. 12-3).

(1) If the palmaris longus tendon is present, the needle is inserted radial to the tendon just proximal to the distal flexion crease of the wrist.

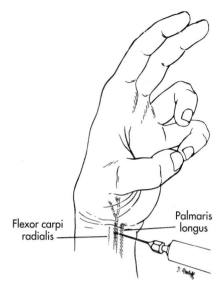

FIG. 12-3 Median nerve block.
(From Rosen P, Sternbach G: *Atlas of emergency medicine,* Baltimore, 1979, Williams & Wilkins.)

    (2) If the palmaris longus tendon is absent, the needle is inserted approximately 1 cm ulnar to the flexor carpi radialis tendon.

    (3) The needle is advanced until resistance by deep fascia is encountered. Then 1 ml of 2% lidocaine is injected.

    (4) The fascia is then penetrated, and an additional 2 ml is injected.

    (5) Paresthesias in the distribution of the median nerve are often elicited as the needle point contacts the nerve. It is preferable to inject the anesthetic around the nerve, since an intraneural injection may produce painful neuritis.

  c. Ulnar nerve block (Fig. 12-4).

    (1) At the wrist, 2 to 3 ml of 2% lidocaine is injected radial to the flexor carpi ulnaris tendon, just proximal to the pisiform bone.

    (2) At the elbow the same amount of anesthetic is injected around the nerve where it is palpable in the olecranon groove along the medial epicondyle of the humerus.

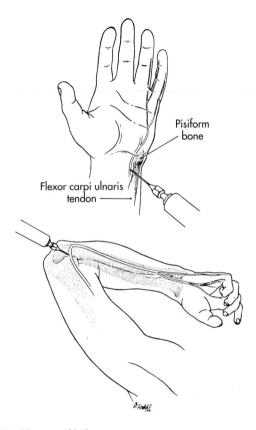

FIG. 12-4 Ulnar nerve block.
(From Rosen P, Sternbach G: *Atlas of emergency medicine,* Baltimore, 1979, Williams & Wilkins.)

      d. Radial nerve block (Fig. 12-5).
          (1) The radial nerve at the wrist has already divided into several sensory branches. A modified field block is thus necessary.
          (2) Some 5 ml of anesthetic is injected over an area extending from a point just radial to the radial artery, across the radial aspect of the wrist, and onto the extensor surface.
   3. Chest, intercostal nerve block (see Chapter 4).

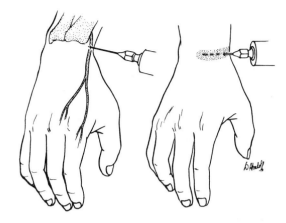

FIG. 12-5 Radial nerve block.
(From Rosen P, Sternbach G: *Atlas of emergency medicine,* Baltimore, 1979, Williams & Wilkins.)

4. Lower extremities.
   a. Sciatic nerve.
      (1) *Distribution.* The block provides anesthesia to the back of the thigh, the lateral aspect and the back of the leg, and the foot (Fig. 12-6).
      (2) *Landmarks.* With the patient lying on the contralateral side and the hip flexed about 40 degrees, anesthetic is injected 3 to 5 cm distal to the midpoint of a line from the posterior superior iliac spine to the proximal border of the greater trochanter. A long needle is used. Paresthesias should be elicited, the needle withdrawn several millimeters, and 7 to 10 ml of 1% anesthetic injected.
   b. Femoral nerve.
      (1) *Distribution.* The block provides anesthesia to the medial thigh, leg, and foot (see Fig. 12-6).
      (2) *Landmarks.* Anesthetic is injected at a point just lateral to the femoral arterial pulse, 2.5 cm distal to the inguinal ligament. From 5 to 15 ml of anesthetic should be injected in a fanwise manner. Paresthesias are rarely elicited.
   c. Lateral femoral cutaneous nerve.
      (1) *Distribution.* The block provides anesthesia to the lateral portion of the thigh (see Fig. 12-6).
      (2) *Landmarks.* Anesthetic is injected 2.5 cm medial and 2.5 cm distal to the anterior superior iliac spine. No

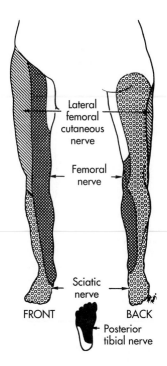

Lateral
femoral
cutaneous
nerve

Femoral
nerve

Sciatic
nerve

FRONT   BACK

Posterior
tibial nerve

FIG. 12-6 Sensory area distribution of nerves in the lower limbs.

paresthesias need to be elicited. The needle should be passed through the fascia lata and 5 to 10 ml of anesthetic injected in a fan pattern.

d. Posterior tibial nerve.

(1) *Distribution.* This block provides anesthesia to most of the sole of the foot except the most proximal and lateral portion (Fig. 12-6).

(2) *Landmarks.* Anesthetic is injected posterior to the posterior tibial pulse at the level of the medial malleolus. Paresthesias are occasionally elicited. From 5 to 10 ml of 1% lidocaine or mepivacaine should be injected.

II. COMPLICATIONS OF REGIONAL ANESTHESIA.

A. Except for the intercostal nerve block during which inadvertent entry into the thoracic cavity may produce a pneumothorax, most of the regional procedures described are rarely associated with significant complications.

B. The priorities in the initial treatment of the complications of regional anesthesia are as follows (see Chapter 3 for a more extensive discussion):

1. Assurance of an adequate airway.
2. Maintenance of adequate respirations.
3. Maintenance of adequate circulation.

C. Toxic reactions.

1. Systemic reactions may well be the most serious complication of regional anesthetic blocks.
2. They usually are associated with the inadvertent introduction of large amounts of local anesthetic into the systemic circulation.
3. The symptoms are proportional to the amount of local anesthetic introduced.
4. They are usually referable to the following:
   a. CNS.
   b. Cardiovascular system.
   c. Respiratory system.
5. A mild toxic reaction may be characterized by nothing more than a feeling of warmth, light-headedness, dizziness, and a sensation of being "high" or intoxicated. It is easily managed by the administration of oxygen and reassurance of the patient.
6. More severe toxic reactions cause a more marked stimulation of the CNS that leads to convulsions. These should be managed as outlined in Chapter 21. IV diazepam is the drug of choice to control such convulsions.
7. CNS depression (general anesthesia) may occur after an initial CNS stimulation. The barbiturates, diazepam, or narcotics can augment the CNS-depressant action. As depression of the CNS increases, the local anesthetic starts to act as a general anesthetic, and unconsciousness may ensue. Local anesthetics have in fact been used as general anesthetics by IV administration.
8. Respiration may be diminished by action on the respiratory center and possible peripheral curarelike effects of the local anesthetic.
9. The local anesthetic can affect the membrane of the myocardial cell and depress cardiac output.
10. Peripherally, the local anesthetics may depress ganglia and smaller blood vessels and cause dilation and hypotension.

D. Management.

1. Respiratory failure.
   a. Establish a patent airway by properly positioning the head and mandible, by inserting an oral or nasal airway, or by inserting an endotracheal tube.

      b. Assist ventilations with a bag mask or a mechanical ventilator system.

  2. Cardiovascular problems.

      a. Occasionally bradycardia may be severe, even progressing to cardiac arrest.

      b. Treatment of bradycardia should be with IV atropine, 0.5 mg. This can be repeated every 5 minutes to a maximum of 2.0 mg. If bradycardia persists, an infusion of isoproterenol, 2 mg in 500 ml of 5% dextrose in water, should be begun and the infusion rate adjusted to maintain a pulse faster than 60 beats per minute.

      c. Hypotension. The patient should be placed in Trendelenburg's position, and 200 to 300 ml of normal saline solution is infused IV over a period of 15 to 20 minutes. If the hypotension is refractory to this, dopamine, 400 mg in 500 ml of 5% dextrose in water, should be infused at a dose of 5 to 15 μg/kg/min or levarterenol, 4 to 8 mg in 500 ml of 5% dextrose, with the dose titrated against the blood pressure response.

E. Hypersensitivity. The response of the patient is very similar to that from a severe systemic reaction. The amount of local anesthetic that was administered may be quite small compared with that for a true systemic reaction. The management of this condition is very similar to that of a severe allergic reaction.

F. Reaction to epinephrine. Epinephrine in small concentrations frequently is used to prolong the duration of a local anesthetic. This is particularly true of lidocaine, which tends to diffuse quickly and be absorbed rapidly. The addition of epinephrine causes vasoconstriction and slows down the absorption and diffusion of the drug. However, absorption of the epinephrine itself, even in minute amounts, can cause tachycardia, mental excitement, and occasionally piloerection.

G. Fear.

  1. The response of an apprehensive patient may well produce a "reaction" to local anesthetics. No matter how hard one tries to allay the patient's fear and explain the procedure, fear of the needle or the effects of the local anesthetic may provoke severe apprehension. Nausea and vomiting are probably the most common manifestations of this psychogenic reaction.

  2. Hypotension, bradycardia, and loss of consciousness may also occur, and these may mimic a severe systemic toxic reaction. These usually respond to elevation of the legs and administration of oxygen. Sedation of the patient may be necessary.

III. SEDATION.

A. It is frequently advantageous to administer sedative or analgesic medication in patients before repairing a laceration or performing other painful procedures. This is especially true for children.

B. When large doses of analgesics or sedatives are anticipated, preparation should be made to ensure adequate monitoring and treatment if necessary. The patient should be kept on a cardiac monitor and pulse oximeter and an IV line established. Airway management equipment and reversal medications (see below) should be immediately available.

C. Elderly patients and those with chronic lung disease are particularly at risk to complication. Lower doses (e.g., a 50% reduction) of analgesic and sedative medications are advisable in such patients.

D. The side effects of parenteral analgesics and sedatives are additive. The dosage of each should be adjusted accordingly when they are used concomitantly.

E. Narcotic analgesics.

1. These agents provide both analgesia and sedation.
2. Disadvantages include potential respiratory suppression, hypotension, and nausea.
   a. Narcotic effect can be reversed with naloxone (Narcan), 0.4 to 0.8 mg IV. The duration of action is 1 to 2 hours.
   b. Inadequate respiration should be assisted with a bag-valve-mask device until pharmacologic narcotic reversal is achieved. Hypotension should be treated with leg elevation and IV fluids as needed.
   c. Nausea can be prevented or treated with antiemetic agents.
3. A number of narcotic preparations are available. They may be given intramuscularly (IM), but the IV route is preferable. Small incremental doses are administered IV every few minutes (e.g., every 5 minutes) until satisfactory effect is achieved. Larger total doses than those listed below can be given, as long as respiratory suppression is precluded by adequate observation and slow IV titration.
   a. Meperidine (Demerol), 75 to 125 mg IM, often mixed with promethazine (Phenergan), 25 to 50 mg, or hydroxyzine (Vistaril) to counteract the emetic effect of meperidine and to provide increased sedation. Meperidine can also be given slowly IV in 25-mg increments.
   b. Morphine, 5 to 10 mg IV in 2- to 5-mg increments, titrated to effect. Morphine can also be given IM 5 to 15 mg. Morphine has a longer analgesic effect than meperidine and is, in general, preferred for conditions with continuing pain, such as renal colic.
   c. Fentanyl (Sublimaze), 100 to 200 μg slowly IV in 50-μg increments. Because of its rapid onset and brief duration of action (20 to 40 minutes), fentanyl is ideal for short, painful procedures such as orthopedic reductions and abscess drainage.

F. Sedatives.
1. The benzodiazepines are the most useful sedatives for emergency department use. Their amnestic effect is particularly advantageous for painful or frightening procedures.
2. As with the narcotics, respiratory suppression is a risk. The dose should be lowered when both are used, in the elderly, and in those with chronic lung disease.
3. Excessive sedation and respiratory suppression can be reversed with the specific benzodiazepine antagonist flumazenil (Romazicon), 0.2 mg IV over 15 seconds, repeated every minute as needed to a total dose of 1 mg.
4. Several benzodiazepine preparations are commonly used.
   a. Diazepam, 5 to 15 mg is given slowly by IV titration in 2- to 5-mg increments. IM absorption is variable and the IV route is recommended.
   b. Midazolam (Versed), 1 to 5 mg IV slowly. The effect may be delayed for several minutes after each injection, and a minimum of 2 to 3 minutes should separate each 0.5- to 1.0-mg dose.

IV. MUSCULAR PARALYSIS.
A. Succinylcholine.
1. This is a short-acting muscle relaxant that may be used to facilitate endotracheal intubation.
2. Its onset of action is within 1 minute, and the duration of action is 5 to 15 minutes.
3. When administered in an IV bolus, the usual dose is 1 to 1.5 mg/kg for adults and children and 1.5 to 2 mg/kg for infants less than 10 kg. Muscular fasciculations precede relaxation.
4. More prolonged muscle relaxation may be attained by continuous IV infusion. A solution containing 1 to 2 mg of succinylcholine per milliliter of IV solution should be mixed. The administration rate should be monitored by the degree of muscle relaxation present.
B. Tubocurarine.
1. This is a longer-acting agent than succinylcholine. The onset of action when administered IV is within 3 minutes, and the duration is 30 to 40 minutes.
2. The usual dose is 15 to 30 mg for adults and 0.2 mg/kg for children. Reversal may be accomplished by the administration of atropine, 0.2 mg/kg, and neostigmine, 0.08 mg/kg. The usual adult dose is 2.5 mg of neostigmine given IV with 1.0 mg of atropine.
C. Nondepolarizing agents.
1. Pancuronium is a more potent muscle relaxant than tubocurarine and has a comparable onset of action and duration.
2. The recommended dose is 0.04 to 0.1 mg/kg IV, with repeated injections as needed. The effects may be reversed

with atropine and neostigmine in the doses given in Section IV, B, 2.
3. Other nondepolarizing agents include vecuronium and atracurium. Both have rapid onsets of action and have shorter durations of action than pancuronium. The dose for vecuronium is 0.08 to 0.1 mg/kg; that for atracurium is 0.4 to 0.5 mg/kg.

13

Laceration Repair

I. GENERAL PRINCIPLES OF WOUND CARE.

A. General surgical principles, including the prevention of infection and tetanus prophylaxis (see Chapter 14), apply to all soft-tissue injuries.

B. Neurovascular status should be assessed, including appropriate pulses and capillary filling (see Chapter 16), sensation, and motor function (see Chapter 9).

C. Sedation is sometimes advisable, especially for children (see Chapter 12).

D. Adequate anesthesia must always be provided. Local infiltration with 1% lidocaine is generally used. (See Chapter 12 for full discussion of local and regional anesthesia.) Lidocaine with epinephrine, 1:1,000, may be appropriate for facial lacerations with bleeding, but epinephrine should not be used in areas where vasoconstriction may compromise circulation, such as the fingers or toes, or close to the nasal or auricular cartilage.

E. The discomfort of lidocaine injection can be reduced by injecting slowly. Other measures include warming the lidocaine in a blanket warmer and adding a small amount of sodium bicarbonate to obtain a more neutral pH. (See Chapter 12.)

F. Hair around the wound may be trimmed closely with scissors, but the eyebrows should not be shaved, since they are valuable landmarks for realignment of tissues and occasionally they will not regrow.

G. The skin surrounding the wound must be prepared with an antiseptic solution, and cleansing should include gentle scrubbing of the wound bed or copious lavage of the wound with a sterile saline solution. High-pressure irrigation methods using a syringe or pulsatile hydrostatic nozzles are most effective. The volume of irrigation fluid used should be dictated by the degree of contamination of the wound.

H. Antiseptics that contain alcohol or iodine should not be used for internal scrubbing or irrigation because they cauterize the healthy wound borders and incite inflammatory reactions in the wound.

I. Draping with towels helps maintain a clean, unobstructed field. The face is often left exposed, especially in children, to reduce patient anxiety and to allow the physician to observe the patient's respiratory effort and level of consciousness if there is potential for compromise.

J. Foreign debris and devitalized tissue are removed; however, debridement should be limited to obviously necrotic tissue, particularly in wounds near the eyelids and nose.

K. Surgical trauma must be minimized and tissue manipulated as atraumatically as possible.

L. Small bleeding points may be controlled by the application of pressure, ligated with fine sutures, or coagulated with electrocautery if necessary.

II. SUTURE MATERIAL.

A. Size.
1. Face: 5-0 or 6-0.
2. Scalp: 4-0 or 5-0.
3. Hand: 5-0.
4. Extremities and trunk: 4-0 or 5-0.

B. Type.
1. Skin.
   a. Nonabsorbable: nylon or polypropylene.
   b. Absorbable: special "rapid absorbing" preparations of gut or polyglycolic acid. These recently introduced materials do not require suture removal.
2. Below the skin and mucosal surfaces.
   a. Polyglycolic acid is strongest and most pliable—ideal for deeper layers and exposed mucosa.
   b. Chromic catgut is less strong but incites less inflammatory response—better for superficial subcutaneous layer of the face.

III. SUTURE TECHNIQUE.

A. Technical aspects (Figs. 13-1 to 13-3).
1. Fine instruments and meticulous care in handling the tissues are basic requirements.
2. Sutures must just approximate tissues without constricting.
3. Tight sutures cause tissue necrosis and delay wound healing; they produce "railroad ties" across the scar.
4. Simple sutures that take in sufficient and equal amounts of subcutaneous and dermal tissue usually give good wound approximation.
5. Skin edges should be everted to ensure appropriate healing.

B. Poor scars result from the following:
1. Suture material that is too heavy.
2. Inclusion of too much tissue in the suture.
3. Sutures that are too tight.
4. Delayed removal of sutures.

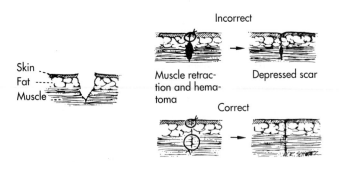

FIG. 13-1 Muscle injury.

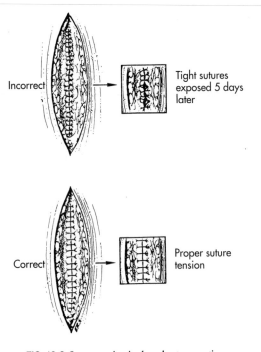

FIG. 13-2 Suture tension in the subcutaneous tissue.

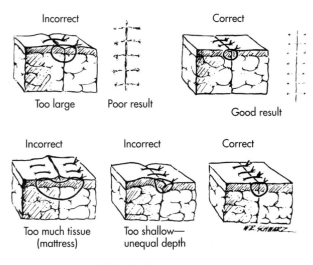

Incorrect

Too large

Poor result

Correct

Good result

Incorrect

Too much tissue
(mattress)

Incorrect

Too shallow—
unequal depth

Correct

W.E. SCHWARZ

FIG. 13-3 Suture technique.

IV. SUTURE REMOVAL.

A. The ideal time for removal of skin sutures depends on location, vascular supply, and wound tension.

B. Sutures should be removed as soon as wound healing permits before the development of a significant inflammatory response to the foreign material.

C. Thin skin such as that of the eyelids heals very quickly; sutures can be removed in 2 to 3 days.

D. The somewhat thicker skin of the rest of the face heals more slowly. Sutures should remain for 4 to 5 days.

E. Scalp sutures should be removed in 7 days.

F. Extremity sutures are removed in 7 to 10 days.

G. Wounds of the trunk or extensor surfaces overlying large joints (i.e., knee, elbow) may require 10 to 12 days.

V. SPECIAL WOUNDS.

A. The untidy wound.

1. The grossly contused, crushed, serrated laceration ("untidy" wound) is often best handled in the following manner:
   a. Wound excision to obtain precise borders.
   b. Undermining of the wound edges if needed, followed by advancement of the overlying skin and careful suturing (Fig. 13-4).

2. Excisional revision cannot be done where a feature such as the eyelid is involved; distortion would result.

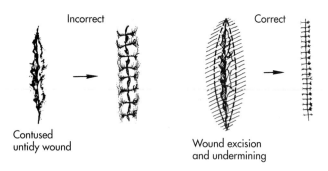

Incorrect

Contused
untidy wound

Correct

Wound excision
and undermining

FIG. 13-4 Skin laceration.

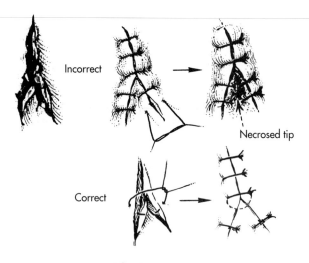

Incorrect

Necrosed tip

Correct

FIG. 13-5 "Corner" suture.

B. Stellate or V-shaped lacerations.

1. These may result in an ischemic skin flap if not properly managed.
2. Care should be taken to avoid strangulation of the tip by sutures.
3. A "corner suture" through the dermis of the tip may help in alignment (Fig. 13-5).

C. Scything wounds with beveled edges.

1. These wounds often heal with contraction along the oblique tract of fibrous tissue and produce a rolled or pouting wound margin.
2. This will be even more apparent in the "trapdoor" wound where the circular scar also contracts to cause further pouting in the wound margin.
3. Trimming the border to produce vertical edges will result in a better scar (Fig. 13-6).

D. Tongue and oral mucosa.

1. Small lacerations of the tongue, buccal mucosa, and lips that are produced by the teeth generally heal satisfactorily without sutures. The frenulum does not require repair.
2. Shallow mucosal injuries require only a single-layer repair. Absorbable suture material is used, and a loose closure is performed to allow for drainage. Epinephrine may be added to lidocaine anesthetic to control bleeding if necessary.
3. Through-and-through lacerations of the cheek or lip require the following:
   a. Careful muscle/capsule approximation.
   b. Precise skin closure.
   c. Approximation of the oral mucosa.
4. Precise alignment of the skin-vermilion border of the lip is most important. This should precede the placement of other sutures (Fig. 13-7).
5. After repair, frequent cleansing of the mouth with 3% hydrogen peroxide will prevent crusting and subsequent purulent collections.
6. Bleeding inside the mouth can often be controlled with cold-water rinsing. The application of ice (a Popsicle is ideal) is also useful. A wet tea bag can also control bleeding because tannic acid has some vasoconstricting effect.

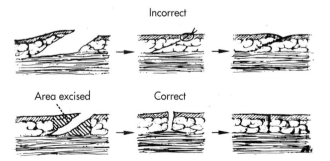

FIG. 13-6 Scything wound.

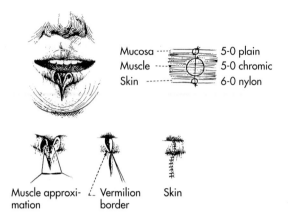

Mucosa ---- 5-0 plain
Muscle ---- 5-0 chromic
Skin ------- 6-0 nylon

Muscle approxi-   Vermilion   Skin
mation   border

FIG. 13-7 Through-and-through lip laceration.

E. Eyelid lacerations.
   1. When repairing eyelid lacerations, the most important land-
      mark is the gray line (ciliary margin). This must be perfectly
      aligned as the first step in eyelid repair. Failure to precisely
      align the ciliary margin will result in notching of the eyelid.
      Such repairs are best performed by facial surgeons if available.
F. Inground foreign material.
   1. Bicycle and motorcycle accidents frequently cause extensive,
      deep abrasions commonly called "road burns."
   2. Failure to remove inground foreign material from such
      wounds not only may lead to infection but also may leave
      permanent pigmentation in the skin, commonly referred to as
      "accidental tattoo."
   3. Foreign material should be removed by irrigation, scrubbing,
      or surgical debridement. Anesthesia of abrasions may be at-
      tained with the topical application of 4% lidocaine before de-
      bridement.
   4. When the discoloration is limited to the wound edges, it may
      be better to debride these areas with a scalpel.
   5. After the abrasion has been treated, it is dressed with topical
      antibiotic, Xeroform, and a gauze dressing applied under
      moderate pressure.

14

Soft Tissue Infections

I. GENERAL CONSIDERATIONS.
A. Types of infections.
1. Cellulitis is the infection of cutaneous and subcutaneous tissue characterized by acute erythema, warmth, swelling, and tenderness. Fever may be present.
2. An abscess is a cavity containing pus. Fluctuance is the hallmark of an abscess, although it is not always detectable. Localized warmth, swelling, and tenderness directly over the abscess cavity are also typical.
3. Lymphangitis is recognized by red streaks overlying the inflamed lymphatic vessels and extending proximally from the infected area.

B. Principles of treatment.
1. Antibiotics are indicated in soft-tissue infections accompanied by cellulitis, acute lymphadenopathy, lymphangitis, or fever.
2. Incision and drainage (I&D) is the proper treatment for abscesses. Antibiotics are added if there are signs of spreading infection such as cellulitis, lymphadenopathy, lymphangitis, or fever. In the absence of systemic infection, localized abscesses adequately drained may not require antibiotics because the drugs generally do not penetrate into abscess cavities.
3. Elevation and application of heat are suggested for any soft-tissue infection.

II. ABSCESS.
A. Principles of treatment.
1. I&D is required. Antibiotics are added if signs of spread are present (see Section I, B, 2).
2. A patient with parenteral drug abuse–related abscess may require admission to the hospital for IV antibiotics if there is any sign of systemic infection such as fever.
3. Patients with cardiac valvular disease or prosthetic valves should be given antibiotics before I&D in accordance with the regimen described in Section III, B, 1, c, (3).

4. Anesthesia for I&D may be difficult to achieve.
   a. Lidocaine should be injected into the skin above the abscess cavity, but injection into the cavity itself is usually ineffective and unnecessarily painful.
   b. Systemic agents may be helpful, such as inhaled nitrous oxide, parenteral narcotics (fentanyl, 2 μg/kg; morphine, 5 to 10 mg; hydromorphone [Dilaudid], 2 mg; or meperidine, 75 mg IM), or benzodiazepines (midazolam, 2 to 5 mg IV).
   c. Cooling sprays are used by some physicians but generally do not provide sufficient local anesthesia for skin incision.
5. Loculations, if present, should be disrupted by blunt dissection with a hemostat.
6. Irrigation should be continued until all pus is drained. Saline, hydrogen peroxide, or povidone-iodine may be used.
7. Drain insertion (with iodinated gauze) will prevent premature closure while the abscess is still draining. Deep cavities may be packed with the same material.
8. Irrigation and drain replacement should be carried out at 1- to 2-day intervals until there is no more pus formation. If the wound has been packed, progressively less packing should be replaced at each visit to allow closure from the inside out.
9. Diabetes may present initially as a nontraumatic infection such as an abscess. Analyzing urine for glucose may be advisable, especially for a recurrent or refractory abscess.

B. Specific abscesses.
1. Felon.
   a. This is an infection of the pulp of the volar pad overlying the distal phalanx of a finger or toe.
   b. Because the infection often leads to the accumulation of pressure and ischemic necrosis, early drainage is indicated.
   c. Under digital block anesthesia, a central longitudinal incision is made in the finger pulp where the abscess is pointing (Fig. 14-1).
   d. The digital septa should not be disrupted. This represents a change from the traditional practice, which has often led to instability of the fingertip.
   e. The wound is irrigated with saline, and a small drain is inserted.
   f. The drain can be removed in 1 to 2 days, the tract irrigated, and the wound allowed to close by granulation.
   g. Antistaphylococcal antibiotic coverage is advisable.
2. Paronychia.
   a. This is an abscess of the skin around the base of the nail. It can extend under the nail plate as well.

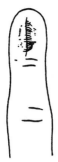

FIG. 14-1 Incision of a felon (distal fat pad infection).
(From Way LW, editor: *Current surgical diagnosis and treatment,* ed 10, Stamford, Conn, 1993, Appleton & Lange.)

  b. An incision is made over the fluctuant area.
  c. The cavity is irrigated and a small drain inserted.
  d. The drain is removed after 1 day and the finger soaked periodically in warm water.
  e. If infection extends under the nail, the lateral third of the nail plate on the side of the paronychia should be removed. Trephination may suffice, however.
  f. After surgical drainage, antibiotics are not indicated unless there are signs of cellulitis, lymphangitis, or felon.
  g. Small paronychia without fluctuance may be treated nonsurgically with warm soaks and an antistaphylococcal antibiotic.
3. Deep infections of the hand.
  a. Infection of the deep palmar space is a major threat to the hand. Hospital admission and surgical consultation are necessary.
  b. Tenosynovitis causes fusiform swelling of the finger and severe pain on passive motion. Surgical drainage in the operating room is mandatory.
  c. Both the above infections require operative intervention by a hand surgeon and should not be treated in the emergency department.
4. Olecranon bursitis.
  a. Often nontraumatic, this disorder is characterized by painful swelling, fluctuance, and erythema of the extensor surface of the elbow overlying the olecranon prominence.
  b. The bursitis may be due to a purely inflammatory process or to a bacterial infection.

    c. Needle aspiration is indicated. Performing a Gram's stain and culture of the aspirate should reveal the causative bacteria if infection is present.

    d. Nonsteroidal antiinflammatory agents are used, such as indomethacin, 25 to 50 mg three times daily.

    e. Antibiotics are added if infection is suggested by fever, elevated serum leukocyte count, or Gram's staining of the aspirate. A cephalosporin or dicloxacillin is appropriate, 250 to 500 mg four times daily.

    f. I&D is not generally performed, especially if the bursitis is purely inflammatory. Unlike most abscesses, olecranon bursitis is often slow to heal after I&D, whereas a trial of antiinflammatory or antibiotic medication is often successful.

III. INFECTIONS COMPLICATING TRAUMATIC WOUNDS.
A. Prevention of tetanus.

  1. General considerations.

    a. *Clostridium tetani* causes serious illness by toxin production even when infection is confined to a circumscribed area of tissue damage.

    b. Tetanus prevention is dependent on the following:

      (1) Primary prophylactic immunization.

      (2) Meticulous surgical care of wounds.

      (3) The proper use of human tetanus antitoxin and tetanus toxoid.

  2. Routine immunization. In patients who have a history of adequate primary immunization, routine booster injections should be given every 10 years.

  3. Injured patients with no evidence of complete toxoid immunization.

    a. Patients who have not had the basic series should receive immunization with diphtheria-tetanus toxoid at the time of injury and subsequent injections at 6 and 24 weeks.

    b. For moderately severe wounds, 250 units of human tetanus immune globulin should also be given. Injuries that are grossly contaminated, major burns, and major open fractures fall into this category.

    c. Tetanus can arise from minor injuries that do not receive good local care in persons who have been inadequately immunized.

  4. Injured patients with a history of complete tetanus toxoid immunization.

    a. These patients should receive a diphtheria-tetanus toxoid booster if they have not had a toxoid booster within the past 5 years. For minor, relatively clean abrasions, a 10-year limit is sufficient.

    b. For a severely contaminated wound, especially if neglected for 24 hours, both toxoid and antitoxin should be given. This may also be appropriate for injured patients who have not had a booster for many decades.

c. Meticulous care of the wound, including vigorous cleansing or irrigation and generous debridement, is important to prevent tetanus and other infections.

B. Wound infection.

1. Prevention of wound infection.

   a. Cleansing and debridement are the most important means of preventing wound infection. Removal of foreign bodies may require irrigation as well, particularly for deep wounds. Care should be taken not to force irrigating fluid into deep tissue planes.

   b. Loose closure of significantly contaminated wounds is suggested to allow adequate drainage.

   c. Prophylactic antibiotics may be useful for contaminated wounds, especially of the hand, and for bite wounds, particularly human and cat (see Section C). In general, however, prophylactic antibiotics are far less important than adequate cleansing and debridement.

      (1) If used, the prophylactic antibiotic should generally be a β-lactamase–resistant agent effective against coagulase-positive *Staphylococcus aureus*. A typical regimen is a 5-day course of a cephalosporin such as cephalexin, 250 to 500 mg four times daily, or dicloxacillin, 250 to 500 mg four times daily. Erythromycin, 250 to 500 mg four times daily, may be used in penicillin-allergic patients.

      (2) Compromised hosts such as patients with diabetes are particularly prone to infection, and prophylactic antibiotics are used more readily in this population.

      (3) Infective endocarditis may be caused by the entrance of bacteria through skin breaks, even in the absence of wound infection. People with prosthetic valves (mechanical or porcine) or valves previously damaged by rheumatic fever are particularly prone to infective endocarditis.

         (a) Antibiotic prophylaxis in such patients would seem prudent if they sustain significant soft-tissue injuries.

         (b) Regimens might include IM cephalosporin at the time of suturing (cefazolin, 1 g IM) plus a 5-day course of cephalexin or dicloxacillin, 250 to 500 mg four times daily.

2. Treatment of wound infections.

   a. Antibiotic therapy for actual infection should generally involve a 10-day course of dicloxacillin or cephalexin, 250 to 500 mg four times daily.

   b. Opening of the sutured wound by removing some or all of the sutures may be required if there is pus, evidence of abscess cavity formation, or failure to respond to antibiotics.

c. A retained foreign body may cause wound infection. Radiologic examination or repeat exploration may be indicated if this possibility exists.

d. Severe wound infections, particularly those of the hand, may require hospital admission for IV antibiotic therapy.

C. Bite wounds.

1. Because of their high incidence of infection, bite wounds deserve special mention.

2. Human bites are most dangerous because they often involve the hand, and because the human mouth is particularly well endowed with bacterial flora.

3. Cat bites present a high risk of infection because the wounds are typically deep punctures that allow little opportunity for adequate irrigation or drainage.

4. Cat scratches are also prone to infection because of the feline predilection for licking paws, thereby contaminating them with oral flora.

5. Dog bites are much less prone to infection. The wounds are usually open tears that can be thoroughly debrided and irrigated.

6. Debridement and irrigation are crucial. Prophylactic antibiotics will not prevent infection if the wound is left contaminated.

7. Although very minor wounds may be left open, any significant bite laceration should be sutured.

   a. Primary closure is indicated for most animal bite wounds.

   b. Delayed primary closure after 2 to 3 days is the treatment of choice for all human and other primate bite wounds, as well as for particularly contaminated bite wounds from any animal. The traditional practice of allowing human bite wounds to heal by secondary intent often results in severe scarring and affords no greater protection from infection than thorough debridement, irrigation, and delayed primary closure.

8. Antibiotic prophylaxis is indicated for human and cat bites and for high-risk dog bites: amoxicillin/clavulanic acid (Augmentin) may be the most effective agent. (See Section C, 11.)

9. Human bite wound infections of the hand should be followed closely and may need to be treated in the hospital with IV antibiotics.

10. Cat and, to some extent, dog bite infections may involve several organisms:

    a. Infections arising within 24 hours of the bite are usually caused by *Pasteurella multocida*, a small aerobic gram-negative rod. This organism is most sensitive to penicillin, 500 mg four times daily, and to doxycycline, 100 mg twice daily. Several weeks of therapy may be necessary. *Pasteurella* is often resistant to erythromycin and sometimes not very susceptible to cephalosporins or dicloxacillin.

b. Infections arising after 24 hours are often caused by *S. aureus, Streptococcus,* or both. A penicillinase-resistant antibiotic can be used, such as dicloxacillin or cephalexin.

TABLE 14-1
Indications for Postexposure Rabies Prophylaxis

Animal species	Condition of animal at time of attack	Treatment of exposed person*
Domestic		
Dog and cat	Healthy and available for 10 days of observation	None, unless animal develops rabies,† then HRIG,‡ and HDCV§
	Rabid or suspected rabid Unknown (escaped)	Consult public health officials. If treatment is indicated, give HRIG‡ and HDCV§
Wild		
Skunk, bat, fox, coyote, raccoon, bobcat, and other carnivores	Regard as rabid unless proved normal by laboratory tests‖	HRIG‡ and HDCV§
Other		
Livestock, rodents, and lagomorphs (rabbits and hares)	Consider individually. Local and state public health officials should be consulted about the need for rabies prophylaxis. Bites of squirrels, hamsters, guinea pigs, gerbils, chipmunks, rats, mice, other rodents, rabbits, and hares almost never call for antirabies prophylaxis	

All bites and wounds should immediately be thoroughly cleaned with soap and water. If antirabies treatment is indicated, both human rabies immune globulin (HRIG) and human diploid cell vaccine (HDCV) should be given as soon as possible, *regardless* of the interval from exposure.

†During the usual holding period of 10 days, begin treatment with HRIG and HDCV at first sign of rabies in a dog or cat that has bitten someone. The symptomatic animal should be killed immediately and tested.

‡If HRIG is not available, use equine antirabies serum (ARS). Do not use more than the recommended dose.

§If HDCV is not available, use duck embryo vaccine (DEV). Local reactions to vaccines are common and do not contraindicate continuing treatment. Discontinue treatment with the vaccine if fluorescent antibody (FA) tests of the animal are negative.

‖The animal should be killed and tested as soon as possible. Holding for observation is not recommended.

TABLE 14-2
Dosages for Postexposure Rabies Prophylaxis*

Prophylaxis	Comments	Dosage	Route	Frequency
HRIG†	Always give, unless prior adequate HDCV course; then give only 2 doses HDCV on days 1 and 4	20 IU/kg	Preferably 50% around wound, remember deep IM injection in buttock or thigh	Once, given even if delay of weeks between exposure and prophylaxis
ARS†	Used only if HRIG unavailable	40 IU/kg	IM	Once
HDCV†	Dosage similar for children and adults; only test for antibody response in immunosuppressed patients	5 1-ml doses	IM, not in same site as for HRIG	Repeated on days 3, 7, 14, 28
DEV†	Used if HDCV unavailable; no longer licensed for use in United States	23 1-ml doses	SC	21 daily doses, then on days 31 and 41

*Thorough cleansing to the depth of the wound with a 20% soap solution significantly (up to 90%) reduces rabies risk, especially if the wound is superficial.
†See Table 14-1.

In penicillin-allergic patients, erythromycin is sometimes effective.

c. Both *Pasteurella* and *Staphylococcus* are often susceptible to combination preparations that include a penicillin such as amoxicillin and clavulanic acid. Because the infecting organism is frequently unknown, such preparations are frequently used to treat animal bite wound infections.

D. Rabies.

1. Rabies is essentially a uniformly fatal illness in humans.

2. Wild carnivorous animals, especially skunks, foxes, raccoons, coyotes, bobcats, and bats, are the most important source of rabies infection in the United States. The presence of rabies in domestic dogs and cats varies from region to region.

3. Every bite wound case must be evaluated individually. Special attention must be paid to the circumstances of the individual exposure, geographic location, species of the animal involved, and prevalence of rabies in that species in the area. Contact with state or local health officials may be helpful.

4. Local treatment of wounds.

   a. Immediate and thorough washing of all bite wounds and scratches may be the most important measure for preventing rabies.

   b. Tetanus prophylaxis and measures to control bacterial infection should be given as indicated.

5. *Immunization.* The recommendations in Tables 14-1 and 14-2 are only a guide. In applying them, take into account the animal species involved, the circumstances of the bite or other exposure, the vaccination status of the animal, and the presence of rabies in the region. Local and state public health officials should be consulted.

PART III

Nontraumatic
Emergencies

15

Cardiac Emergencies

This chapter discusses acute ischemic chest pain, myocardial infarction, cardiogenic pulmonary edema, dysrhythmias, cardiac arrest, and implanted pacemakers and cardioverter/defibrillators.

For cardiac arrest in children, see Chapter 30.

I. ISCHEMIC CHEST PAIN AND ACUTE MYOCARDIAL INFARCTION.

A. Definition.
Acute cardiac ischemia is caused by an imbalance between the O_2 demands of the myocardium and its arterial blood supply. In angina pectoris the ischemia resolves without myocardial necrosis. In acute myocardial infarction (AMI), myocardial necrosis is usually due to the occlusion of an atherosclerotic coronary artery by thrombus.

B. Risk factors.
Cardiac ischemia, with or without acute infarction, must be suspected in all persons with chest pain, especially all men over 40 and all postmenopausal women. It also can occur in young men and in menstruating women. Risk factors of particular significance include:

1. A history of death or AMI in family members at a relatively young age.
2. Specific disorders such as diabetes mellitus and hyperlipidemias.
3. Gross obesity.
4. Heavy smoking.
5. Hypertension.

C. Evaluation.

1. History.

a. The symptoms of angina and AMI may be identical except that anginal pain usually resolves after several minutes of rest.

b. The classic symptom of cardiac ischemia is crushing substernal chest pain radiating into the left shoulder and arm, accompanied by sweating and nausea.

c. However, chest pain may be relatively mild, burning, sharp, or pleuritic. It may radiate to the jaw, shoulder, left or right arm, wrist, back, or epigastrium, or it may not radiate at all. Chest pain may be entirely absent, particularly in the elderly or patients with diabetes. Weakness or dizziness may be the only complaint.

   d. Other symptoms may include dyspnea, nausea, and abdominal discomfort.

   e. Stoic or frightened patients may minimize their symptoms; language and cultural barriers may lead to misinterpretation of the historical information.

2. Physical examination. The physical examination in acute ischemia reveals an anxious patient in significant discomfort. Diaphoresis and dyspnea may be apparent. Rales and distended neck veins may reflect congestive heart failure (CHF).

3. ECG.

   a. The ECG of the patient with angina may be normal or nonspecific, or it may reveal depressed ST segments.

   b. The early ECG in AMI may also be nonspecific and rarely even normal. Half the patients with a final diagnosis of AMI have a nondiagnostic initial ECG in the ED. Some of these patients had unstable angina that then deteriorated to infarction. Others were infarcting on presentation, but their ECG had not yet become diagnostic. A repeat ECG within 20 to 30 minutes of the first one is thus indicated in patients with continuing chest pain.

   c. The ECG will become abnormal with AMI and will reveal ST segment elevation, perhaps "hyperacute" T wave peaking, and later Q waves, all in leads corresponding to the site of myocardial necrosis.

   d. However, a preexisting left bundle-branch block pattern makes it difficult to diagnose AMI electrocardiographically. A change in pattern from prior tracings is suspicious for AMI.

4. Enzymes.

   a. The serum levels of several cardiac enzymes become elevated in AMI. Unfortunately, this occurs over several hours, rendering all of them insufficiently sensitive to be relied on during the ED phase of care. Thus a normal enzyme level *does not* rule out AMI during the first hours in the ED.

   b. Total creatine kinase (CK), and the more cardiospecific MB bands (CK-MB), may take as much as 3 to 6 hours to reach abnormal levels after the onset of AMI.

   c. Myoglobin may rise within 1 to 3 hours but is less specific than CK-MB.

   d. Troponin I and T have a time course similar to that of CK-MB but are more specific for AMI than either CK-MB or myoglobin.

5. Differential diagnosis.

   a. The crucial issues to be decided are:

     (1) Cardiac vs. noncardiac cause.

     (2) If cardiac, AMI vs. unstable angina.

   b. Thoracic aortic dissection typically causes a constant, "tearing" pain radiating to the back. Blood pressure in the left arm may be lower than that in the right. Chest x-ray may show a widened or distorted mediastinum, pleural cap, and other stigmata of a leaking dissection.

c. Pulmonary emboli cause primarily dyspnea (as does CHF). If present, chest pain is pleuritic (as is the pain of some AMIs). But unlike MI pain, that caused by pulmonary emboli is generally not present between breaths when the chest is not moving.

d. Esophageal spasm causes pain very similar to that of cardiac ischemia and AMI. It is often described as substernal pressure–and it may be relieved by nitroglycerine, a smooth muscle relaxant. The symptoms are sometimes exacerbated by swallowing.

e. Esophageal reflux causes a burning substernal pain and is often relieved by antacid. *Caution:* If relief with antacid is not obtained within 1 to 2 minutes, cardiac causes should be strongly considered. Esophageal reflux may lead to esophageal spasm as well.

D. General measures and initial treatment of possible cardiac ischemia.

1. Immediate continuous cardiac rhythm monitoring, IV line insertion, and oxygen by nasal cannula or mask.

2. Continuous nursing surveillance and immediate physician availability.

3. 12-lead ECG with immediate evaluation.

4. If there is any significant possibility of AMI or other serious medical problem such as aortic dissection or pulmonary embolus, blood should be drawn for CBC, cardiac enzymes, electrolytes, and coagulation studies. A portable chest x-ray should be strongly considered.

5. Nitroglycerine may be used as follows to reduce pain and myocardial strain: sublingual spray or tablet (0.4 to 0.6 mg repeated every 10 minutes), followed by an IV infusion if pain persists (5 to 25 μg/min).

6. Morphine sulfate may be administered IV in 2-mg increments to relieve pain and reduce anxiety. In patients with chronic lung disease, morphine may cause an altered level of consciousness or respiratory suppression and may require reversal with naloxone, 0.8 mg by IV push.

7. Nitroglycerine and morphine may cause hypotension as a result of either afterload reduction (arterial vasodilation) or excessive preload reduction (venodilation). Particularly in patients with inferior AMI who also have right ventricular infarcts, preload reduction causes hypotension. Drug-induced hypotension is treated with leg elevation and if necessary small increments of IV fluids: 200 ml over 5 to 10 minutes, paying careful attention to the neck veins, lung bases, and the appearance of an S_3 gallop for evidence of incipient cardiac failure.

E. Specific treatment of myocardial infarction.

The goal of treating AMI is to stabilize the patient, to dissolve the thrombus as rapidly as possible, and to prevent reocclusion. *Time is crucial.*

1. Aspirin (not enteric coated) should be given immediately, 180 to 325 mg PO, to help prevent reocclusion and possibly to act synergistically with thrombolytic agents to dissolve clot.
2. Thrombolytic therapy.
   a. Unless there are contraindications, alteplase (t-PA) or streptokinase (SK) should be given within 30 to 60 minutes to all patients with obvious AMI. Alternatively, some patients may undergo immediate angioplasty if this can be done rapidly.
   b. Cautions and contraindications.
      (1) These drugs should be avoided in patients with active internal bleeding; history of stroke; recent (within 2 months) intracranial or intraspinal surgery or trauma; intracranial neoplasm, arteriovenous malformation, or aneurysm; known bleeding diathesis; or severe uncontrolled hypertension (persistent BP > 180 systolic or 110 diastolic despite nitroglycerine, nitroprusside, etc.).
      (2) Risks may be increased but should be considered against the significant potential benefits of thromboytic therapy, in patients with conditions such as recent (within 10 days) major surgery, trauma, or gastrointestinal or genitourinary bleeding.
      (3) Although any history of stroke is still technically a contraindication as of publication date, t-PA has now been approved for use in selected patients with acute ischemic stroke, and many centers are giving t-PA to AMI patients with a remote (>6 months) history of ischemic (nonhemorrhagic) stroke.
   c. The following regimens may be used:
      (1) t-PA (Activase), 15 mg IV bolus, followed by 0.75 mg/kg (up to 50 mg) infused over 30 minutes, followed by 0.5 mg/kg (up to 35 mg) infused over the next 60 minutes, or:
      (2) Streptokinase (Streptase, Kabikinase), 1.5 million U/hr IV, often preceded by diphenhydramine 50 mg IV to prevent allergic reaction.
      (3) Time is crucial because myocardial tissue continues to necrose until blood flow is reestablished. In patients with obvious AMI, the thrombolytic agent should be administered within 30 to 60 minutes of arrival at the ED.
   d. Two other thrombolytic agents are available. Both offer the convenience of bolus dosing, but their cost is equivalent to that of t-PA.

(1) Anistreplase (Eminase) 30 U IV over 2 to 5 minutes is equivalent to streptokinase in effectiveness.

(2) Reteplase (Retavase) 10 U IV, repeated in 30 minutes, is at least as effective as streptokinase and may be as effective as alteplase (t-PA).

3. Anticoagulation. Heparin is used to prevent reocclusion and is started during or immediately after the t-PA infusion. The standard regimen is a 5000 U IV bolus, followed by an infusion at 1000 U/hr, adjusted to maintain the partial thromboplastin time (PTT) at 1.5 to 2 times baseline. A weight-based regimen may be more likely to achieve the desired PTT level: 80 U/kg bolus followed by 18 U/kg/hr, adjusted as necessary. Heparin is often, but not always, given when streptokinase is used.

4. β-blockade has been shown to reduce mortality in patients with AMI. The following regimens may be used:

a. Metoprolol, 5 mg IV bolus every 5 minutes to a total of 15 mg, or:

b. Esmolol, 0.5 mg/kg IV bolus followed by infusion at 0.05 mg/kg/min.

c. Esmolol is short acting and is thus preferable for patients in whom β-blockade should be administered cautiously if at all, for example, those with CHF, heart block, or bronchospasm.

5. Angioplasty and surgery.

a. Pharmacologic thrombolytic therapy successfully dissolves the acute coronary artery thrombosis in most cases. Whereas many of these patients may eventually require percutaneous transluminal coronary angioplasty (PTCA) or coronary artery bypass grafting (CABG) to address the underlying atherosclerotic lesion, these measures are less dangerous and more successful when delayed until after the pharmacologically recanalized artery has healed.

b. Immediate PTCA or CABG is indicated, however, when pharmacologic thrombolytic therapy is contraindicated or unsuccessful, or in cardiogenic shock.

c. Although PTCA or CABG should be deferred if the vessel has recanalized with pharmacologic thrombolytic therapy, some centers are performing PTCA instead of administering thrombolytic agents. The relative superiority of these alternative treatment regimens is controversial, but what is undisputed is that time is crucial. Any delay in administering a thrombolytic drug, or in performing angioplasty or surgery, results in increased myocardial necrosis and mortality.

6. AMI with complications. Common ED complications include cardiogenic shock, pulmonary edema, dysrhythmias, and cardiac arrest. These are discussed later in this chapter.

F. **Cardiac ischemia without acute infarction.**

1. Even if the patient is not acutely infarcting, it is important to recognize symptoms resulting from myocardial ischemia. Mortality is high in patients with unstable angina, and early intervention may be life-saving.

2. An increase in anginal severity, frequency, or duration, or a lowering of the threshold for its occurrence, are diagnostic of unstable angina—a condition often called *preinfarction angina* for good reason.

3. Symptoms of angina are similar to those of AMI but are transient. The ECG may show ST segment depression or may be nondiagnostic. Cardiac enzymes are normal (as they may also be early in the course of AMI).

4. Whereas patients with stable, resolved angina are sometimes discharged from the ED if they can be followed closely as outpatients, patients with unstable angina should be admitted to the hospital. Thrombolytic therapy is not effective for such patients, but PTCA, CABG, or medical therapy with heparin and/or β-blockade may prevent the impending MI.

II. CARDIOGENIC SHOCK.

A. **Definition.**

1. Cardiogenic shock is caused by poor cardiac contractility resulting from AMI. It has a mortality of 80% or more. It can occur in any AMI patient but is more likely with very large infarcts, anterior infarcts, and combined anterior-inferior infarcts.

2. Tachydysrhythmias and bradydysrhythmias can cause hypotension, but this is generally not called cardiogenic shock.

B. **Diagnosis.**

1. Evidence of AMI.

2. Presence of shock as reflected by hypotension, diaphoresis, clammy skin, and signs of end-organ hypoperfusion such as altered level of consciousness and decreased renal output (see Chapter 1).

3. Persistence of evidence of poor cardiac output after treating pain, anxiety, dysrhythmias, and a trial of volume expansion (see below).

C. **Treatment.** See Chapter 1 for full discussion of shock.

1. Pain relief, reassurance, and continuous nursing surveillance.

2. Treatment of dysrhythmias (see Section IV).

3. Preload enhancement.

   a. Leg elevation.

   b. Fluid challenge of 200 to 500 ml IV normal saline. Monitor neck veins and the CVP, and remember that the CVP may not accurately reflect left-sided pressures. Stop fluids if the CVP rises. Continue cautious fluid bolusing as needed if the CVP is unchanged and the clinical state is not deteriorating.

    c. Fluid challenge is especially important for patients with inferior AMI because many such patients have concomitant right ventricular (RV) infarction. (The same artery may supply both regions.) Patients with RV infarction and hypotension may not have true cardiogenic shock and may require only preload augmentation with fluids to reverse the hypotension. RV infarct patients are thus particularly sensitive to preload reduction with nitroglycerine or morphine, and blood pressure should be monitored carefully.

4. Inotropic agents. Dopamine, 200 mg in 250 ml D_5W to provide 5 to 15 µg/kg/min. Remember that dopamine at high dosage functions as an adrenergic stimulant; therefore start with 5 to 8 µg/kg/min. Dobutamine, 200 mg in 250 ml D_5W, is also useful with a starting dose of 2 to 10 µg/kg/min. Both drugs are sometimes administered together.

5. Afterload reduction. One compensatory mechanism the body uses to combat shock is arterial vasoconstriction (see Chapter 1). In patients with AMI, however, the resulting excessive afterload may be counterproductive by forcing the ischemic heart to use more oxygen as it pumps against a higher-resistance vasculature. In such patients, cardiac output may be improved by reducing arterial resistance, thereby reducing myocardial oxygen demand. This is generally done in the intensive care setting with appropriate hemodynamic monitoring of pulmonary artery wedge and intraarterial pressures.

6. Whereas thrombolytic therapy may be administered in cardiogenic shock, immediate PTCA or CABG is more effective, and even their success is limited because of the amount of myocardial damage in cardiogenic shock. If invasive therapy must be delayed because of transfer to another hospital, thrombolytic therapy should be initiated before transfer.

III. CARDIOGENIC PULMONARY EDEMA.
A. Definition.

1. Pulmonary edema is the accumulation of liquid and solute in the extravascular tissues and spaces of the gas-exchanging areas of the lung. Noncardiac pulmonary edema is caused by abnormal pulmonary capillary permeability and is discussed in Chapters 17 and 27.

2. Cardiogenic pulmonary edema is due to increased hydrostatic pressure within the pulmonary circulation. Causes include the following:

    a. Elevated intravascular volume, often due to excessive sodium intake or reduced renal excretion. This is the most common cause of pulmonary edema and is usually not accompanied by AMI.

    b. Severe, acute systemic hypertension.

      c. Complications of AMI such as papillary muscle infarct with acute mitral regurgitation, intraventricular septal rupture, or severe left ventricular pump failure.

B. Diagnosis.

1. Whereas low-grade CHF may be a slowly progressive or chronic condition, pulmonary edema is an acute event characterized by the sudden onset of dyspnea. Rales are heard on chest auscultation. Neck veins are usually distended, a reflection of the elevated CVP that follows elevation of pulmonary capillary wedge pressure.

2. The chest radiograph is diagnostic, but x-ray findings may lag behind the clinical state. Early findings include redistribution of blood flow to the upper lobes, followed by evidence of increased interstitial fluid. Eventually, alveolar infiltrates will be seen, often particularly prominent in the perihilar regions.

3. ABGs will show hypoxemia and hypocarbia. Hypercarbia may be present resulting from increased CO_2 retention caused by fatigue or concomitant bronchospasm.

C. Treatment.

1. Allow the patient to assume the most comfortable position: sitting upright allows optimal ventilation/perfusion matching, and dangling the legs reduces preload.

2. Administer high-flow oxygen by cannula or mask. Rarely, endotracheal intubation may be necessary. Continuous positive airway pressure (CPAP) may preclude the need for intubation in severely hypoxic patients but is often not well tolerated. Newer devices such as nasal biphasic positive airway pressure (BiPAP) may be more easily tolerated than CPAP.

3. In the absence of hypotension, give nitroglycerine, 0.4 mg (1/150 g) sublingually, followed if necessary by an IV nitroglycerine infusion starting at 10 μg/min, increasing by 5 to 10 μg/min to a maximum of 250 to 500 μg/min. Nitroglycerine paste, 1 to 2 inches, may be applied to the skin in milder cases or if blood pressure is marginal.

4. IV morphine sulfate in 2-mg increments may be given to reduce both anxiety and preload (venodilation). Beware of possible respiratory suppression, particularly in patients with COPD.

5. Administer diuretic therapy such as furosemide, 40 mg IV. If the patient is currently taking this drug, give 80 mg. Double the initial dose if there is no response in 30 minutes. (Furosemide also helps by reducing preload.)

6. Dysrhythmia treatment. For pulmonary edema caused by a dysrhythmia, speed of treatment is important. (See Section IV for full discussion of dysrhythmias.)

      a. Consider cardioversion for tachycardias such as acute rapid atrial fibrillation, flutter, or other supraventricular rhythms, and for ventricular tachycardia. Less severe tachydysrhythmias may be treated pharmacologically.

b. For bradydysrhythmias, give atropine 0.5 to 1.0 mg IV. β-adrenergic drugs such as isoproterenol should be used only with great caution because they increase myocardial oxygen consumption. Refractory bradycardias may require a pacemaker. If available, external pacing in the ED may be quite effective until a transvenous pacer can be inserted.

7. For significant bronchospasm, as may occur in pulmonary edema patients who also have COPD, administer albuterol 2.5 to 5 mg by inhalation.

8. Endotracheal intubation may be required for patients with very severe pulmonary edema or for those in whom the combination of hypoxia and exhaustion has reduced respiratory effort.

9. Phlebotomy removal of 250 to 500 ml of blood may rapidly reduce fluid overload and reverse pulmonary edema. This is rarely needed but may be especially useful in patients with chronic renal failure.

IV. CARDIAC DYSRHYTHMIAS.
A. General considerations.

1. Patients with dysrhythmias need careful assessment of their volume status, electrolyte levels, acid-base balance, medication intake, and a search for underlying disease.

2. Particular attention should be paid to those patients who have a baseline diminished vascular supply to the brain, myocardium, and kidneys. Slight reductions in blood flow may severely damage these organs.

3. Pharmacologic therapy of dysrhythmias is appropriate unless the patient is acutely unstable. Immediate cardioversion or pacing may be required if the dysrhythmia is causing significant hypotension, decreased level of consciousness, or severe chest pain.

4. Immediate cardioversion should be considered for any unstable tachycardia, regardless of the specific type.

5. Immediate external pacing should be considered for any unstable bradycardia, regardless of the specific type.

6. Wide-complex tachycardias may be supraventricular with aberration or ventricular. If there is any doubt, consider a wide-complex tachycardia to be ventricular and treat appropriately.

B. Sinus tachycardia (Fig. 15-1).
1. ECG.
a. Atrial rate, 100 to 160/min.
b. Ventricular rate, 100 to 160/min.
c. P waves normal.
d. P-R interval normal.
e. QRS complex normal.
2. Causes.
a. Fever.

    b. Hypotension, hypovolemia.

    c. Emotional factors, pain.

    d. Hypoxia.

    e. MI, pulmonary embolism, heart failure.

    f. Drugs having β_1-adrenergic effect such as epinephrine and other bronchodilators, atropine, caffeine, nicotine, and thyroid medication.

  3. Treatment. Evaluate for the aforementioned causes and treat accordingly.

C. Paroxysmal supraventricular tachycardia (PSVT) (Fig. 15-2).

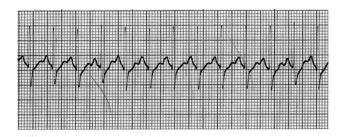

FIG. 15-1 Sinus tachycardia, rate 176. (usually below 160).
(From Stapczynski JS: Dysrhythmias. In Rund DA et al, editors: *Essentials of emergency medicine,* ed 2, St Louis, 1996, Mosby.)

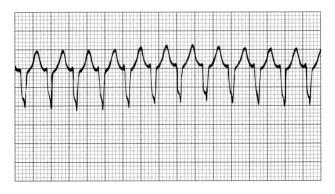

FIG. 15-2 Supraventricular tachycardia.
Exact origin of rhythm cannot be determined. (From Stapczynski JS: Dysrhythmias. In Rund DA et al, editors: *Essentials of emergency medicine,* ed 2, St Louis, 1996, Mosby.)

1. *ECG.*
   a. Atrial rate, 150 to 230/min (usually 160 to 190/min).
   b. Ventricular rate, 150 to 230/min (usually 160 to 190/min).
   c. P waves often not seen.
   d. P-R interval normal when present.
   e. QRS segment normal or widened.
   f. Carotid sinus massage (CSM) has either no effect or terminates the episode. It does not merely slow the abnormal rhythm.
2. *Causes.*
   a. May occur in the absence of structural heart disease.
   b. May be precipitated by caffeine, alcohol, stress, or exertion.
   c. Underlying Wolff-Parkinson-White (WPW) syndrome, rheumatic heart disease, AMI.
3. *Treatment* (Box 15-1).
   a. As with any tachycardia, if the patient is unstable (ischemic chest pain, hypotension, or losing consciousness), consider immediate synchronized cardioversion beginning with 50 J and increasing as needed. Sedation and/or anesthesia should be used in conscious patients. If the patient is stable, proceed as follows.
   b. Vagal stimulation may be considered but is often unsuccessful. Modalities include CSM, gagging, face or hands in ice water, and Valsalva's maneuver. CSM should be used with caution in older patients and is contraindicated in the presence of carotid bruits. Ice water should be avoided in patients with ischemic heart disease. All these measures have limited success.

BOX 15-1

Treatment Sequence as Needed: Narrow-Complex Supraventricular Tachycardia

Vagal maneuvers (see contraindications)
Adenosine, 6 mg
Adenosine, 12 mg
Adenosine, 18 mg

EITHER

Verapamil, 2.5-5 mg
Verapamil, 5-10 mg

OR

Diltiazem, 10-20 mg
Diltiazem, 25 mg

c. Adenosine, 6 mg rapid IV push over 1 to 3 seconds, is the most effective treatment. If unsuccessful, give 12 mg 1 to 2 minutes later, and another 12 to 18 mg 1 to 2 minutes after that if necessary.

d. If adenosine is unsuccessful, or if PSVT recurs, the calcium channel blockers verapamil or diltiazem may be administered.

    (1) Verapamil, 2.5 to 5 mg IV over 1 to 2 minutes. If unsuccessful, 5 to 10 mg may be given 15 to 30 minutes later. If hypotension occurs, treat with Trendelenberg's position, fluids, and/or calcium chloride, 0.5 to 1 g IV slowly. Pretreatment with calcium chloride may prevent verapamil-induced hypotension.

    (2) Diltiazem, 10 to 20 mg IV over 2 minutes. If unsuccessful, 25 mg may be given 15 minutes later. Diltiazem has less hypotensive effect than verapamil.

    (3) Calcium channel blockers should be avoided in patients with wide-complex QRS (unless the rhythm is known with certainty to be supraventricular). They are also best avoided in PSVT patients with a history of Wolff-Parkinson-White syndrome. Also, they should not be used in patients receiving IV β-blockers.

e. Digoxin may be helpful in refractory cases, 0.25 to 5 mg IV push, followed by an additional 0.25 mg 1 hour later if needed.

f. If PSVT is not abolished by the above measures, cardioversion can be performed. An alternative is *extremely* cautious β-blockade with, for example, esmolol (500 μg/kg IV over 1 min, followed if necessary by infusion at 50 μg/kg/min to a maximum of 300 mg/kg/min), or propranolol (1 mg IV to a maximum of 5 mg). (See Section IV, 3, d.)

D. Multifocal atrial tachycardia (MAT) (Fig. 15-3).

  1. ECG.

    a. Atrial rate, greater than 100/min.

    b. Ventricular rate, greater than 100/min.

    c. P waves have varying morphology from at least three different foci.

    d. P-R interval varies.

    e. QRS complex is normal.

  2. Causes.

    a. Severe pulmonary disease.

    b. Severe cardiac disease of any type.

    c. Metabolic and electrolyte imbalances, infection.

    d. Drugs: alcohol, bronchodilators.

  3. Treatment.

    a. Evaluate for underlying causes and treat accordingly.

    b. Calcium channel blockers, lidocaine, procainamide, or magnesium sulfate may sometimes control the dysrhyth-

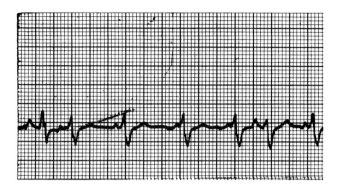

FIG. 15-3 Multifocal atrial tachycardia.
Note that baseline shows no evidence of atrial fibrillation. (From Stapczynski JS: Dysrhythmias. In Rund DA et al, editors: *Essentials of emergency medicine,* ed 2, St Louis, 1996, Mosby.)

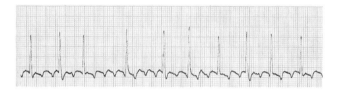

FIG. 15-4 Atrial flutter.
(From Stapczynski JS: Dysrhythmias. In Rund DA et al, editors: *Essentials of emergency medicine,* ed 2, St Louis, 1996, Mosby.)

mia. However, MAT is a sign of serious underlying disease that must be treated.

E. Atrial flutter (Fig. 15-4).

   1. ECG.

      a. Atrial rate, 200 to 400/min.

      b. Ventricular rate, 50 to 300/min, depending on atrioventricular (AV) conduction.

      c. P waves occur in a saw-toothed or sine wave pattern.

      d. QRS complex has normal shape and duration unless there is aberrant conduction.

      e. Relationship of P waves to QRS complex usually varies from 1:1 to 4:1.

      f. CSM often transiently increases AV block.

2. *Causes.*
    a. Chronic heart disease.
    b. Hypoxia, stress, trauma, thyrotoxicosis, alcohol, pulmonary embolus.
3. *Treatment* (Box 15-2).
    a. Evaluate for possible underlying cause and treat accordingly.
    b. Cardioversion should be considered if the patient is clinically unstable or if the atrial flutter does not respond to pharmacologic therapy. Use 50 J initially, and if unsuccessful, double the energy for the next shock.
    c. Calcium channel blockers may be used to slow the ventricular rate in atrial flutter.
        (1) Diltiazem, 10 to 20 mg IV over 2 minutes. If unsuccessful, 25 mg may be given 15 minutes later. Diltiazem has less hypotensive effect than verapamil.
        (2) Verapamil, 2.5 to 5 mg IV over 1 to 2 minutes. If unsuccessful, 5 to 10 mg may be given 15 to 30 minutes later. If hypotension occurs, treat with Trendelenberg's position, fluids, and/or calcium chloride, 0.5 to 1 g IV slowly. Pretreatment with calcium chloride may prevent verapamil-induced hypotension.
        (3) Calcium channel blockers are contraindicated in patients with atrial flutter or fibrillation and underlying

---

BOX 15-2
Treatment Alternatives: Atrial Flutter and Fibrillation

Either calcium channel blockers such as:
    Verapamil, 2.5-5 mg, repeated at 5-10 mg if needed
    Diltiazem, 10-20 mg, repeated at 25 mg if needed
Or β-blockers such as:
    Esmolol, 0.5 mg/kg IV to start, followed by an infusion of 0.05 mg/kg/min
    Metoprolol, 5 mg IV over 2-5 minutes, repeated every 5 minutes to a total of 15 mg
    Atenolol, 5 mg IV over 5 minutes, repeated 10 minutes later
    Propranolol, 1-3 mg IV over 2-5 minutes, repeated every 2 minutes or by infusion to a maximum dose of 0.1 mg/kg, the rate of administration not to exceed 1 mg/min
Other measures may include:
    Digoxin, 0.25 to 0.5 mg IV push, followed by 0.25 mg every 1-4 hours for 1-3 doses
    Procainamide, 30-50 mg/min IV to a maximum of 17 mg/kg

Wolff-Parkinson-White syndrome because they may cause accelerated AV conduction in such patients.

   d. β-blockers are also effective in slowing the ventricular rate, but β-blockers and calcium channel blockers should generally not both be used IV during the same episode because of additive side effects. Contraindications to β-blockers are asthma, severe congestive heart failure, and AV block. Esmolol, metoprolol, and atenolol are relatively β_1 selective and thus have less tendency toward β_2 bronchospasm than propranolol. Esmolol is very short acting, and its effect is rapidly terminated if complications arise.

     (1) Esmolol, 0.5 mg/kg IV to start, followed by an infusion of 0.05 mg/kg/min.

     (2) Metoprolol, 5 mg IV over 2 to 5 minutes, repeated every 5 minutes to a total of 15 mg.

     (3) Atenolol, 5 mg IV over 5 minutes, repeated 10 minutes later.

     (4) Propranolol, 1 to 3 mg IV over 2 to 5 minutes, repeated every 2 minutes or by infusion to a maximum dose of 0.1 mg/kg. The rate of administration should not exceed 1 mg/min.

   e. Digoxin, by increasing the AV block, may convert atrial flutter to atrial fibrillation with a slowed ventricular rate. Give 0.25 to 0.5 mg IV push, followed by 0.25 mg every 1 to 4 hours for 1 to 3 doses. (The usual digitalizing dose is 1 to 1.5 mg.) Digoxin should not be given to patients with WPW syndrome.

F. Atrial fibrillation (Fig. 15-5).

   1. ECG.

    a. Atrial rate, greater than 400/min.

    b. Ventricular rate, 100 to 200/min (irregularly irregular).

    c. P waves not identifiable—wavy baseline.

    d. QRS complex usually normal.

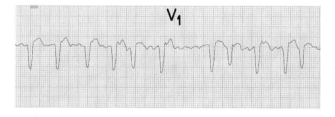

FIG. 15-5 Atrial fibrillation.
(From Stapczynski JS: Dysrhythmias. In Rund DA et al, editors: *Essentials of emergency medicine,* ed 2, St Louis, 1996, Mosby.)

2. *Causes.*
   a. Myocardial disease of any cause.
   b. Precipitation by alcohol or stress.
   c. MI.
   d. Electrolyte imbalance, especially hypokalemia.
   e. Thyrotoxicosis, pulmonary embolism, WPW syndrome.
3. *Treatment.*
   a. For hemodynamically compromised patients with acute atrial fibrillation, synchronized cardioversion is indicated. Using IV sedation and/or anesthesic if the patient is conscious, begin cardioversion with 100 J and increase power until successful.
   b. Evaluate for underlying cause and treat accordingly.
   c. In stable patients the ventricular rate may be slowed with either diltiazem or digoxin. Both are contraindicated in patients with atrial fibrillation or flutter who have underlying WPW syndrome.
      (1) Diltiazem, 10 to 20 mg IV over 2 minutes. If unsuccessful, 25 mg may be given 15 minutes later. Diltiazem has less hypotensive effect than verapamil.
      (2) Digoxin, 0.25 to 0.5 mg IV push, followed by 0.25 mg every 1 to 4 hours for 1 to 3 doses. (The usual digitalizing dose is 1 to 1.5 mg.)
   d. In patients with WPW syndrome, procainamide, quinidine, or disopyramide can be used. However, cardioversion is a better alternative, especially in hemodynamically compromised patients.

G. Sinus bradycardia (Fig. 15-6).
   1. *ECG.*
      a. Atrial rate, less than 60/min.
      b. Ventricular rate, less than 60/min.
      c. P wave normal.
      d. P-R interval normal.
      e. QRS complex normal.

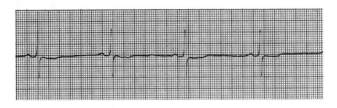

FIG. 15-6 Sinus bradycardia, rate 45.
(From Stapczynski JS: Dysrhythmias. In Rund DA et al, editors: *Essentials of emergency medicine,* ed 2, St Louis, 1996, Mosby.)

2. *Causes.*
   a. Vagal stimulation resulting from Valsalva's maneuver, CSM, vomiting, raised intracranial pressure, anxiety.
   b. MI, especially inferior.
   c. Drugs: digoxin, morphine, β-blockers, quinidine.
   d. Sinus node disease, for example, arteriosclerotic cardiovascular disease (ASCVD), rheumatic fever.
   e. Hypothyroidism, hypothermia, hypokalemia.
3. *Treatment* (Box 15-3).
   a. In asymptomatic patients, no treatment except observation, for example, in AMI.
   b. In patients who show hemodynamic compromise:
      (1) Atropine, 0.5 to 1 mg IV every 3 to 5 minutes up to 2 mg.
      (2) If atropine is unsuccessful or the patient is deteriorating, apply an external pacemaker and prepare for insertion of a transvenous pacemaker. External pacing may require sedation with a benzodiazepine.
      (3) If pacing is delayed, unavailable, or unsuccessful, the following agents may be used.
         (a) Dopamine, 5 to 20 μg/kg/min, or:
         (b) Epinephrine, 2 to 10 μg/min in severe clinical situations.
         (c) Isoproterenol should be used with caution, if at all. Although it is a good chronotrope, it also dilates peripheral vessels and increases myocardial oxygen consumption—both deleterious effects with symptomatic bradycardia.

H. Atrioventricular block.

1. *ECG.*
   a. *First-degree AV block.* P-R interval greater than 0.20 seconds is of little clinical significance and needs no treatment (Fig. 15-7).
   b. *Second-degree AV block.* Atrial rhythm is usually sinus but can be any SV rhythm. Ventricular rate is less than the atrial rate, that is, there are more P waves than QRS com-

---

BOX 15-3
Treatment Sequence as Needed: Sinus Bradycardia and Atrioventricular Block

---

Atropine, 0.5-1 mg IV every 3-5 minutes up to 2 mg
External pacing
Dopamine, 5-20 μg/kg/min
Epinephrine, 2-10 μg/min
Possibly isoproterenol (see precautions in Sections IV, G and H)

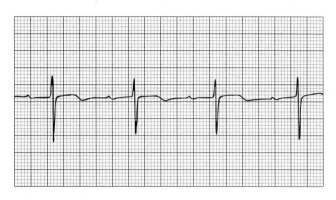

FIG. 15-7 First-degree atrioventricular block.
(From Stapczynski JS: Dysrhythmias. In Rund DA et al, editors: *Essentials of emergency medicine,* ed 2, St Louis, 1996, Mosby.)

plexes. There is a definite relationship between the P's and QRS's. There are two types of second-degree AV block, defined by that relationship:

(1) Wenckebach (Mobitz I). P waves are normal. The P-R interval progressively lengthens, and the R-R interval progressively shortens with each beat until one QRS is "dropped." The cycle then repeats. The QRS complex is normal (Fig. 15-8).

(2) Mobitz II. P waves are normal. The P-R interval is normal and identical for all conducted beats. The QRS complex is normal (Fig. 15-9).

c. *Third-degree AV block (complete heart block).* Atrial rhythm is usually sinus but can be any SV rhythm. Ventricular rate is less than the atrial rate, that is, there are more P waves than QRS complexes. Unlike second-degree block, there is no relationship between the P's and QRS's, that is, there is complete AV dissociation. The QRS may be wide or narrow, depending on whether the escape focus is ventricular or junctional (Fig. 15-10).

2. *Causes.*
a. ASCVD, especially AMI.
b. Drugs: digitalis, antihypertensives, β-blockers.

3. *Treatment* (see Box 15-3).
a. New-onset second-degree and third-degree blocks in the setting of AMI often require pacing.
(1) Mobitz I (Wenckebach) second-degree block with inferior MI may revert to sinus rhythm and require only temporary pacing.

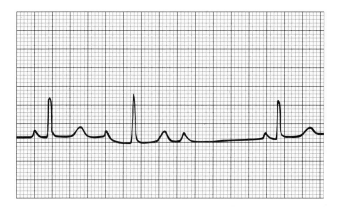

FIG. 15-8 Second-degree atrioventricular block. Mobitz type I (Wenckebach). (From Stapczynski JS: Dysrhythmias. In Rund DA et al, editors: *Essentials of emergency medicine,* ed 2, St Louis, 1996, Mosby.)

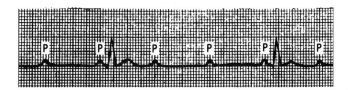

FIG. 15-9 Second-degree atrioventricular block. Mobitz type II. (From Goldberger AL, Goldberger E: *Clinical electrocardiography,* ed 4, St Louis, 1990, Mosby.)

 (2) Mobitz II and complete heart block occur more often with anterior MI, imply more severe disease of the conducting system, and usually require permanent pacing. In this setting, Mobitz II block often progresses to complete block.

 b. Treatment of all symptomatic bradycardias is similar, but there has been recent evidence that atropine may be deleterious in the setting of Mobitz II or complete heart block with ventricular escape. In general, treat symptomatic AV block as follows:

 (1) Atropine, 0.5 to 1 mg IV every 3 to 5 minutes up to 2 mg. Use atropine with caution in patients with Mo-

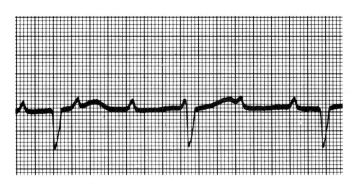

FIG. 15-10 Complete third-degree AV block.
(From Stapczynski JS: Dysrhythmias. In Rund DA et al, editors: *Essentials of emergency medicine,* ed 2, St Louis, 1996, Mosby.)

bitz II or new third-degree block with ventricular escape (wide QRS).

(2) If atropine is unsuccessful or if the patient is deteriorating, apply an external pacemaker and prepare for insertion of a transvenous pacemaker. External pacing may require sedation with a benzodiazepine. If pacing is delayed, unavailable, or unsuccessful, the following agents may be used:

(3) Dopamine, 5 to 20 µg/kg/min, or:

(4) Epinephrine, 2 to 10 µg/min in unstable clinical situations.

(5) Isoproterenol should be used with caution, if at all. Although it is a good chronotrope, it also dilates peripheral vessels and increases myocardial oxygen consumption—both deleterious effects with symptomatic bradycardia.

I. Premature ventricular complexes (PVCs) (Fig. 15-11).

  1. ECG.

   a. Atrial rate, 60 to 100/min.

   b. Ventricular rate, usually 60 to 100/min but irregular pulse.

   c. P waves normal.

   d. P-R interval normal for basic rhythm, no P wave for PVC.

   e. Normal QRS interspersed with wide (>0.12 seconds), bizarre-shaped QRS complexes.

   f. Frequent, coupled, or multifocal PVCs may portend ventricular tachycardia (VT) or ventricular fibrillation (VF), especially in the setting of AMI. However, VF or VT may occur without "warning" PVCs.

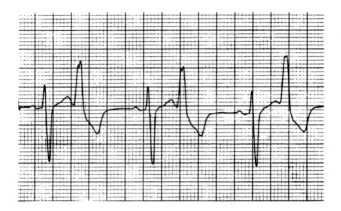

FIG. 15-11 Premature ventricular complexes.
(From Stapczynski JS: Dysrhythmias. In Rund DA et al, editors: *Essentials of emergency medicine,* ed 2, St Louis, 1996, Mosby.)

2. Causes.
   a. Coronary artery disease.
   b. Hypoxia.
   c. Metabolic disturbances, especially acidosis.
   d. Electrolyte imbalance, especially hypokalemia.
   e. Drugs: catecholamines, isoproterenol, tricyclic anti-depressants, caffeine, alcohol, tobacco, digitalis, quinidine, procainamide.
   f. Benign PVCs may occur in the absence of cardiac disease.
3. Treatment (Box 15-4).
   a. Evaluate for underlying cause and treat accordingly. Specifically, correct hypoxia or abnormal metabolic states and discontinue any precipitating drugs.
   b. PVCs with sinus bradycardia may represent "escape beats." Use atropine, 0.5 to 1.0 mg IV, to increase the sinus rate and consider pacing if bradycardia persists.
   c. The new onset of frequent, coupled, or multifocal PVCs requires immediate treatment, especially in the setting of AMI.
      (1) Lidocaine, 1.0 to 1.5 mg/kg (usually 100 mg IV push) followed by either repeated boluses (half the first dose) every 5 to 10 minutes to a maximum dose of 3 mg/kg, or an IV infusion at 2 to 4 mg/min.
         (a) Consider reducing the bolus and maintenance dose by as much as half for patients with significant cardiac failure or liver disease.

      (b) Use lidocaine only for truly premature ventricular activity. Do not use lidocaine for escape ventricular complexes that are compensating for a supraventricular bradycardia or heart block. Abolishing the escape rhythm may lead to cardiac arrest.

    (2) Procainamide, 20 to 30 mg/min to a maximum of 1 g in the average-sized person.

    (3) Bretylium, 5 to 10 mg/kg over 10 minutes.

    (4) Overdrive pacing may be indicated in selected cases.

J. Ventricular tachycardia (Fig. 15-12).

   1. ECG.

     a. Atrial rate variable.

     b. Ventricular rate, 100 to 200/min.

     c. P wave usually not seen.

     d. QRS complex, bizarre-shaped and widened, greater than 0.12 seconds.

   2. Causes are the same as for PVCs (see Section I).

   3. *Treatment* (see Box 15-4). VT is a potentially very dangerous rhythm. Perfusion may be adequate or may be so minimal that blood pressure is essentially nonexistent. VT frequently deteriorates to VF. Therapy of VT thus depends on the impact of this rhythm on the patient's condition.

BOX 15-4

Treatment Sequence as Needed: Ventricular Ectopy and Stable Ventricular Tachycardia

---

Lidocaine, 1.0-1.5 mg/kg, followed by half the first dose every 5-10 minutes to a maximum dose of 3 mg/kg, *or* an IV infusion at 2 to 4 mg/min

Procainamide, 20-30 mg/min to maximum of 17 mg/kg

Bretylium, 5-10 mg/kg over 10 minutes

Note: For stable wide-complex tachycardia of uncertain type, adenosine may be tried after lidocaine in case the rhythm is supraventricular tachycardia with aberration. Unstable tachycardias should be converted electrically.

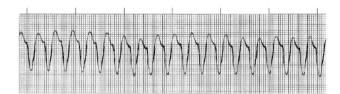

FIG. 15-12 Ventricular tachycardia, rate 170.
(From Stapczynski JS: Dysrhythmias. In Rund DA et al, editors: *Essentials of emergency medicine*, ed 2, St Louis, 1996, Mosby.)

   a. If the patient is fully conscious and only mildly sympto-
      matic, administer lidocaine, 1.0 to 1.5 mg/kg (usually 100
      mg IV push) followed by either repeated boluses (half the
      first dose) every 5 to 10 minutes to a maximum dose of 3
      mg/kg or an IV infusion at 2 to 4 mg/min. If conversion
      does not occur, resort to the following treatments.
   b. If the patient is hypotensive or becomes confused, con-
      sider cardioversion immediately with an energy of 100 J
      and double the energy level with each unsuccessful
      attempt.
   c. After conversion, follow with either lidocaine or
      bretylium, 5 to 10 mg over 10 min.
   d. If cardioversion is successful but VT recurs, repeat the
      shock at the energy level that was previously successful.
   e. Resistant or recurring VT may require the following:
      (1) Procainamide, 20 to 30 mg/min to maximum of 17
          mg/kg.
      (2) Bretylium, 5 to 10 mg/kg over 10 minutes if the pa-
          tient is stable, or 5 mg IV push if the patient is unsta-
          ble, with 10 mg given 5 minutes later if still unstable.
      (3) Amiodarone (Cordarone) for hemodynamically unsta-
          ble VT if refractory to other therapy: 150 mg IV over 10
          minutes (15 mg/min), followed by 360 mg over next 6
          hours (1 mg/min), followed by maintenance infusion
          of 540 mg over remaining 18 hours (0.5 mg/min). Com-
          plications of amiodarone may include hypotension,
          bradycardia and heart block, and ventricular dysrhyth-
          mias including torsades de pointes and VF.
   f. Correct hypoxia or abnormal metabolic state and stop ad-
      ministration of any precipitating drugs.
K. Torsades de pointes (Fig. 15-13).
   1. ECG.
      a. Atrial rate, P waves usually not seen.
      b. Ventricular rate of 160 to 280 and usually long Q-T interval.
      c. Irregular ventricular rhythm with cycles of alternating elec-
         trical polarity and QRS peaks rotating around isoelectric
         line.
      d. Ventricular amplitude varies in sinusoidal pattern.
   2. Causes.
      a. Antiarrhythmic agents that prolong repolarization (espe-
         cially quinidine, procainamide, and disopyramide), phe-
         nothiazines, and tricyclic antidepressants.
      b. Hypokalemia, hypomagnesemia, and hypocalcemia.
   3. Treatment (Box 15-5).
      a. Patients are usually without major hemodynamic compro-
         mise. Withdrawal of offending agent or correction of elec-
         trolyte imbalance is necessary and sometimes sufficient.
      b. If treatment is desired, and certainly if the patient is he-
         modynamically compromised, the following measures

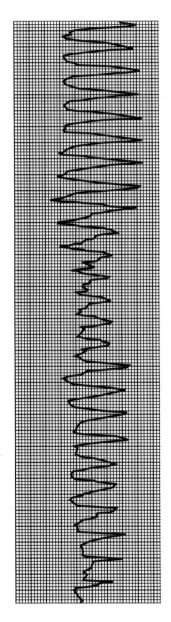

FIG. 15-13 Torsades de pointes.
(From *Advanced cardiac life support*, Dallas, 1994, American Heart Association.)

BOX 15-5
Treatment Sequence as Needed: Torsades de Pointes

Magnesium sulfate, 1-2 g IV over 1-2 minutes, followed by the same
  amount per hour
Isoproterenol, 2 to 8 μg/min
Pacing or cardioversion

---

may be successful. The underlying cause must still be
corrected.
  (1) Magnesium sulfate is often effective, 1 to 2 g IV over 1
     to 2 minutes, followed by the same amount per hour.
  (2) Isoproterenol, 2 to 8 μg/min may abolish torsades by
     overdriving the ventricles.
  (3) Pacing or cardioversion may be required in persistent
     cases.
  c. Avoid quinidine, disopyramide, and procainamide.

V. CARDIAC ARREST.
A. General considerations.
  1. Cardiac arrest is the clinical state in which cardiac output is
     effectively zero. Although it is usually due to VF, asystole, or
     pulseless electrical activity (PEA), it can be produced by other
     dysrhythmias that occasionally result in totally ineffective car-
     diac output. These include profound bradycardias and VT.
  2. For most cardiac arrests, the evaluation and treatment plan
     should follow the principles and details described in this sec-
     tion. However, in special cases, specific procedures may be
     life-saving if performed immediately. Such cases include the
     following:
     a. Pericardial tamponade requiring needle or open pericar-
        diotomy.
     b. Tension pneumothorax requiring immediate needle de-
        compression followed by chest tube insertion.
     c. Refractory hypothermia requiring rewarming as described
        in Chapter 27.
     d. Refractory electrocution requiring direct internal defibril-
        lation.
     e. Massive pulmonary embolus, which might respond to im-
        mediate embolectomy or to t-PA, 100 mg IV over 2 hours,
        followed by heparin, 10,000 units IV.
  3. Witnessed ventricular fibrillation should be defibrillated im-
     mediately. Cardiopulmonary resuscitation (CPR) should be
     performed with repeated evaluation of perfusion (carotid or
     femoral pulses) and oxygenation (breath sounds, oximetry,
     capnometry, blood gases).

BOX 15-6

Treatment Sequence: Ventricular Fibrillation and Pulseless Ventricular Tachycardia

Defibrillation up to 3 times with increasing energy: 200 J, 200-300 J, 360 J
Epinephrine, 1 mg IV push, repeated every 3-5 min
Repeated defibrillation at 360 J after each medication
Lidocaine, 1.0-1.5 mg/kg IV push, repeated as needed to maximum dose of
  3 mg/kg
Bretylium, 5 mg/kg IV push, repeated in 5 minutes if needed at 10 mg
Magnesium sulfate, 1-2 g IV
Procainamide, 30 mg/min to maximum dose of 17 mg/kg

---

    4. Closed-chest cardiac compression is effective in most situations. Emergency thoracotomy and internal cardiac compression may be considered if there are no pulses with good external compression technique, or if VF is refractory to external defibrillation. Indications for ED thoracotomy and internal cardiac compression include cardiac arrest in the following situations:

      a. Exsanguinating hemorrhage from any cause (e.g., trauma, ruptured ectopic pregnancy or ovarian cyst, gastrointestinal bleeding). The aorta is compressed just above the diaphragm to preserve blood flow to the vital organs (see Chapter 4).

      b. Pericardial tamponade unresponsive to pericardiocentesis. Pericardiotomy is performed to decompress the pericardial space (see Chapter 4).

      c. Penetrating chest injuries with suspected great vessel or cardiac trauma (see Chapter 4).

      d. Severe hypothermia with refractory ventricular fibrillation requiring direct rewarming of the heart. (Infusion of warm saline through bilateral tube thorocostomies or cardiopulmonary bypass are options to open thoracotomy.) (See Chapter 27.)

      e. Electric shock with refractory ventricular fibrillation requiring internal defibrillation beginning with 10 J.

B. Evaluation and treatment (Boxes 15-6 and 15-7).

    1. It is assumed that the reader is familiar with basic CPR techniques. The airway must be secured, ventilation established, and external compressions begun if immediate defibrillation is not available or is unsuccessful.

    2. Bag-valve-mask ventilation should be initiated, and if ventilation is successful by this route, endotracheal intubation may be delayed until initial measures have been taken.

Box 15-7
Treatment Sequence: Asystole and Pulseless
Electrical Activity

Epinephrine, 1 mg IV push every 3-5 minutes
Atropine, 1 mg IV push every 3-5 minutes to a total of 0.04 mg/kg (3 mg in the average person) for asystole and for PEA with underlying bradycardia

---

3. An IV line is established and drugs are administered according to the following protocols.
4. *Ventricular fibrillation and pulseless ventricular tachycardia* (Fig. 15-14; see Fig. 15-12 and Box 15-6).
   a. Defibrillate immediately up to 3 times with increasing energy: 200 J, 200 to 300 J, 360 J. If unsuccessful, continue with the following:
   b. Epinephrine, 1 mg IV push, repeated every 3 to 5 minutes.
   c. Repeated defibrillation as needed at 360 J.
   d. The following drugs may be helpful, with defibrillation at 360 J attempted after each drug administration:
      (1) Lidocaine, 1.0 to 1.5 mg/kg IV push, repeated as needed to maximum dose of 3 mg/kg.
      (2) Bretylium, 5 mg/kg IV push, repeated in 5 minutes if needed at 10 mg.
      (3) Magnesium sulfate, 1 to 2 g IV.
      (4) Procainamide, 30 mg/min to maximum dose of 17 mg/kg.
      (5) Amiodarone may also be effective for treatment and prophylaxis of recurrent VF if other measures are unsuccessful. See Section V, J, 3, e, (3) for discussion of dosage and precautions.
5. *PEA and asystole* (Fig. 15-15; see Box 15-7).
   a. PEA and bradyasystolic rhythms are usually due to deterioration of VF, MI, or hypoxia. Other causes include hypovolemia, cardiac tamponade, tension pneumothorax, hypothermia, massive pulmonary embolus, drug overdose, acidosis, and hyperkalemia.
   b. Treatment.
      (1) Correction of any underlying precipitating disorder.
      (2) Epinephrine, 1 mg IV push every 3 to 5 minutes.
      (3) Atropine, 1 mg IV push every 3 to 5 minutes to a total of 0.04 mg/kg (3 mg in the average person) for asystole and for PEA with underlying bradycardia.

VI. IMPLANTED PACEMAKERS AND CARDIOVERTER/DEFIBRILLATORS.

The presence of these devices may not preclude the need for cardiac resuscitation. They may fail to operate as expected, or the heart

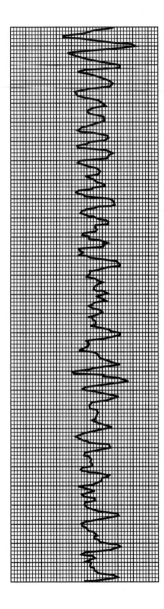

FIG. 15-14 Coarse ventricular fibrillation.
Note high amplitude waveforms, which vary in size, shape, and rhythm, representing chaotic ventricular electrical activity. There are no normal-looking QRS complexes. (From *Advanced cardiac life support*, Dallas, 1994, American Heart Association.)

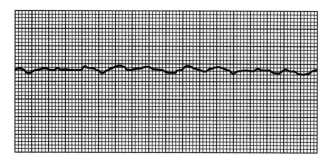

FIG. 15-15 Fine ventricular fibrillation ("coarse" asystole).
In comparison with Fig. 15-14, amplitude of electrical activity is much reduced. Note complete absence of QRS complexes. Slow undulations like this are virtually indistinguishable from asystole. (From *Advanced cardiac life support,* Dallas, 1994, American Heart Association.)

may not respond. The protocols discussed in this chapter should be initiated as needed. If defibrillation or cardioversion is performed, place the paddles well away from the implanted device.

A. Implanted permanent pacemakers.
　1. Patients may be symptomatic from a malfunctioning pacemaker.
　2. Review a 12-lead ECG for pacemaker activity. A chest radiograph may be helpful in identifying electrode position.
　3. If pacemaker activity is present, there should be appropriate capture, that is, a pacemaker spike should be followed by a P wave or a QRS complex. Also, there should be appropriate sensing, that is, a native P wave or a QRS complex should inhibit a demand pacemaker.
　4. If no pacemaker activity is present on the 12-lead ECG, there are three possibilities:
　　a. The patient's native rhythm is faster than the set rate of the demand pacemaker.
　　b. There is oversensing of the T wave or myopotential inhibition, both of which inhibit pacemaker activity.
　　c. There is complete battery failure with no output.
　5. If no pacemaker activity is apparent on ECG, apply a magnet over the pacemaker for 20 seconds and observe the ECG tracing.
　　a. If the pacemaker is functioning, it will fire at a fixed rate, often called the *magnet rate.* If pacemaker activity is now present, the patient was either in a native rhythm faster than the set rate or there was oversensing.
　　b. If there is no activity when the magnet is applied to the pacemaker, complete battery failure has occurred.

      c. Because magnet use carries a small risk of dangerous dysrhythmias, its application should be limited to a short period (20 seconds) for diagnosis only.

B. Implanted cardioverter/defibrillators.

    1. If the device is functioning properly, it should deliver a shock within 30 seconds of dysrhythmia occurrence. If the device does not discharge after 30 seconds of VF, it is not operable. In this case, or if the dysrhythmia is not abolished by the device, the VF protocol should be initiated.

    2. There is no danger if the implanted defibrillator does discharge while the rescuer's hands are on the chest, although a mild shock might be felt.

16

Vascular Emergencies (Traumatic and Nontraumatic)

I. ACUTE ARTERIAL ISCHEMIA.

A. The following findings may be present individually or as a full constellation in the event of acute arterial occlusion or injury. All should be sought in the physical examination and documented in the medical record.

B. Early symptoms and signs.
1. Sudden onset of severe pain in an extremity.
2. Paresthesias followed by the gradual loss of sensation.
3. Gradual loss of motor function.
4. Coolness of the skin below the obstruction.
5. Pallor of the extremity with diminished capillary filling of the fingers or toes.
6. Absence of pulses distal to the anatomic block. The Doppler ultrasound stethoscope is extremely useful for auscultating pulses that are not palpable.

C. Late symptoms and signs.
1. Violaceous hue of skin.
2. Increased size of an extremity with firm consistency of muscle on palpation.
3. Gangrene.
4. Paralysis.
5. Absence of pain or sensation in a distal extremity.
6. Systemic bacteremia.

II. ARTERIAL EMBOLIZATION.

A. Most arterial emboli arise from an intracardiac thrombus. Atrial fibrillation, mitral stenosis, or a recent MI is frequently associated with the formation of cardiac thrombus. Rarely a left atrial myxoma may present as an acute arterial embolus. Atherosclerotic major vessels and aneurysms are also sites from which particles may embolize.

B. The embolus commonly lodges at major vessel bifurcations. The findings of acute ischemia are present.

C. The pulse above a distal extremity obstruction is usually stronger than a pulse in the normal contralateral limb.

D. Arteriography is useful in anatomic localization. In the elderly, it may reveal associated obstruction secondary to arteriosclerosis obliterans.

E. Treatment is directed toward expeditious extraction of the clot in the operating room. An initial dose of 5000 U of heparin should be administered intravenously.

III. ARTERIOSCLEROSIS OBLITERANS.

A. Occlusion in this arterial disease of aging is a gradual, progressive process. It is usually accompanied by the development of collateral circulation. Occasionally, the narrow-vessel lumen will become thrombotic suddenly or be obstructed by an embolus, thereby causing acute ischemia.

B. The lower extremity is most commonly involved. In addition to the findings characteristic of acute ischemia, the patient often has a history and signs of the following:

1. Leg claudication.
2. Atrophic skin changes.
3. Ulceration.
4. Areas of gangrene.

C. Management. When the diagnosis of arterial occlusion is made, the patient should be admitted to the hospital. Arrangements should be made for immediate arteriography.

IV. ACUTE VENOUS DISEASE.

A. Ruptured varicosities.

1. Hemorrhage of a thin, dilated superficial vein in patients with varicose veins of a lower extremity may occur spontaneously or after injury.
2. The area where the greater saphenous vein crosses the medial malleolus is most commonly involved.
3. Subcutaneous and intradermal rupture of a varix results in an ecchymotic patch or a hematoma that, if untreated, can lead to a stasis ulcer.
4. Blood loss is usually minimal but may be extensive enough to require a transfusion. Bleeding is usually controlled by the application of a compression dressing and an elastic bandage from the toes to the tibial tubercle.

B. Thrombophlebitis. Venous stasis is a major cause of thrombophlebitis. Conditions that predispose to thrombophlebitis include immobility (such as due to bed rest or extremity casting), obesity, pregnancy, the use of oral contraceptive agents, and malignancy.

1. Acute superficial thrombophlebitis.
   a. The lesions are painful, erythematous cords that follow the

course of superficial veins. The inflammatory reaction usually subsides in 7 to 18 days.

b. Treatment includes bed rest with elevation of the extremity and warm, moist packs and nonsteroidal antiinflammatory agents.

2. Deep thrombophlebitis.

a. The urgent nature of this condition stems from the complication of pulmonary embolism.

b. Thrombophlebitis most commonly involves the deep veins
of the calves, the iliofemoral system, and the pelvic veins.

c. Signs and symptoms.

(1) There is usually a rapid onset of pain and swelling of
the limb.

(2) There is diffuse tenderness on manual compression.

(3) Forcible dorsiflexion of the foot causes pain in the
calf. There may be increased resistance to such passive
dorsiflexion (Homans' sign).

(4) Calf tenderness on palpation and a firmness of the calf
muscles may be the only signs.

(5) Iliofemoral thrombophlebitis causes swelling of the
thigh and tenderness along the common femoral vein
beneath the inguinal ligament.

(6) The calf and thigh circumferences of the involved extremity may exceed those of a normal contralateral extremity by 2 cm or more.

d. Diagnosis.

(1) Venography is the definitive diagnostic procedure, but
it is invasive and involves the potential complications
of radiographic contrast material.

(2) Radioactive fibrinogen scanning is useful in the diagnosis of *fresh* calf vein thrombosis. It is not useful in
the diagnosis of thrombi of the upper part of the thigh
or pelvis, which are the most likely to cause embolization to the pulmonary circulation.

(3) Impedance plethysmography is a noninvasive technique for the diagnosis of popliteal, femoral, and
iliac vein thrombosis. It is not useful for calf vein
thrombosis.

(4) Doppler ultrasonography and duplex Doppler scanning
are the most accurate noninvasive tests for detecting
interference with venous flow. However, they are more
useful for venous obstruction above the knee than
below.

e. Treatment.

(1) The patient should be admitted to the hospital and
restricted to bed rest with the involved extremity elevated.

(2) Blood should be drawn for a baseline activated PTT.

(3) The patient should then be anticoagulated with IV

heparin to maintain the activated PTT at 1.5 to 2.0 times the baseline level.

    (a) A standard dosing regimen is a 5000-U IV priming dose followed by 1000 U/hr by infusion pump.

    (b) Weight-based heparin dosing may achieve a therapeutic effect more reliably. Administer 80 U/kg as an initial dose, followed by 18 U/kg/hr.

    (c) With either regimen the dose of heparin should be adjusted in accordance with the PTT.

  (4) Low-molecular-weight heparin has recently become available in the United States, and studies have shown that subcutaneous administration of this agent may be more effective and safer than conventional heparin for treatment of deep vein thrombosis (DVT).

V. AORTIC DISEASE.

A. Thoracic aortic dissection.

1. The most common underlying condition is hypertension. Conditions causing cystic medial necrosis (e.g., Marfan's syndrome, Ehlers-Danlos syndrome) and congenital disorders, such as bicuspid aortic valve, and coarctation of the aorta, also predispose.

2. Dissection results when blood enters an intimal tear. There is then extravasation into the vascular media and dissection of the hematoma between the layers of the vessel. Dissection may proceed distally and involve the subclavian, renal, or iliac vessels or proceed proximally and cause aortic insufficiency or cardiac tamponade. The dissection may rupture into a bronchus and cause hemoptysis, into the gastrointestinal tract and result in hematemesis, or into the left pleural space.

3. *Clinical presentation.* Most patients with aortic dissection experience pain. The pain is usually in the anterior chest or the epigastrium, is excruciatingly severe, and may radiate to the interscapular area. Occasionally the event is painless; the patient may have syncope or signs of hypovolemic shock. If dissection involves the left subclavian artery, the amplitudes of the pulses in the arms may differ. A murmur of aortic insufficiency or signs of cardiac tamponade may be present. Most patients in whom a rupture has not yet occurred are hypertensive. When hypotension is present, it may be due to hypovolemia or cardiac tamponade.

4. *Diagnosis.* The diagnosis is suggested by a widened mediastinal silhouette on the chest radiograph. Additional findings are a double aortic shadow, hazy aortic contour, or left pleural effusion.

    a. Traditionally, definitive diagnosis has been via aortography, but this is time-consuming, and false-negatives occasionally occur.

        b. Excellent diagnostic options are transesophageal echocardiography, CT, or magnetic resonance imaging (MRI).

   5. *Treatment.*

        a. Hypovolemic shock or cardiac tamponade should be treated appropriately (see Chapter 1), if present.

        b. If the patient is hypertensive, the blood pressure should be reduced to a systolic level of 110 to 120 mm Hg. The agent of choice is sodium nitroprusside, 40 mg in 250 ml of 5% dextrose in water. It should be infused via infusion pump, the infusion rate titrated to the effect on the blood pressure.

        c. In addition, propranolol (Inderal) should be administered to reduce the pulsatile force of aortic flow. Propranolol should be given intravenously 1 mg every 2 to 5 minutes to attain a heart rate of 60/min (to a maximum total dose of 0.1 mg/kg).

        d. A vascular surgeon should be consulted.

B. Abdominal aortic aneurysm.

   1. An abdominal aortic aneurysm is seen predominantly in older men with atherosclerotic vascular disease. Many are initially asymptomatic, with a pulsatile mass found on routine physical examination.

   2. Rupture of an aortic aneurysm is generally retroperitoneal. This results in the abrupt onset of severe, constant, middle- or lower-abdominal pain, with radiation into the back or groin. A pulsatile abdominal mass may or may not be palpable. Hypotension or shock may be present.

   3. The walls of the aneurysm frequently calcify, and the aneurysm may be visible on a lateral radiograph of the abdomen. The presence of an aneurysm can also be determined by CT or abdominal ultrasonography.

   4. *Treatment.* The patient should be treated for hypovolemic shock (see Chapter 1) and prepared for emergency surgery.

VI. TRAUMA.

   A. Laceration, perforation, or contusion of the vessel wall may result in the acute cessation of arterial flow.

   B. If the artery is completely severed, the vessel retracts into the surrounding tissues. Usually, constriction of the open vessel edges by contraction of the circular coats of muscle in the media prevents extensive blood loss.

   C. A partially transected major artery tends to gape widely and may result in severe hemorrhage.

   D. Arterial perforations from knives, ice picks, or low-velocity missiles may not be apparent immediately if the surrounding tissues are filled with blood. Distal pulses may be palpable, and the circulation may appear intact on clinical evaluation. However, if these injuries are untreated, arteriovenous fistulas or pulsating hematomas (false aneurysms) may result.

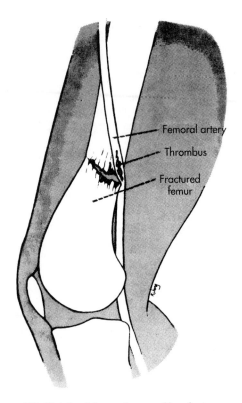

FIG. 16-1 Arterial contusion caused by a fracture.

E. Arterial contusions commonly are caused by the following:
1. Crushing blunt trauma.
2. Fractures (Fig. 16-1).
3. Shock wave trauma from high-velocity missiles passing in close proximity to the vessel.
    a. There is damage to the vessel wall, with a hematoma developing between the intima and the media.
    b. As the clot enlarges, the lumen of the vessel gradually becomes occluded (Fig. 16-2).
F. In rapidly decelerating vehicular accidents, the origin of the left subclavian artery may be subjected to a shearing force. An absent left radial pulse may be the first indication of injury to the descending thoracic aorta.

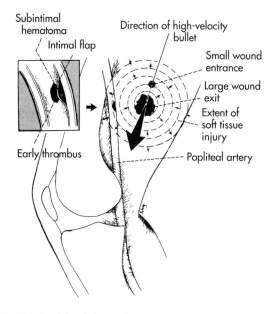

FIG. 16-2 Arterial occlusion produced by high-velocity penetrating injury.

G. Treatment.
   1. Intravascular volume must be restored and hypoxia and acidosis corrected.
   2. Arterial bleeding from a limb wound should be controlled by direct application of pressure or application of bulky compression dressings reinforced with an elastic bandage.
   3. No attempt should be made to control bleeding by blindly clamping in the depths of the wound.
      a. Tourniquets should be used only if absolutely necessary because they occlude collateral circulation and promote distal intravascular thrombosis.
      b. If a tourniquet is the only way to stop the bleeding, it must be released every 20 minutes.
   4. To avoid additional injury to adjacent vessels, fractures should be stabilized by splinting before the patient is moved.
   5. Preliminary arteriography may be helpful to show the extent and exact point of injury. This should be obtained in consultation with a surgeon.
   6. If there is any question of arterial integrity, the patient should undergo surgical exploration. Exploration should also be con-

sidered for an injury in which a high-velocity missile penetrates an area adjacent to a major vessel.

7. Arterial repair should be performed in an operating room where adequate anesthesia, light, instruments, and assistance are available.

H. Venous trauma.

1. Major vein injury is usually associated with arterial trauma. Occasionally, however, a penetrating wound may involve a large vein exclusively.

2. As in arterial trauma, active bleeding is controlled by compression dressings; blind clamping in the depths of the wound should be avoided.

3. Since operative repair of injured veins has been introduced, the incidence of posttraumatic extremity edema and phlebitis has markedly decreased. A vascular surgeon should be consulted.

17

Respiratory Emergencies

I. **GENERAL CONSIDERATIONS.** Oxygenation depends on a clear airway, adequate ventilatory effort to move air in and out of the lungs, and adequate diffusion of gases between alveoli and blood. Interference with any of these parameters can result in an acute respiratory emergency. As with any patient, the first priority is to secure the ABCs, beginning with airway and then breathing. Once these are secured, other specific respiratory problems can be addressed.

Respiratory disorders can often be differentiated on the basis of auscultated breath sounds and may be categorized as follows:

A. **Obstruction of airflow.**

1. Upper airway obstruction interferes primarily with inspiratory effort and is characterized by *inspiratory stridor.* Obstruction may be extrinsic because of a foreign body or intrinsic caused by the tongue, epiglottis, or larynx.

2. Lower airway obstruction interferes primarily with expiration and is characterized by *expiratory wheezing. Diminished breath sounds* may also occur. Interference with airflow in the lower airway occurs with bronchospasm of any cause, including asthma, anaphylaxis, or COPD.

B. **Fluid in the airways.**

1. Thick fluid in the larger airways causes a "thick" sound on auscultation often called *rhonchi.* This sound is frequently heard with bronchitis.

2. Thinner fluid in the smaller airways causes *rales.* These are heard with pneumonia, pulmonary edema, and atelectasis.

C. **Obstruction of blood flow.**

Interference with blood flow does not alter breath sounds, which are therefore normal in pulmonary embolus.

D. **Disorders of respiratory drive.**

1. Hypoventilation causing decreased breath sounds may be due to obtundation or coma of any cause, including drug overdose, head injury, hypoxia, or suppression of respiratory drive by excess oxygen administration in some people with COPD.

2. Hypoventilation may also result from spinal cord transection at the thoracic or cervical levels, which decreases ventilation by interrupting innervation to the intercostal muscles. High cervical cord transection blocks diaphragmatic motion as well and may lead to total respiratory arrest.

3. Hyperventilation is caused by any stimulus to the cerebral respiratory drive, such as hypoxia, fear, or pain. Metabolic acidosis (e.g., diabetic ketoacidosis) induces a compensatory respiratory alkalosis, another cause of hyperventilation. The condition known as the "hyperventilation syndrome" is due to acute anxiety.

E. Violation of the pleural space.

1. Breath sounds may be diminished if either air or fluid is introduced into the pleural space.

2. Pneumothorax also causes tympany to percussion.

3. Fluid in the pleural space causes dullness to percussion. Examples are hemothorax, pleural effusion, and empyema.

II. ASSESSMENT OF OXYGENATION.

A. Physical examination.

1. Inadequate oxygenation may be obvious because of cyanosis, stridor, or inadequate ventilatory effort apparent on visualization or auscultation.

2. In such cases, immediate clearing of the airway and mechanical assistance of ventilation should be instituted.

3. If inadequate airway and ventilation are not initially obvious, other diagnostic modalities may be helpful. These include transcutaneous oxygen saturation monitoring, ABGs, chest radiograph, radioisotope scanning, and pulmonary arteriography. The first two are addressed in this section and the others elsewhere in this chapter.

B. Transcutaneous (TC) oxygen saturation monitoring.

1. This is an extremely useful and rapid guide to overall oxygenation. Circulation must be adequate in the finger, ear, or forehead, the most common sites for monitoring.

2. An O_2 saturation of 90% corresponds roughly to a PO_2 of 60 mm Hg. A common mistake is to confuse O_2 saturation values with PO_2 values: an O_2 saturation below 90% reflects significant hypoxia.

C. ABGs.

1. The PO_2, PCO_2, and pH are directly measured. The bicarbonate and base excess values are calculated.

2. Blood gas analysis is significantly more accurate than transcutaneous oxygen saturation monitoring.

3. A PO_2 below 60 represents significant hypoxia. However, a normal PO_2 in the presence of a low PCO_2 indicates that the patient is having to breathe excessively to maintain adequate oxygenation.

4. Several formulas are useful for interpreting blood gas results:
   a. *Age-correction formula.* Expected $PO_2 = 103 - (0.4 \times$ age).
   b. Correlation.
      (1) *Acute.* For each 10–mm Hg deviation from normal in PCO_2, there is an expected inverse change of 0.07 in pH.
      (2) *Chronic.* For each 10–mm Hg deviation from normal in PCO_2, there is an expected inverse change of 0.03 in pH.
   c. Respiratory compensation of acute metabolic acidosis. For every fall in serum bicarbonate concentration of 1 mEq/L, there is an expected 1–mm Hg fall in PCO_2.
   d. Calculation of alveolar-arterial PO_2 gradient.
      (1) Calculated alveolar $PO_2 = 150 - (PCO_2 \times 1.2)$.
      (2) Gradient = calculated $PAO_2 - PO_2$ (measured).
      (3) Normally, the gradient is less than 15 mm Hg.
      (4) Hypoxemia may occur in all the following: hypoventilation, ventilation-perfusion (V/Q) mismatch, shunting, and diffusion impairment. There is an increased alveolar-arterial PO_2 gradient in persons with all these abnormalities *except* hypoventilation. The application of high-flow oxygen can significantly correct hypoxia in all persons *except* those with arteriovenous shunting. This must be done with care in the patient in whom the hypoxia may be due to COPD.

D. Treatment.

1. If the patient is breathing adequately but appears hypoxic on the basis of history, physical examination, TCO_2 saturation, or ABG measurement, supplemental oxygen should be administered.
2. For the patient without CO_2 retention, oxygen should be adjusted so that the PO_2 is maintained at 60 to 70 mm Hg. This may be done via nasal prongs at flow rates of 2 to 6 L/min, or by face mask. Prongs usually cannot deliver more than 40% oxygen at even high flow rates. A nonrebreathing mask is necessary for delivery of more than 60% oxygen.
3. For the patient with CO_2 retention, oxygen should be administered with care, beginning with a 24% Venturi mask or nasal prongs at a 0.5 to 2.0-L/min flow. The PO_2 should be maintained at 50 to 60 mm Hg.
4. If oxygenation cannot be maintained with either nasal prongs or nonrebreathing mask, CPAP or BiPAP devices may be useful if the patient is spontaneously breathing.

5. If ventilation must be actively assisted, however, initiate bag-valve-mask ventilation with supplemental oxygen and prepare for endotracheal intubation.

6. Endotracheal intubation may be necessary if hypoventilation cannot rapidly be reversed (e.g., with naloxone for narcotic overdose). (See Chapter 12 for discussion of rapid-sequence intubation and use of paralyzing agents.)

III. UPPER AIRWAY OBSTRUCTION.
A. Etiology.
1. Exogenous causes include foreign bodies such as small toys, broken teeth, dentures, or vomitus.
2. Endogenous obstruction is more common, however, with the tongue being the most frequent offender. Epiglottitis (see Chapter 30) and laryngospasm (discussed below) can also cause airway obstruction.

B. Symptoms. Choking and panic.
C. Signs. Inspiratory stridor is the hallmark of obstructed airway. Aphonia occurs with total obstruction.
D. Treatment.
1. Airway obstruction is an extreme emergency. The ABCs must be secured immediately.
2. Position the mandible and carefully clear any oral obstructions apparent. Suction secretions, blood, or vomitus as indicated.
3. The Heimlich maneuver may be attempted. However, ED treatment involves a laryngoscope and forceps to remove foreign bodies. Care must be exercised not to force the object deeper into the airway.
4. If the obstruction cannot be cleared and respiratory arrest has occured or is imminent, needle or surgical cricothyrotomy should be performed as described in Chapter 4.

IV. ACUTE VENTILATORY FAILURE.
A. Etiology. Hypoventilation may be due to interference with central respiratory drive or to spinal trauma, as discussed in Section I, D.
B. Diagnosis.
1. The patient with suppression of the cerebral respiratory center is usually obtunded. Cyanosis may be present.
2. Spinal cord transection is accompanied by paralysis and loss of intercostal muscle contraction.
3. Transcutaneous oxygen saturation is low. Blood gases reveal low PO_2 and high PCO_2.

C. Treatment.
1. If the patient is breathing spontaneously, nasal prongs or mask oxygenation may be sufficient.
2. In more significant cases, BiPAP or CPAP may suffice.

3. Severe hypoventilation requires assisted ventilation with a bag-valve-mask device, followed by endotracheal intubation.
4. Before intubation, pharmacologic reversal should be attempted if drug overdose is suspected (see Chapters 21 and 27).

V. BRONCHOSPASM: ASTHMA, ANAPHYLAXIS, COPD.
A. Etiology.
1. Spasm of the muscles in the walls of the bronchioles may be due to asthma, anaphylaxis, or COPD.
2. As exhalation progresses, the abnormally constricted airway becomes more problematic, and interference with airflow becomes more severe.
3. Tidal volume decreases, resulting in alveolar and eventually arterial hypoxia.

B. Symptoms. Dyspnea and sometimes chest tightness.
C. Signs.
1. Expiratory wheezing is the hallmark of bronchospasm. Inspiratory wheezing may also be heard.
2. The expiratory phase of ventilation is prolonged.
3. Accessory muscle use and intercostal or periclavicular contractions may be seen.
4. Breath sounds may be diminished because of the overall decreased volume of airflow. In severe cases, wheezing may be minimal or absent. Greatly diminished or absent breath sounds is an ominous finding, indicating minimal airflow.
5. As the patient deteriorates, obtundation may occur.

D. Treatment. (See Chapter 30 for discussion of asthma in children.)
1. All patients with respiratory distress feel more comfortable sitting up because V/Q matching is optimized. Do not force the patient to lie down.
2. Oxygen should be given by nasal cannula or if necessary by nonrebreathing mask. An initial flow rate of 6 L/min by nasal cannula is typical, but this level may suppress ventilatory drive in patients with COPD, for whom an initial rate of 0.5 to 2 L/min is advised.
3. A β_2-adrenergic bronchodilator should be administered by metered dose inhaler, hand-held nebulizer, or if necessary, positive pressure. Albuterol is most commonly used, 2.5 to 5 mg (0.5 to 1 ml of a 0.5% solution in 2 to 3 ml saline) every 20 to 30 minutes if necessary for three doses. Albuterol may be administered continuously as well (2.5 to 7.5 mg/hr). Excessive tachycardia is the primary side effect. However, increasing tachycardia could also be a sign of worsening hypoxia.
4. Steroids are now recognized as a major component of therapy. For significant bronchospasm, treatment should be

initiated in the ED, for example, prednisone 60 mg PO, hydrocortisone (Solu-Cortef), 250 mg IV, or methylprednisolone (Solu-Medrol), 125 mg IV. (See Table 17-1 for comparison of various steroid preparations.)

5. If the acute bronchospastic attack responds to treatment, the patient may be discharged. Inhaled bronchodilators should be continued, and any significant episode should be treated with a brief course of steroids. Various regimens are used, for example, prednisone or prednisolone, 60 to 120 mg/day in divided doses for 3 days or tapered over 10 days.

6. Epinephrine, 0.3 ml of 1/1000 dilution may be given SC for severe cases of bronchospasm. Although epinephrine is particularly effective in anaphylaxis, its use has declined significantly as more effective inhaled agents have become available. Epinephrine is rarely necessary with asthma and should be used with great caution, if at all, in older patients with COPD.

7. Anticholinergic therapy with ipratropium bromide, 0.5 mg mixed with albuterol may be of some use in certain COPD patients with acute bronchospasm.

8. Magnesium sulfate, 2 to 3 g IV over several minutes may possibly be of help in severe cases of bronchospasm.

9. Methylxanthine therapy has been used less frequently as more effective, less toxic agents have become available. However, severe cases may respond to aminophylline, 5 to 6 mg/kg IV over at least 20 minutes, followed by 0.5 to 0.9 mg/kg/hr IV infusion. The dose should be reduced in the elderly, in those with liver or heart failure, and in patients taking oral theophylline preparations or certain medications (such as erythromycin, ciprofloxacin, and cimetidine).

10. As the patient improves, airflow increases, along with peak expiratory flow rate and forced expiratory volume. Wheezes generally decrease as well, although as formerly closed alveoli begin to open, there may be a transient increase in wheezing.

E. Specific causes of bronchospasm.

1. Asthma.

a. Now recognized as due to an underlying chronic eosinophilic bronchitis, asthma is a disorder consisting of recurrent episodes of acute bronchospasm, often precipitated by infection or allergy.

b. Although there are several subtypes, asthma patients presenting to the ED may be of any age, from infant to elderly.

c. Steroids are particularly helpful in asthmatic patients, and most should be discharged from the ED with a short oral course as described above. An inhaled steroid may also be used.

TABLE 17-1
Relative Potencies of Commonly Used Corticosteroids

Generic name	Trade name		Relative antiinflammatory potency (glucocorticoid effect)	Relative sodium-retaining potency (mineralocorticoid effect)	Equivalent dose for antiinflammatory effect (mg)
	Oral preparations	Intravenous preparations			
Hydrocortisone	Cortef	Solu-Cortef	1	1	80
Prednisolone	Prelone, Pediapred	—	4	0.8	20–25
Prednisone	Prednisone	—	4	0.8	20–25
Methylprednisolone	Medrol	Solu-Medrol	5	0.5	16–20
Betamethasone	Celestone	Celestone	25	0	2–3
Dexamethasone	Decadron	Decadron	25	0	2–4

    d. If acute bronchospasm is accompanied by acute bronchitis, antibiotics may be prescribed. This is particularly common in children.

2. Anaphylaxis.

    a. Bronchospasm may be triggered by an allergic reaction. True anaphylaxis is a severe allergic reaction consisting of any combination of bronchospasm, laryngospasm, or hypotension resulting from loss of normal vascular tone (see Chapter 1).

    b. As with any allergic reaction, treatment consists of sympathomimetic and antihistamine medications.

    c. Epinephrine, 0.3 ml of 1/1000 dilution is given SC or IM, with significant caution in the middle-aged or elderly. For severe cases, epinephrine may be administered IV, 0.1 mg (1 ml of a 1/10,000 solution) diluted in 10 ml saline over 5 minutes.

    d. Parenteral antihistamines are also given, for example, diphenhydramine (Benadryl), 50 mg IM or IV. Histamine$_2$ blockers may be added to the H_1 agent for significant cases, for example, cimetidine (Tagamet), 300 mg IV or ranitidine (Zantac), 50 mg IV.

    e. Parenteral steroid is also administered, for example, hydrocortisone, 250 mg IV or methylprednisolone, 125 to 250 mg IV.

    f. The general antiallergic measures above are supplemented with specific treatment as indicated:

        (1) For bronchospasm and laryngospasm, albuterol is administered as described previously in this section. Inhaled epinephrine is also effective.

        (2) For laryngospasm, IV lidocaine, 1 mg/kg has been reported to be effective in some cases.

        (3) For hypotension, 1 to 2 L of IV saline or lactated Ringer's solution is infused rapidly. Severe cases may respond to the MAST (PASG) suit or to an IV α-adrenergic agent such as norepinephrine (Levophed), 2 to 12 μg/min, phenylephrine (Neo-Synephrine), 100- to 180-μg/min infusion or 0.1- to 0.5-mg bolus q 10-15 min, or high-dose dopamine, 10 to 20 μg/kg/min. (See Chapter 1 for discussion of distributive shock.)

3. COPD.

    a. COPD is usually the result of chronic smoking. The condition consists of either or both of the following:

        (1) Chronic bronchitis caused by destruction of pulmonary cilia, resulting in chronic inflammation with frequent superimposed episodes of acute bronchitis.

        (2) Emphysema caused by destruction of alveoli, resulting in coalescent, distended air sacs, with enlargement of the lungs and often the entire chest cavity.

   b. COPD patients are prone to both acute infection and acute bronchospasm, either of which may precipitate a visit to the ED.
   c. Acute bronchospasm is treated as described previously in this section. There are several aspects relevant to COPD patients, however:
      (1) Chronic CO_2 retention in emphysema patients results in diminished sensitivity of their CO_2 receptor, which normally controls breathing. Administration of oxygen may inactivate their backup O_2 receptor, resulting in respiratory arrest. Supplemental oxygen should thus be given carefully, beginning with 0.5 to 2 L/min by nasal cannula as described previously. However, oxygen should not be denied to the hypoxic patient. If necessary, ventilation should be assisted as discussed in Section III.
      (2) COPD patients are generally elderly, and epinephrine is rarely used, if at all, in this age-group.
      (3) Ipratroprium bromide may be helpful in some COPD patients with bronchospasm.

VI. INFECTION.
A. General considerations.
   1. Pulmonary infections may range from mild bronchitis to fatal pneumonia.
   2. The definitions of bronchitis vs. pneumonia vary, but in general *bronchitis* causes a cough without significant systemic symptoms. Rhonchi are frequently auscultated. Leukocytosis and infiltrate on chest radiograph are both usually absent.
   3. *Pneumonia* is characterized by systemic symptoms such as fever and myalgias in addition to coughing. Dyspnea, pleuritic chest pain, and occasionally gastrointestinal symptoms may also be present. Rales, leukocytosis, and infiltrate on chest radiograph are also characteristic.
   4. Especially in the elderly and in infants, symptoms may be vague and cough may be absent.
   5. Pneumonia is sometimes classified as "typical" or "atypical," outdated terms that should be discarded. However, these are somewhat different types of infection and are therefore described below:
      a. "Typical" pneumonia involves a relatively sudden onset of fever, a productive cough with purulent sputum, often pleuritic chest pain, and physical signs of pulmonary consolidation such as rales, dullness to percussion, bronchial or tubular breath sounds, and egophony. *Streptococcus pneumoniae* and *Haemophilus influenzae* are the most common causes of "typical" pneumonia.

b. "Atypical" pneumonia symptoms usually begin more gradually and include a dry, nonproductive cough and often significant extrapulmonary symptoms such as headache, sore throat, vomiting, and diarrhea. Physical examination may not be very revealing, but an infiltrate is apparent on chest radiograph. *Mycoplasma pneumoniae* is the most common cause of "atypical" pneumonia.

c. Organisms responsible for atypical pneumonia are generally difficult to culture and not readily seen by sputum Gram's stain. Their frequency has thus been greatly underestimated. It is now recognized, however, that they are a very common cause of pneumonia in all age-groups. In fact, they are not at all "atypical."

6. Diagnostic modalities that may be of use in evaluating pneumonia include chest radiograph, TcO_2, ABGs, sputum Gram's stain, and sputum and blood cultures.

B. Etiologic organisms. *Note: The antibiotics discussed in this section are generally effective, but see Section VI, D for specific empiric treatment regimens.*

1. Bronchitis is often viral, whereas pneumonia is more often bacterial, except in young children and immunosuppressed patients, in whom both viral and bacterial pneumonias are frequent.

2. Common bacterial causes of bronchitis and "typical" pneumonia include:

a. *Streptococcus pneumoniae* (pneumococcus).
    (1) Large, lancet-shaped gram-positive cocci in pairs and short chains.
    (2) The most common cause of bacterial pneumonia requiring hospitalization.
    (3) Traditionally most sensitive to penicillin and erythromycin, but increasingly resistant to penicillin.

b. *Haemophilus influenzae.*
    (1) Small, pleiomorphic gram-negative coccobacilli.
    (2) Common in alcoholics, smokers, the elderly, and in children under 6 who have not been vaccinated against it.
    (3) Traditionally sensitive to amoxicillin but increasingly resistant. Still often sensitive to trimethoprim-sulfamethoxazole (TMP/SMX) and the newer macrolides (clarithromycin and azithromycin). Also usually effective: β-lactam/β-lactamase inhibitor combinations (amoxicillin/clavulanate, ampicillin/sulbactam), second- and third-generation cephalosporins, and quinolones (ciprofloxacin, ofloxacin).

c. *Moraxella catarrhalis.*
    (1) A gram-negative bacterium formerly called *Neisseria catarrhalis* or *Branhamella catarrhalis.*

      (2) Common among the elderly and debilitated.

      (3) Frequently sensitive to macrolides, tetracyclines (doxycycline), TMP/SMX, third-generation cephalosporins, and β-lactam/β-lactamase inhibitor combinations.

  d. *Streptococcus pyogenes* (streptococcus).

      (1) The etiologic agent of "strep throat." This gram-positive, chain-forming coccus is a relatively uncommon cause of lower respiratory tract infection.

      (2) Often causes empyema with pneumonia.

      (3) Usually most sensitive to penicillin.

  e. *Staphylococcus aureus.*

      (1) Gram-positive cocci grouped in clusters.

      (2) Staphylococcal pneumonia is generally either a superinfection after influenza or a result of hematogenous seeding of the lungs from contaminated needles in drug users.

      (3) Hematogenous spread results in scattered, focal infiltrates throughout the lung fields on chest radiograph.

      (4) Sensitive to nafcillin, methicillin, or first- and second-generation cephalosporins. Third-generation cephalosporins are usually effective, but activity may be inconsistent. Quinolones are also effective.

  f. *Klebsiella pneumoniae.*

      (1) A gram-negative bacillus found most often in elderly nursing home patients, alcoholics, and people with COPD. Also a very common cause of nosocomial pneumonia in hospitalized patients.

      (2) Third-generation cephalosporins are especially effective, as are carbapenem-cilastatin combinations (imipenem/cilastatin) and monobactams (azotreonam).

3. Common "atypical" organisms include:

  a. *Mycoplasma pneumoniae.*

      (1) Because the organism has no cell wall, it is not sensitive to penicillin and does not retain Gram's stain. It thus cannot be seen on routine sputum microscopy.

      (2) Mycoplasma pneumonia is common between ages 5 and 30 but is now recognized as also common in any age-group.

      (3) Macrolides and tetracyclines are effective.

  b. *Chlamydia pneumoniae.*

      (1) A small bacterium with an obligate intracellular phase of its life cycle, this organism is an increasingly recognized cause of atypical pneumonia in young adults.

      (2) It is difficult to isolate by culture but is sensitive to macrolides and tetracyclines.

   c. *Legionella pneumophila.*
     (1) A gram-negative bacillus, this organism may nevertheless be difficult to identify on standard smears.
     (2) There is no person-to-person spread, but cases often occur in clusters because of contaminated heating or air-conditioning systems.
     (3) Gastrointestinal symptoms are particularly common.
     (4) Although usually benign, Legionnaires'disease may be fatal in the elderly.
     (5) *Legionella* is sensitive to macrolides.

4. Parasitic pneumonia: *Pneumocystis carinii.*
   a. This parasitic infection is common in immunosuppressed patients, particularly those with acquired immunodeficiency syndrome (AIDS).
   b. There is no person-to-person spread or risk.
   c. The primary symptom is usually dyspnea, with cough being less prominent.
   d. Signs of consolidation are often absent on examination, but the infiltrate is obvious on radiograph.
   e. TMP/SMX is the most common agent used for pneumocystis pneumonia. Pentamidine may be effective for resistant cases.

5. Mycobacterial pneumonia: *Mycobacterium tuberculosis* and Mycobacterium avium complex (MAC) *(M. avium and/or M. intracellulare).*
   a. Once rare in the developed world, these bacilli are now very common among AIDS patients.
   b. Risk of spread to health care workers is significant, and special masks and ventilation should be available in the ED for suspected cases.
   c. Tuberculosis should always be considered in AIDS patients with pneumonia (along with pneumocystis).
   d. Treatment of mycobacterial pneumonia is beyond the scope of this book.

C. Antibiotics for lung infections.
1. Varying bacterial susceptibilities are found in the literature. There are several reasons:
   a. Differences between in vitro and in vivo activity.
   b. Differences between various drugs in the same category.
   c. Lack of full clinical testing against all organisms as of the time of publication.
   Note: Only a few examples are listed below for each drug category. Other agents in the same category may also be appropriate.

   2. β-Lactams.
     a. **Penicillins.**
       (1) Drugs:
         Penicillin VK, 250 to 500 mg PO qid
         Amoxicillin, 250 to 500 mg PO tid
         Ampicillin, 500 to 1000 mg IV qid

    (2) Activity:

        Non–lactamase-forming gram-positive cocci

        S. pneumoniae, S. pyogenes

        Non–lactamase-forming gram-negative bacilli
            (amoxicillin and ampicillin only)

        H. influenzae

    (3) Recent emergence of resistance:

        H. influenzae is now often resistant to amoxicillin and ampicillin (and has been to penicillin for decades).

        S. pneumoniae has become increasingly resistant to all the penicillins.

b. **First-generation cephalosporins.**

    (1) Drugs:

        Cephalexin (Keflex), 250 to 500 mg PO qid

        Cefadroxil (Duricef, Ultracef), 1 g PO/day in 1 or 2 doses

        Cefazolin (Ancef, Kefzol), 500 mg to 1 g IV q6-12h

    (2) Activity: Gram-positive cocci (including penicillinase-producing strains). Limited activity against gram-negative bacteria. Therefore *not* appropriate for empiric treatment of pneumonias.

c. **Second-generation cephalosporins.**

    (1) Drugs:

        Cefuroxime (Ceftin, Zinacef, Kefurox), 250 to 500 mg PO bid; 750 mg to 1.5 g IV q8h

        Cefaclor (Ceclor), 250 to 500 mg PO q8h

        Cefoxitin (Mefoxin), 6 to 8 g IV/day in divided doses.

    (2) Activity: Active against organisms covered by first-generation cephalosporins such as gram-positive cocci, including penicillinase-producing strains. Also active against *H. influenzae* (including ampicillin-resistant strains). Variable activity against other gram-negative bacteria, but generally effective against those causing pneumonia. Good CNS penetration. Good empiric treatment for community-acquired pneumonia in older patients.

        S. pneumoniae

        S. aureus (including penicillinase-producing strains)

        H. influenzae (including ampicillin-resistant strains)

        Often *K. pneumoniae*

        Oral anaerobes

        M. catarrhalis

d. **Third-generation cephalosporins.**

    (1) Drugs:

        Cefixime (Suprax), 400 mg/day PO

        Cefotaxime (Claforan), 1 to 2 g IV q8h

Ceftriaxone (Rocephin), 1 to 2 g IV q day

Ceftizoxime (Cefizox), 1 g IV q8h

Ceftazidime (Fortaz, Tazicef, Tazidime), 0.5 to 1 g IV q8-12h

Cefoperazone (Cefobid), 1 to 2 g IV q12h

(2) Activity: Less active against staphylococci than first-generation cephalosporins. However, expanded spectrum of activity against gram-negative bacteria compared with both first- and second-generation cephalosporins. β-lactamase resistant. Good CNS penetration. Good empiric treatment for community-acquired pneumonias in older patients.

S. pneumoniae

Usually *S. aureus* (including penicillinase-producing strains)

H. influenzae (including ampicillin-resistant strains)

K. pneumoniae

Oral anaerobes

M. catarrhalis

e. **Carbapenem-cilastatin combinations.**

(1) Drugs:

Imipenem-cilastatin (Primaxin), 500 mg IV q6-8h

(2) Activity: Cilastatin blocks renal metabolism of imipenem. Broad activity against gram-negative and gram-positive bacteria. Appropriate for serious infections.

S. aureus

S. pneumoniae

H. influenzae

Klebsiella species

Pseudomonas aeruginosa

Bacteroides species

f. **Monobactams.**

(1) Drugs:

Aztreonam (Azactam), 1 to 2 g IV q8-12h

(2) Activity: Excellent for gram-negative pneumonias. No activity against gram-positive or anaerobes. Therefore *not* appropriate for empiric therapy of pneumonia.

g. **Combination β-lactam/β-lactamase inhibitors.**

(1) Drugs:

Amoxicillin-clavulanate (Augmentin), 250 to 500 mg PO tid

Ampicillin-sulbactam (Unasyn), 1 to 2 g ampicillin IV q6h

Ticarcillin-clavulanate (Timentin), 3 g ticarcillin IV q4-6h

(2) Activity: These agents inactivate the β-lactamases of both gram-positive and gram-negative bacteria by

combining clavulanic acid or sulbactam with a β-lactam antibiotic. They are effective against the usual spectrum of the antibiotic, including those organisms that have developed β-lactamase.

3. Macrolides.

  a. Drugs:

    Erythromycin, 250 to 500 mg PO qid, 500 mg IV q6h

    Clarithromycin (Biaxin), 250 to 500 mg PO q12h

    Azithromycin (Zithromax), 500 mg PO to start, then 250 mg PO qd 3 4 more days

  b. Activity: All the macrolides are active against the gram-positive bacteria (except S. aureus), as well as the "atypical" organisms. Clarithromycin and azithromycin are better tolerated orally than erythromycin, and are also effective against Haemophilus. Gastrointestinal side effects of erythromycin often limit the dose to 1 g/day, which is usually sufficient for mild or moderate infections. Enteric-coated preparations are preferred.

    S. pneumoniae

    S. pyogenes

    M. pneumoniae

    C. pneumoniae

    L. pneumophilia

    H. influenzae (clarithromycin and azithromycin only)

4. Fluoroquinolones.

  a. Drugs:

    Ciprofloxacin (Cipro), 500 to 750 mg PO q12h, 400 mg IV q12h

    Ofloxacin (Floxin), 400 mg PO or IV q12h

  b. Activity: Inhibition of DNA gyrase. Broad spectrum against gram-negative bacteria, but activity is only moderate at best against *S. pneumoniae* and *M. pneumoniae*. The fluoroquinolones are thus not ideal agents for treating pulmonary infections, and drugs in this class other than those above are not used at all for this purpose.

D. Treatment.

  1. The antibiotics discussed in the previous section are generally effective for the particular organisms listed. However, antibiotic resistance is increasing rapidly, and the choice of antibiotic should ideally be based on culture and sensitivity (C&S) testing.

  2. Emergency patients, however, must be treated before C&S results are known. Gram's stain of a sputum sample may suggest the offending organism, and an appropriate antibiotic is selected for empiric therapy.

  3. A proper sputum sample for Gram's staining reveals less than 10 epithelial cells and more than 25 leukocytes per low-power field (100× magnification).

4. Unfortunately, many organisms have been developing resistance to the antibiotics that have historically been effective. Penicillin-resistant *S. pneumoniae* is an ominous example. Recent guidelines of the American Thoracic Society have therefore deemphasized the sputum Gram's stain and have recommended more broad-spectrum empiric antibiotic therapy for pneumonia as follows.

   a. Outpatients under age 60 without comorbidity:

      (1) A macrolide: erythromycin (or a second-generation macrolide [clarithromycin, azithromycin] for *H. influenzae* coverage in smokers or alcoholics).

      (2) Alternatively, a tetracycline (e.g., doxycycline).

   b. Outpatients over age 60 or with comorbidity:

      (1) Second-generation cephalosporin, TMP/SMX, or a β-lactam/β-lactamase inhibitor combination.

      (2) Addition of a macrolide is optional.

   c. Patients requiring hospitalization, not severely ill:

      (1) Second- or third-generation cephalosporin or a β-lactam/β-lactamase inhibitor combination.

      (2) Addition of a macrolide is optional.

   d. Patients requiring hospitalization who are severely ill:

      (1) A macrolide plus either a third-generation cephalosporin or another agent with anti-*Pseudomonas* activity such as imipenem/cilastatin or ciprofloxacin.

5. Section VI, C summarizes appropriate dosages for the various antibiotics used to treat pulmonary infections.

VII. NONCARDIOGENIC PULMONARY EDEMA AND THE ADULT RESPIRATORY DISTRESS SYNDROME (ARDS).

A. Definitions.

1. Noncardiogenic pulmonary edema is the accumulation of interstitial and alveolar fluids in the absence of left ventricular failure. Hydrostatic pressure is normal, but the pulmonary capillaries "leak" fluid into the alveoli.

2. ARDS is a form of noncardiogenic pulmonary edema caused by an inflammatory process that activates neutrophils, leading to the release of highly active oxidants that damage the lung and destroy surfactant. This results in alveolar collapse in addition to pulmonary edema. ARDS often develops about 12 to 36 hours after the initial insult and is thus not often present during the ED phase of care. Avoidance of overhydration in the ED, however, will decrease the possibility of ARDS developing.

B. Etiology.

1. Noninflammatory causes of pulmonary edema include the following:

   a. High-altitude pulmonary edema.

   b. Drug overdose (e.g., narcotics, salicylates).

   c. Cerebral edema.

2. Inflammatory causes include the following:
   a. Sepsis.
   b. Major trauma.
   c. Inhalation injury.
      (1) Toxic gases (pulmonary "burn").
      (2) Near drowning.
      (3) Gastric content aspiration.
   d. Fat embolus.
3. Inflammation (ARDS) may develop after a noninflammatory process.

C. Diagnosis.

1. Dyspnea is the principal symptom.
2. Chest auscultation reveals rales. Neck veins, CVP, and pulmonary capillary wedge pressure are all normal.
3. Chest radiograph demonstrates alveolar fluid but not the hallmarks of increased left ventricular pressure. Absent are increased upper lobe vascularity, perihilar prominence, and cardiac enlargement.

D. Treatment.

1. Although reduction of preload (venodilators, diuretics) is very effective for cardiogenic pulmonary edema (see Chapter 15), such measures are usually of little use if left ventricular failure is not the cause.
2. Oxygenation must be maintained and alveoli kept open while surfactant is regenerated. Early application of positive pressure ventilation is very helpful: CPAP or BiPAP in mild cases and endotracheal intubation with PEEP for significant ARDS.
3. The underlying cause (e.g., sepsis) of pulmonary edema or ARDS must be corrected before the lung process can resolve.
4. Experimental treatments include inhaled surfactant and agents to stabilize neutrophils or counteract the superoxidants they release.

VIII. PULMONARY EMBOLISM.

A. Etiology.

1. The source of most pulmonary emboli (PE) is thrombi in the deep venous systems of the pelvis or thighs.
2. Venous stasis is the major predisposing factor to thrombosis. Patients subjected to prolonged bed rest or immobilization (e.g., casted extremity) are at greatest risk.
3. Other predisposing factors are malignancy, recent MI, CHF, polycythemia vera, and sickle cell anemia. Persons who are obese, pregnant, postpartum, or taking oral contraceptive agents are also at risk.

B. Diagnostic findings and studies.

1. Tachypnea is the principal symptom. Dyspnea, pleuritic chest pain, hemoptysis, fever, or a pleural friction rub may also occur.

2. Pleuritic chest pain may take hours or a day or two to develop. Its absence by no means rules out PE.
3. Massive PE can cause obstructive shock (see Chapter 1).
4. ABG measurements usually indicate hypoxemia, but the Po_2 may be greater than 90 mm Hg. Therefore a normal Po_2 does not rule out a pulmonary embolus.
5. Whereas the ECG may be abnormal, the changes are usually nonspecific. The ECG is therefore generally of little help. Among the changes that may occur are sinus tachycardia and right ventricular and atrial prominence (e.g., right axis deviation).
6. Chest radiograph findings are normal in most cases. Elevation of a hemidiaphragm, infiltrate, pleural effusion, and platelike atelectasis are the most common abnormal findings. The loss of vascular markings in a portion of the lung (Westermark's sign) strongly suggests PE but is frequently difficult to distinguish.
7. The diagnosis of PE is often very difficult because of the inadequate sensitivity or specificity of the various diagnostic modalities available.
8. V/Q scanning.
   a. A normal perfusion scan essentially excludes the diagnosis of PE. However, very few perfusion scans are totally normal.
   b. V/Q scanning has a greater likelihood of providing a diagnosis but only when there are segmental or lobar defects seen by perfusion scanning that are not matched by ventilation defects. Significant lung disease or major abnormalities on chest radiograph are likely to result in nondiagnostic scans.
9. Pulmonary angiography.
   a. This is the definitive diagnostic study; it is the gold standard. However, it is invasive and involves a significant dye load.
   b. Morbidity and mortality are relatively low but are increased in patients with underlying cardiac or renal insufficiency.
10. Lower-extremity color duplex ultrasonography.
    a. A positive finding of DVT strongly reinforces the diagnosis of PE.
    b. A negative finding strongly suggests the absence of PE but does not rule it out.
11. D-dimer.
    a. A breakdown product of clot, d-dimer level has been advocated as an indicator of PE.
    b. Although quite sensitive, d-dimer measurement is very nonspecific, and this modality is thus not very helpful.

C. Diagnostic strategy.

1. A diagnostic pathway has been suggested that combines the various modalities into a coherent strategy.

2. A normal or "near-normal" perfusion scan rules out PE, especially when the clinical suspicion is low.
3. A high-probability V/Q scan combined with a high or intermediate clinical suspicion can be considered diagnostic of PE.
4. All other combinations of clinical suspicion and V/Q scanning are not diagnostic and should be followed by pulmonary angiography.
5. Unfortunately, most patients fall into the category of low- or intermediate-probability V/Q scan, or of "discordance" between the clinical suspicion and the scan results. Most authorities recommend pulmonary angiography in such patients to confirm the diagnosis.
6. Pulmonary angiography without prior scanning may be reasonable in the presence of CHF or parenchymal lung disease that interferes with perfusion scanning.
7. Some authorities (but not all) suggest that serial lower-extremity color duplex ultrasonography may be substituted for pulmonary angiography in patients without high probability of PE based on V/Q scanning and clinical suspicion.
8. An accurate diagnosis of PE is important for two reasons:
   a. Failure to treat PE may result in further, potentially fatal embolization.
   b. Treatment of PE can cause major hemorrhage, which would be particularly unfortunate if the PE were not really present.

D. Treatment.

1. Anticoagulation.

   Anticoagulants are used to prevent propagation of the underlying thrombus and migration of additional clot to the lungs:

   a. Heparin.
      (1) The standard regimen is a 5000 to 10,000 U IV bolus, followed by an infusion at 1000 U/hr, adjusted to maintain the PTT at 1.5 to 2 times baseline.
      (2) A weight-based regimen may also be used: 80 U/kg bolus followed by 18 U/kg/hr, adjusted as necessary.
   b. Coumadin.
      Oral anticoagulation is begun during hospitalization and is continued for 3 to 6 months in most patients.
   c. Low-molecular-weight heparin.
      This product has recently been introduced. It can be given subcutaneously once or twice a day in a standard dose and may result in a therapeutic PTT without need for actual testing.

2. Thrombolysis.

   Thrombolytic therapy may be used for massive PE, but most cases can be managed without such treatment. The

dosages below are standard, but the optimal regimens for each agent have not yet been determined.
   a. t-PA: 100 mg IV over 2 hours.
   b. Streptokinase: 250,000 U IV over 30 minutes, followed by an infusion at 100,000 U/hr over 24 hours.
   c. Urokinase: 4400 U/kg IV over 10 minutes, followed by 4400 U/kg/hr for 12 to 24 hrs.
3. Surgical embolectomy. Embolectomy is a last resort for massive, life-threatening PE in patients for whom thrombolytic therapy is ineffective or contraindicated.
4. Vena caval interruption. An umbrella filter may be placed inside the inferior vena cava via a percutaneous approach to prevent further embolization in patients with life-threatening PE, in patients with contraindications to anticoagulation, or in those who embolize despite anticoagulation.

IX. THE HYPERVENTILATION SYNDROME.
A. Hyperventilation may be caused by anything that stimulates the cerebral respiratory center: hypoxia, acidosis, fever, pain, or anxiety.
B. The "hyperventilation syndrome" is due to anxiety and consists of tachypnea, hyperpnea, or both.
C. Symptoms may include dyspnea, dizziness, nausea, chest pressure, a feeling of panic or impending doom, and syncope.
D. Respiratory alkalosis shifts the balance of ionized and bound calcium, often causing a characteristic pattern of muscle cramping involving the hands and/or feet known as carpal-pedal spasm. The metacarpal-phalangeal joints are flexed with the interphalangeal joints extended, and the ankles are plantar flexed.
E. Treatment consists of reassurance and if necessary, pharmacologic sedation (e.g., diazepam, 10 mg PO).
F. Breathing into a paper bag to increase the inspired PCO_2 has fallen out of favor because it is not overly effective and can actually cause hypoxia.
G. The cause of hyperventilation in the frightened patient may not be mere anxiety. Remember that hypoxia (e.g., pulmonary embolus) or acidosis (e.g., ketoacidosis) may also be associated with anxiety and normal breath sounds.
H. Although the hyperventilation syndrome is not a serious condition, it is exceedingly uncomfortable. These patients are truly suffering and should be treated sympathetically.

X. PNEUMOTHORAX.
Although most pneumothoraxes are traumatic, spontaneous pneumothorax is not uncommon. See Chapter 4 for discussion of pneumothorax.

XI. INHALATION DISORDERS.
A. **Pulmonary "burn"** (see Chapter 27).
   1. Fires and industrial exposure may result in the inhalation of toxic gases, including carbon monoxide, sulfur oxide, nitrogen oxide, hydrogen chloride, phosgene, and chlorine.

2. Prolonged inhalation, especially in an enclosed area, is particularly likely to result in injury.

3. Although the upper airway may sustain thermal injury, damage to the lungs from fire is usually the result of inhalation of toxic fumes rather than heat injury per se. The exception is exposure to steam, which can cause epithelial necrosis and edema in the tracheobronchial tree.

4. Burns on the face and nasal hairs, hoarseness, and carbon particles in the sputum indicate that respiratory injury may have taken place. However, significant lung injury can occur even in the absence of any of these signs. Pulmonary injury should be suspected if there is evidence on the basis of history, physical findings, or signs of respiratory distress.

5. The major result of such injury is chemical pneumonitis, with loss of surfactant leading to atelectasis, and leakage of fluid across damaged pulmonary capillary membranes leading to pulmonary edema. This results in the inflammatory form of noncardiogenic pulmonary edema known as ARDS (see Section VII).

6. The onset of respiratory symptoms and chest x-ray abnormalities may be delayed for 24 hours.

7. Diagnostic evaluation includes ABGs, chest x-ray, and carboxyhemoglobin (COHg) level.

8. Treatment of ARDS is described in Section VII, D and involves early positive pressure ventilation with PEEP via an endotracheal tube.

9. Early endotracheal intubation should also be considered for patients with extensive thermal burns of the face or mucous membranes because the development of edema will render the procedure more difficult subsequently.

B. Carbon monoxide (CO) poisoning.

1. CO is released from the incomplete combustion of organic material. Fires and automobile exhaust are common sources, along with natural gas leaking from home heating systems.

2. The toxic effect of CO is caused by its greater affinity for hemoglobin compared with oxygen, resulting in the inhibition of oxygen transport, delivery, and utilization.

3. The clinical manifestations of CO poisoning include visual and auditory impairment, diminished cognitive and psychomotor performance, and cardiac ischemia and arrhythmias. Delayed CNS effects may include parkinsonism, mental retardation, disorientation, and psychosis.

4. Signs and symptoms approximately correlate with levels of COHg:

   a. COHg less than 10%: usually no symptoms.

   b. COHg 10% to 20%: frontal and temporal bandlike headache.

   c. COHg 30% to 40%: headache, weakness, visual impairment, nausea, vomiting.

  d. COHg 40% to 50%: impaired consciousness.

  e. COHg 50% to 60%: coma, convulsions.

  f. COHg greater than 60%: cardiorespiratory depression, death.

 5. The aforementioned should be used only as a guide because significant clinical findings may occur at levels lower than these. Cherry-red coloration of the skin and mucous membranes is not a sensitive index of poisoning.

 6. Treatment.

  a. Determine the COHg level. Arterial P_{O_2} levels may be normal in persons with CO poisoning because P_{O_2} measures total oxygen content and not merely that portion bound to hemoglobin, which is the effective form of oxygen in the blood, and which is displaced by carbon monoxide.

  b. Apply high-flow oxygen while awaiting the COHg result. Increasing the inspired concentration of oxygen helps displace CO from hemoglobin and hastens its elimination from the body.

  c. Oxygen via mask at 100% should be administered to all symptomatic patients with a COHg level greater than 10%.

  d. Patients with significant mental impairment or COHg greater than 40% should be treated in a hyperbaric chamber if one is available.

  e. Patients with cardiac dysfunction, those who were rendered unconscious, and those with COHg levels higher than 25% should be admitted to the hospital for cardiac monitoring and oxygen administration.

C. Gastric aspiration.

 1. Obtunded patients are prone to aspiration of gastric contents into the lungs.

 2. The aspirated material may include food particles and stomach acid, both highly inflammatory to the lungs.

 3. Whereas (usually right-sided) rales or rhonchi may be auscultated and an infiltrate seen on chest film, these findings become more apparent as an inflammatory capillary-leak syndrome develops over the ensuing hours. The process may be localized or may progress to ARDS with spread to the entire lung or even both lungs.

 4. Treatment consists of antibiotics and early positive pressure ventilation if ARDS is developing (see Section VII, D).

 5. Steroids are controversial, but if used, they should be given within the first hour.

D. Near drowning. See Chapter 27 for discussion.

18

Abdominal Emergencies

I. **GENERAL CONSIDERATIONS.** *See Chapter 19 for discussion of genitourinary tract emergencies and Chapter 20 for discussion of gynecologic emergencies.*

   A. **Symptoms.** Along with nausea, vomiting, and diarrhea, pain is a frequent symptom in patients with acute abdominal emergencies. Assessing the quality of pain is most helpful in determining the etiology.

   1. Steady pain is suggestive of solid organ pathology (e.g., spleen, liver, pancreas).

   2. Cramping, colic type pain is characteristic of hollow viscus pathology (e.g., gallbladder, intestine).

   3. Generalized pain suggests an intestinal source.

   4. Localized pain suggests a specific localized organ.

      a. Right upper quadrant (RUQ): gallbladder and liver.

      b. Left upper quadrant (LUQ): stomach and spleen.

      c. Epigastrium: pancreas and stomach.

      d. Left lower quadrant (LLQ): ovary, fallopian tube, left colon (e.g., diverticulitis).

      e. Right lower quadrant (RLQ): ovary, fallopian tube, right colon (e.g., appendicitis).

      f. Lower central abdomen: bladder.

      g. Shoulder or periscapular pain, often pleuritic: diaphragmatic irritation (e.g., gallbladder, gastrointestinal [GI] gas, or lung pathology).

      h. Back pain at the costovertebral angle: kidney (e.g., pyelonephritis or stone, or aorta/ileac artery dissection or rupture).

      i. Central back pain radiating from the epigastrium: pancreas, posterior gastric/duodenal ulcer, or aortic dissection or rupture.

   5. Pain increased with movement is characteristic of peritoneal irritation (e.g., appendicitis, ruptured viscus).

   6. Loss of appetite is frequent with any abdominal problem, but especially with intestinal disorders (e.g., appendicitis, gastroenteritis).

7. Severe nonlocalized pain with minimal findings on abdominal palpation may reflect acute mesenteric or other intraabdominal vascular occlusion.

B. Physical examination.

1. Bowel sounds may be diminished with any abdominal disorder, absent with viscus perforation or ileus, hyperactive with gastroenteritis, or include the "rushes, pings, or tinkles" characteristic of bowel obstruction.
2. Palpation should be performed very gently, starting farthest from localized areas of pain. Peritoneal involvement may be reflected by the presence of rebound tenderness, psoas or obturator signs, or significant pain when moving between supine and sitting positions or with walking or coughing.
3. Tympanitic distention suggests air distention of gut or sometimes viscus perforation. Distention with dullness to percussion may be caused by free fluid such as ascites.

C. Diagnostic studies.

1. Elevated WBC count may be of help but is often nonspecific and insensitive.
2. Elevated serum amylase may reflect pancreatic inflammation or obstruction.
3. Elevated bilirubin and liver enzymes may be due to gallbladder or liver disorders.
4. Pyuria is characteristic of urinary tract infection. Hematuria may be caused by urinary tract stone. However, pyuria may be seen with ureteral irritation caused by appendicitis, hematuria is often found with pyuria in cystitis, and renal colic may sometimes not cause hematuria.
5. Three-way abdominal radiographs may reveal the air-fluid levels characteristic of bowel obstruction or ileus, or excess stool suggestive of obstipation.
6. IVP, ultrasonography, or spiral CT are all useful for diagnosing genitourinary (GU) tract obstruction.
7. Standard CT scanning and ultrasonography may be helpful in finding other pathology such as cholelithiasis or pancreatitis.
8. Other GI studies using radiocontrast material such as barium or radionuclide tracers have less utility for rapid ED evaluation.

D. Concerns.

1. The concern with solid organ pathology (e.g., spleen) is rupture and hemorrhage.
2. The concern with obstruction of hollow visci is rupture and spillage of intraluminal contents (e.g., stool with large bowel perforation).
3. Always of major concern is delay in diagnosing acute vascular pathology caused by aortic dissection, aortic rupture, or mesenteric vascular occlusion.

4. Patients and their families should be informed that many serious abdominal problems appear benign early in the course. For example, if there is any possibility of early appendicitis, they should be so informed and urged to be reevaluated in several hours unless symptoms resolve.

5. Analgesics have traditionally been withheld pending diagnosis for fear of impairing the physical findings or masking deterioration. It is now generally felt that judicious use of parenteral analgesic agents is reasonable for patients in significant pain. Once the diagnosis has been established, more complete pain relief should be attempted.

II. SPECIFIC ABDOMINAL DISORDERS.
A. Appendicitis.
1. Symptoms.
   a. Increasingly severe pain over several hours to 1 to 2 days.
   b. The classic pattern is nonlocalized or periumbilical pain, followed by nausea, then localization of pain to the RLQ, then fever, and finally leukocytosis. Anorexia is usually present; its absence points away from appendicitis.
   c. *However, the pattern of symptoms is very often atypical.*

2. Physical examination.
   a. RLQ tenderness on palpation is usually present, even before the subjective symptoms localize. *However, this finding may be nonspecific early in the course. It may also be absent with retrocecal location of the appendix or in pregnancy.*
   b. As the serosal surface of the appendix becomes inflamed, peritoneal signs will be found on examination.

3. Diagnostic studies.
   a. Leukocytosis of moderate degree is frequent (e.g., 11 to $14 \times 10^3/\text{mm}^3$).
   b. Urinalysis is generally negative, although white cells may sometimes be found with ureteral inflammation.
   c. Ultrasonography or CT may sometimes be useful in difficult cases.

4. Treatment. Treatment is surgical appendectomy. Broad-spectrum antibiotics to cover gram-negative organisms are frequently begun preoperatively.

B. Cholecystitis and cholelithiasis. Stones form in the gallbladder over time and eventually lodge in the outflow tract (cystic duct), causing the pain of acute cholelithiasis/cholecystitis. Stone impaction and inflammation are usually both present in the acute phase of the disorder.
1. Symptoms.
   a. Cramping RUQ pain, often referred to the shoulder or periscapular region. Pain is often intermittent and frequently pleuritic.
   b. Nausea is common.

   c. Often a history of fatty-food intolerance and a family history of cholecystitis. More frequent in women, in people with Native American lineage (from either North or Latin America), and with obesity.

2. *Physical examination.*

   a. RUQ tenderness on palpation, sometimes with liver percussion tenderness as well.
   b. Fever reflects significant inflammatory or infectious component.

3. *Diagnostic studies.*

   a. Elevated bilirubin and often liver enzymes. Leukocytosis if significant inflammation or infection is present.
   b. Ultrasonography is usually diagnostic.

4. *Treatment.*

   a. Antibiotics and hospitalization if significant fever and leukocytosis are present.
   b. Surgical cholecystectomy.

C. Pancreatitis. Most frequently a long-term sequela of chronic alcoholism, often after a bout of drinking. It may also be caused by gallstones in the common duct.

   1. *Symptoms.* Steady, severe epigastric pain, usually referred to the back.

   2. *Physical examination.* Epigastric tenderness on palpation. Rebound tenderness if significant leakage of pancreatic enzymes.

   3. *Diagnostic studies.*

   a. Elevated serum amylase.
   b. Ultrasonography or CT if diagnostic problem.

   4. *Treatment.*

   a. Nasogastric suction is traditional, although some authorities believe this may actually increase symptoms.
   b. IV hydration and analgesics. Hospitalization is usually required.

D. Peptic disorders.

   1. Peptic disorders include mucosal inflammation (gastritis, duodenitis, and esophagitis), erosion (ulcer), and complications of ulcer such as hemorrhage or perforation. (See Chapter 15 for discussion of esophagitis and esophageal spasm.)

   2. It is now recognized that the underlying pathology of ulcer disease not related to nonsteroidal inflammatory drugs (NSAIDs) is usually infectious, resulting from the bacterium *Helicobacter pylori*. NSAIDs affect the stomach; *H. pylori* can infect either the stomach or duodenum.

   3. *Symptoms.*

   a. Burning epigastric pain, often diminished with antacids.
   b. Pain may be referred to the back with posterior wall ulcer.
   c. Postprandial fullness or emesis may occur with outlet obstruction.

   d. Hemorrhage causes melena and often hematemesis.
   e. Perforation causes peritoneal symptoms.
4. *Physical examination.*
   a. Relatively mild epigastric tenderness on palpation is most common but may be absent.
   b. Hemorrhage causes guaiac-positive stools (unless extremely acute) and if severe, other signs of hemorrhage such as tachycardia and hypotension (see Chapter 1).
   c. Perforation causes rebound tenderness and diminished or absent bowel sounds.
5. *Diagnostic studies.*
   a. Stool guaiac, and if indicated, CBC and guaiac of nasogastric aspirate or emesis.
   b. Three-way abdominal radiographs to look for free air if perforation is suspected.
   c. Eventually endoscopy or upper GI radiocontrast studies.
6. *Treatment.*
   a. Peptic disorders are treated with agents to lower GI acid concentration.
      (1) Antacids have traditionally been used, such as magnesium or aluminum hydroxide preparations (e.g., Maalox, Mylanta, Riopan), 30 ml before meals, at bedtime, and as needed.
      (2) Histamine$_2$ blockers, which decrease acid production, are now generally prescribed, often along with the antacids above. These include ranitidine (Zantac), famotidine (Pepcid), nizatidine (Axid), and cimetidine (Tagamet). The low-dose preparations available without a prescription may be effective for occasional "heartburn," but prescription-strength dosage is necessary for treatment of significant gastritis or ulcer disease.
      (3) Proton pump inhibitors are also very effective in lowering acid production. Omeprazole (Prilosec) may be used instead of histamine$_2$ blockers.
      (4) The prostaglandin analog misoprostol (Cytotec) is not as effective as the histamine$_2$ blockers or proton pump inhibitors in treating acute ulcers but is sometimes prescribed prophylactically in patients at risk for gastric side effects when NSAIDs must be used.
      (5) Although it does not affect acid concentration, sucralfate (Carafate) may help protect the mucosa from the effect of acid. It is probably as effective as lowering acid production.
   b. Upper GI hemorrhage is treated with nasogastric suction and lavage and fluid resuscitation as indicated, along with blood transfusion for significant hemorrhage (see Chapter 1). Surgery may sometimes be required to stop the bleeding.

    c. Gastric or duodenal perforation is treated with nasogastric suction and immediate surgery.

    d. Definitive treatment of non–NSAID-related ulcer disease usually involves eradication of *H. pylori.* A number of antibiotic regimens may be used, but such therapy is generally initiated after the ED phase of care.

E. Bowel obstruction. Small bowel obstruction (SBO) secondary to adhesions from prior surgery is the most common cause. Large bowel obstruction (LBO) is less common but is often due to cancer.

    Serious complications of bowel obstruction include both bowel perforation and strangulation LBO with vascular compromise leading to bowel necrosis.

1. Symptoms.

    a. Generalized abdominal cramping, often intermittent, but increasingly severe. Nausea and vomiting are particularly common with SBO.

    b. Although stool and rectal gas may be passed for some time after the onset of obstruction, passage of both will eventually cease.

2. Physical examination.

    a. Tympanitic distention increases over time.

    b. Characteristic bowel sounds are often described as "rushes, pings, or tinkles."

3. Diagnostic studies.

    a. The three-way abdominal radiograph series is usually diagnostic, revealing distended bowel with the characteristic multiple air fluid levels of SBO.

      (1) These findings are confined to the small bowel in SBO and to the colon in LBO unless an incompetent ileocecal valve allows reflux into the small bowel.

      (2) Ileus may also cause air fluid levels, but these are generally seen throughout both large and small bowel, and bowel sounds are of course absent.

      (3) Supine abdominal films may not reveal air fluid levels. Upright and/or decubitus views should be obtained if bowel obstruction is suspected.

      (4) Free air indicates rupture of the bowel.

    b. The presence of leukocytosis or fever are of concern because they may reflect ischemic or necrotic bowel caused by strangulation.

4. Treatment.

    a. Nasogastric suction, especially for SBO.

    b. IV hydration and analgesia.

    c. Surgery if signs of strangulation or perforation, or if obstruction is not relieved by medical therapy.

F. Diverticulitis. Diverticulitis is an acute inflammation superimposed on underlying diverticulosis.

1. ***Symptoms.*** Localized LLQ pain, only occasionally with nausea.
2. ***Physical examination.***
   a. LLQ tenderness on palpation, sometimes with mild local rebound.
   b. Major rebound tenderness, rigidity, or other peritoneal signs may reflect perforation.
3. ***Diagnostic studies.***
   a. Leukocytosis is common except early in the course.
   b. Three-way abdominal radiographs should be considered if there are significant peritoneal signs, to look for the free air characteristic of viscus perforation.
4. ***Treatment.***
   a. Antibiotic therapy usually cures the acute condition. Surgery is needed only for perforation.
   b. A typical outpatient regimen includes ciprofloxacin, 500 to 750 mg bid plus metronidazole, 500 mg qid.

G. Diarrhea, vomiting, and gastroenteritis.

1. *General considerations.*
   a. Although many abdominal disorders may cause nausea, vomiting, and diarrhea, the presence of these symptoms in the absence of underlying significant pathology usually reflects infectious gastroenteritis.
   b. The term *gastroenteritis* technically implies inflammation of both the stomach (vomiting) and intestine (diarrhea). But the term is often used loosely to indicate an acute, temporary, infectious condition causing either vomiting or diarrhea or both.
   c. Gastroenteritis may be due to viral, bacterial, or protozoal pathogens.
   d. Drinking impure water while camping and traveling in underdeveloped countries are frequent precursors to infectious diarrhea.
   e. A cluster of cases with the same food exposure suggests "food poisoning." Such clusters should be reported to the local health authorities.
   f. Diarrhea may also be caused by inflammatory bowel disease such as ulcerative colitis, Crohn's disease, or human immunodeficiency virus (HIV) infection.
2. *Infectious diarrhea and gastroenteritis.*
   a. Symptoms: vomiting and diarrhea—either alone or in combination, and often accompanied by generalized, intermittent, cramping abdominal pain.
   b. Physical examination.
      (1) Often hyperactive bowel sounds.
      (2) Relatively mild abdominal tenderness, if any, on palpation.
      (3) Signs of dehydration if significant fluid loss: dry mucous membranes, orthostatic dizziness, and possibly orthostatic hypotension.

    c. Diagnostic studies.
       (1) Leukocytosis may be present or absent.
       (2) Serum electrolyte levels and BUN may reflect fluid and mineral loss in severe cases.
       (3) Fecal leukocytes suggest bacterial diarrhea as opposed to viral.
       (4) Stool for culture and ova and parasite studies may reveal the pathogen.
    d. Treatment.
       (1) Nausea may be controlled with parenteral, rectal, or oral agents as discussed below.
       (2) Antidiarrheal medication as discussed below may also be used for a day or two if there is no evidence of toxic megacolon or significant dysentery.
       (3) Dehydration should be corrected. Antiemetic medication may allow oral rehydration, but IV fluid may be required.

3. Nausea and vomiting. Regardless of the cause, adults with these symptoms may be treated with a variety of agents such as the following (see Chapter 30 for children):
    a. Parenteral.
       (1) Prochlorperazine (Compazine), 5 to 10 mg IV or IM.
       (2) Droperidol (Inapsine), 0.625 to 1.25 mg IV.
       (3) Hydroxyzine (Vistaril), 25 to 100 mg IM only.
       (4) Promethazine (Phenergan), 25 to 50 mg IM.
    b. Rectal suppository.
       (1) Promethazine, 25 to 50 mg PR.
       (2) Trimethobenzamide (Tigan), 200 mg PR.
    c. Oral.
       (1) Prochlorperazine, 5 to 10 mg PO.
       (2) Promethazine, 25 to 50 mg PO.

4. Diarrhea.
    a. Symptomatic therapy.
       (1) Uncomplicated diarrhea may be controlled with antimotility agents such as loperamide (Imodium) or diphenoxylate with atropine (Lomotil).
       (2) Such therapy should generally not be used in the presence of dysentery as evidenced by significant bloody diarrhea and high fever.
       (3) In general, no more than 2 days of antimotility therapy should be prescribed from the ED. Persistent symptoms require more thorough work-up.
    b. Antibiotic therapy.
       (1) Most minor or moderate cases of diarrhea are caused by viruses, for which antibiotics are not indicated.
       (2) The presence of WBCs in the stool, however, strongly suggests a bacterial source. Common bacterial pathogens include *Campylobacter,* enterotoxigenic *E. coli* (travelers' diarrhea), *Salmonella,* and *Shigella.*

(3) If WBCs are present in the stool, or if the diarrhea is particularly severe, antibiotic therapy may be initiated in the ED (or may await stool culture results). Effective antibiotics include the following:

    (a) Ciprofloxacin (Cipro), 500 mg bid (effective against all of the common pathogens).

    (b) Erythromycin, 250 mg qid (effective against *Campylobacter*).

    (c) Trimethoprim-sulfamethoxazole (Bactrim, Septra), 1 double-strength tablet (160 mg/800 mg) bid (effective against *E. coli* and *Shigella*).

(4) Current or recent antibiotic use may lead to overgrowth of *Clostridium difficile* in the gut. This "pseudomembranous colitis" can be diagnosed by testing for *C. difficile* toxin in the stool. Treatment is a 10-day course of either metronidazole (Flagyl), 500 mg tid or vancomycin, 125 mg qid.

(5) As discussed above, diarrhea can also be caused by HIV and inflammatory bowel disorders such as colitis and Crohn's disease.

H. Gastrointestinal hemorrhage.

1. General considerations.

a. Upper GI (UGI) bleeding may be caused by peptic ulcer disease, gastritis, esophagitis, esophageal varices, or carcinoma. Risk factors include NSAIDs, smoking, and alcohol abuse.

b. Lower GI (LGI) bleeding may be caused by colon polyps or carcinoma, hemorrhoids, rectal varices, or diverticular disease.

c. Fresh blood is red. The longer it sojourns inside the GI tract, the darker it becomes.

    (1) Bright red hematemesis reflects active UGI bleeding. "Coffee grounds" emesis indicates more subacute UGI hemorrhage.

    (2) Bright red blood from the colon suggests a rectal source. The darker the bloody stool, the higher up the source. Melanotic stools may reflect a UGI source.

2. Symptoms.

a. Abdominal pain is often absent.

b. Dizziness may be a presenting complaint if there has been significant bleeding. *Caution:* The blood may still be intraluminal and not immediately apparent.

3. Physical examination.

a. Abdominal tenderness may not be very significant.

b. Signs of significant blood loss may be present: cool skin, rapid pulse, narrow pulse pressure, low orthostatic or supine blood pressure, or frank shock (see Chapter 1).

4. Diagnostic studies.

a. CBC, coagulation studies, liver enzymes, electrolytes, renal function tests, stool guaiac, and blood for type and crossmatch should be obtained for any significant bleed.

b. Endoscopy should be considered after stabilization.

5. *Treatment.*

   a. A nasogastric tube should be inserted for UGI bleeds and the stomach lavaged until clear. Suction is then maintained.

   b. IV fluid resuscitation and blood replacement are administered as indicated (see Chapter 1).

   c. Parenteral histamine$_2$-blocking agents may be helpful for UGI bleeding (e.g., ranitidine, 50 mg IV).

   d. Most bleeds will stop spontaneously, but some require surgery or intravascular embolization hemostasis via catheterization.

I. GI gas.

1. *Symptoms.* Upper abdominal or diaphragmatic (shoulder or periscapular) pain that is pleuritic, sometimes intermittent, and relieved by belching.

2. *Signs.* Sometimes mild upper abdominal tenderness on palpation.

3. *Diagnostic studies.*

   a. Diagnosis is by exclusion, either clinically or by testing, of other potential causes such as PE, pneumonia, or gallstones.

   b. If studies are necessary, gastric or colon gas will be apparent below the diaphragm on upright x-rays of the chest or abdomen.

4. *Treatment.* Simethicone (Mylicon) or a carbonated beverage to induce belching.

J. Constipation and fecal impaction. Particularly common in the elderly and the debilitated.

1. *Symptoms.*

   a. Constipation may cause surprisingly intense, generalized abdominal cramping.

   b. Fecal impaction usually leads to a defecatory urge and a feeling of fullness at the rectum, often with some incontinence of loose stool.

2. *Signs.*

   a. Bowel sounds are often hyperactive.

   b. The abdomen may be somewhat tender to palpation, often with some distention and palpable loops of bowel.

   c. Rectal examination may reveal impacted stool, or the vault may be empty.

3. *Diagnostic studies.* If the diagnosis is questionable, abdominal x-rays will show an excessive amount of stool in the colon.

4. *Treatment.*

   a. Mineral or oil retention enemas or suppositories.

   b. Laxatives such as Milk of Magnesia or cathartics such as magnesium sulfate solutions.

   c. Digital disimpaction of the rectal vault if necessary.

K. Perirectal abscess.
1. *Symptoms.* Rectal pain.
2. *Physical examination.* Tender perianal mass, often with fluctuance and erythema.
3. *Diagnostic studies.* If necessary, needle aspiration to confirm pus.
4. *Treatment.* If very early and nonfluctuant, warm sitz baths may suffice. If obvious abscess, I&D is indicated. Although large abscesses may need to be drained under general anesthesia, many can be done in the ED.
   a. Consider parenteral narcotic analgesics such as morphine, hydromorphone, or fentanyl (see Chapter 12).
   b. Local anesthetic injection.
   c. Incision, drainage, irrigation, and packing with gauze.
   d. Warm sitz baths and reevaluation in 24 hours.
   e. Antibiotics if significant cellulitis is also present.

L. Thrombosed external hemorrhoid.
1. *Symptoms.* Pain and mass at anus, often with bright red rectal blood.
2. *Signs.* Tender, hard, dark, perianal mass, usually somewhat protuberant, as opposed to perirectal abscess, which arises from deeper tissues.
3. *Diagnostic studies.* If any question of diagnosis, needle aspiration will confirm absence of significant blood, thus eliminating nonthrombosed hemorrhoid (which should not be drained). Aspiration of pus confirms abscess, which should be drained.
4. *Treatment.* If small or not thrombosed, warm sitz baths and bismuth suppositories (e.g., Anusol) may suffice. Rubber banding to necrose the hemorrhoid is also sometimes effective. If the external hemorrhoid is quite painful and thrombosed, I&D is indicated. Although large or internal hemorrhoids may need to be drained under general anesthesia, many can be done in the ED.
   a. Consider parenteral narcotic analgesics such as morphine, hydromorphone, or fentanyl (see Chapter 12).
   b. Local anesthetic injection.
   c. Elliptical excision of overlying skin and evacuation of the clot.
   d. Dressing with topical antibiotic ointment and gauze.
   e. Warm sitz baths and reevaluation in 24 to 48 hours.

M. Abdominal aortic aneurysm and dissection. See Chapter 16.
N. Mesenteric occlusion. See Chapter 16.
O. Acute gynecologic emergencies. See Chapter 20.
1. *Ectopic pregnancy.*
2. *Ovarian cyst.*
3. *Pelvic inflammatory disease.*

      4. Ovulatory pain.
      5. Endometriosis.
      6. Obstetric emergencies.
P. Urologic emergencies. See Chapter 19.
      1. Renal colic.
      2. Urinary tract infection.

19

Genitourinary Tract Emergencies

I. GENITOURINARY TRACT INFECTIONS.
A. Acute cystitis.
1. Cystitis is more common in women than in men. When present in men or if frequent in women, cystitis may reflect an underlying congenital GU tract anomaly.
2. Symptoms may include frequency or urgency of urination, dysuria, suprapubic discomfort, backache, or hematuria.
3. Clean-catch, midstream urinalysis will usually reveal WBCs and often RBCs and bacteria as well.
4. Simple cystitis does not require a culture, but C&S should be ordered for patients with frequent or recurrent urinary tract infections (UTIs), pyelonephritis, or significant underlying disorders such as diabetes.
5. Treatment.
   a. Uncomplicated cystitis is most often treated with trimethoprim 160 mg/sulfamethoxazole, 800 mg (Bactrim DS, Septra DS) bid for 3 days.
   b. Alternative regimens may include nitrofurantoin (Macrobid) or a fluoroquinolone such as ciprofloxacin (Cipro), ofloxacin (Floxin), or norfloxacin (Noroxin). Cephalosporins may also be used.
   c. Analgesia may be indicated for significant symptoms. Dysuria can be treated with a local urinary anesthetic such as phenazopyridine (Pyridium), 200 mg three times a day, after meals. Anticholinergic agents such as hyoscyamine (Cystospaz), 1 to 2 g four times a day, can be prescribed for the suprapubic pain of bladder spasm.

B. Acute pyelonephritis.
1. Symptoms of cystitis are usually present, along with flank pain, fever, chills, and often myalgias.
2. Costovertebral angle tenderness is prominent.

3. Outpatient treatment may be sufficient for mild pyelonephritis.
   a. The urine should be cultured.
   b. The same antibiotics used for uncomplicated cystitis are usually effective against pyelonephritis (with the exception of nitrofurantoin); however, a 10- to 14-day course is necessary.
   c. An initial parenteral dose of an aminoglycoside such as gentamicin (Garamycin), 160 to 240 mg (1.5 to 3 mg/kg), or a broad-spectrum cephalosporin such as ceftriaxone (Rocephin), 1 g, is suggested for frank pyelonephritis before discharge from the ED.
4. Admission to the hospital and parenteral antibiotics may be indicated for significantly ill or septic patients.

C. Urethritis in the male. (See Chapter 20 for discussion of sexually transmitted diseases in women.)

1. The main symptom of urethritis is dysuria, usually accompanied by penile discharge.
2. Because dysuria is also the most common symptom of bladder infection, urethritis must be distinguished from cystitis.
3. Cystitis (as opposed to urethritis) is not uncommon in older men with sluggish urinary flow resulting from prostatic hypertrophy. Cystitis may also occur in men of any age with prostatitis, but in the absence of prostatic abnormality, cystitis in men is usually the result of congenital anomalies of the urinary tract.
4. Thus any sexually mature man with dysuria, especially with a discharge, who has no underlying congenital or prostatic abnormality probably has urethritis rather than cystitis.
5. Obtaining a sample of the urethral discharge for gonorrheal and chlamydial studies is preferred. The patient should be asked not to urinate until the discharge specimen has been obtained, since urination may wash out any discharge from the urethra. If a discharge is collected, urine studies are unnecessary in the absence of symptoms of epididymitis or prostatitis.
6. The epididymis should be evaluated for tenderness, and the prostate may be examined for tenderness or fluctuance (see Sections D and E).
7. The common pathogens causing urethritis are *Neisseria gonorrhoeae* and *Chlamydia trachomatis. Ureaplasma urealyticum* is also frequent.
8. Because gonococcal and nongonococcal infections often coexist, patients are generally treated for both infections:
   a. Ceftriaxone, 125 mg IM, to cover gonorrhea, plus:
   b. Either azithromycin, 1 g PO in a single dose, *or* doxycycline, 100 mg PO $\times$ 7 days, to cover nongonococcal organisms.

    c. An alternative to the ceftriaxone portion of the regimen is ofloxacin 400 mg PO in a single dose. An alternative to the azithromycin or doxycycline portion of the regimen is ofloxacin, 300 mg bid × 7 days.

  9. Because patients may be infected simultaneously with several sexually transmitted diseases, serologic testing for syphilis is often recommended for patients with urethritis.

D. Epididymitis.

1. Acute epididymitis is most commonly a sexually transmitted disease secondary to urethritis. Older men may acquire epididymitis from a urinary pathogen.

2. The condition is usually unilateral with marked scrotal swelling, pain, heat, tenderness to palpation, and erythema. The testis may be involved and may be enlarged and tender. Epididymitis must be distinguished from testicular torsion, in which the pain usually begins more abruptly than with epididymitis (see Section III, A).

3. If a discharge is present, it should be evaluated as explained previously. A urine culture is helpful, especially if no discharge can be obtained.

4. Treatment includes scrotal support, ice, bed rest, antibiotics, analgesics, and an antiinflammatory agent.

5. Antibiotic treatment for sexually transmitted epididymitis is:
    a. Ceftriaxone, 250 mg IM, plus:
    b. Doxycycline, 100 mg bid for 10 days.
    c. An alternative to the combined treatment regimen of ceftriaxone plus doxycycline is floxacin 300 mg bid × 10 days.

6. If the infection is felt not to have been sexually transmitted (e.g., older men with prostatic hypertrophy or after GU instrumentation), treatment should cover urinary pathogens. Fluoroquinolones are often used.

E. Acute prostatitis.

1. The prostate may be seeded from a remote source of infection, but more commonly the source is the epididymis and urethra. Like epididymitis, prostatitis may be caused by a urinary pathogen in older men or after GU instrumentation. Prostatitis is more often gonococcal or chlamydial in younger men.

2. Symptoms usually include dysuria, urgency, and frequent urination, often accompanied by a discharge and perineal or suprapubic pain.

3. Physical examination reveals a tender, boggy prostate.

4. If a discharge is present, it should be studied as for urethritis. The urine should be cultured.

5. Treatment is similar to that for epididymitis as described previously.

F. Penile rashes and lesions. (See Chapter 20 for discussion of genital herpes and fungal infections.)

II. URINARY TRACT OBSTRUCTION.

A. Renal colic.

1. Renal or ureteral colic is due to the passage of a stone from the kidney through the ureter, with stretching of the ureteral smooth muscle and hyperperistalsis proximal to the site of obstruction by the stone.

2. The pain begins suddenly, is severe, radiates from flank to groin, and is often accompanied by nausea and vomiting.

3. Abdominal examination is usually unremarkable, but costovertebral angle tenderness is commonly present.

4. Urinalysis typically reveals RBCs. However, complete obstruction of the ureter may yield a normal urinalysis.

5. Emergency IVP, ultrasonography, or spiral CT scanning can determine the degree of obstruction and confirm the diagnosis. Recurrent stones may not require repeating these diagnostic studies unless the diagnosis is unclear or the stone does not pass within a day or two.

6. *Caution:* Aortic dissection or rupture can cause flank pain, which may be mistaken for renal colic.

7. Treatment is usually conservative and consists of a narcotic analgesic (e.g., morphine IV, titrated for relief) and a prostaglandin inhibitor to decrease ureteral peristalsis (e.g., ketorolac, 60 mg IM or 30 mg IV, half these doses being given to patients over age 65 or those with renal failure).

8. Instrumentation and lithotripsy require general anesthesia and are usually not indicated for acute renal colic.

9. The urine is strained so that the calculus can be chemically analyzed.

10. Pyuria indicates infection caused by obstruction. The urine should be cultured, urologic consultation obtained, and antibiotics begun. Surgical extraction by cystoscopy may be required if there is significant infection.

11. Although most patients can be discharged from the ED with a urine strainer and analgesic prescription, hospital admission may be necessary for control of persistent pain or vomiting or for significant infection.

B. Urinary retention.

1. Acute urinary retention may be caused by benign prostatic hypertrophy, prostatic carcinoma, urethral stricture, acute prostatic infection, vesical or urethral calculus, hemorrhage and clot formation within the bladder, or neurogenic disturbance of bladder function.

2. Immediate relief is achieved by inserting a catheter through the urethra into the bladder.

3. If a catheter cannot be passed via the urethra, a suprapubic cystostomy can be performed with a commercially available suprapubic catheter apparatus.

III. EXTERNAL GENITALIA DISORDERS.

A. Torsion of the spermatic cord.

1. Torsion of the spermatic cord, more frequently called *torsion of the testis*, is a twisting of the spermatic cord that constricts the testicular blood supply. If untreated, this torsion results in testicular necrosis. It is more common in children and young adults and in men with undescended testes.

2. The patient experiences the acute onset of pain and scrotal swelling and sometimes nausea, vomiting, and fever. The involved testis may be palpably rotated compared with the other one. However, this is not a reliable sign.

3. Differentiating torsion from epididymitis may be quite difficult. Both may be associated with pain and swelling. Symptoms resulting from torsion usually begin more abruptly, often during sleep or after exercise. Epididymitis is more likely to begin more gradually and cause fever, pyuria, and scrotal erythema; however, these may be absent (refer to Section I, D for a discussion of epididymitis). The differential diagnosis also includes strangulated hernia and testicular tumor.

4. Doppler ultrasonography and nuclear scanning may be useful, but neither is fully sensitive, and scanning frequently requires an excessive amount of time.

5. Treatment consists of prompt surgical intervention when torsion is suspected. The testis is untwisted and anchored to the parietal layers of the scrotum. Because of the risk of future torsion on the opposite side, orchiopexy is usually performed on the contralateral side as well.

B. Paraphimosis.

1. Paraphimosis is caused by retraction of tight preputial skin behind the glans penis, which then cannot be pulled forward to cover the glans. Failure to bring the skin forward results in

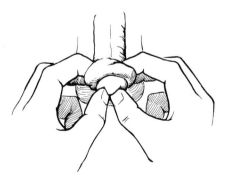

FIG. 19-1 Manual reduction for paraphimosis.

edema of the glans because of constriction by the prepuce at the coronal sulcus.

2. The patient has pain, an edematous prepuce and glans, and a tight ring at the corona.

3. Treatment is manual reduction of the prepuce (Fig. 19-1). The thumbs are placed on the glans, with the index and middle fingers of each hand behind the point of constriction. As the glans is pushed backward, the skin is pulled forward until complete reduction is achieved.

4. If edema is excessive, this type of reduction may be impossible and a dorsal slit may be required. Recurrences are prevented by elective circumcision at a later date.

20

Gynecologic and Obstetric Emergencies

I. INTRODUCTION.

A. Gynecologic problems must be differentiated from urinary tract (see Chapter 19) and gastrointestinal tract (see Chapter 18) disorders, many of which may cause abdominal discomfort. Pelvic and rectal examinations should be considered for all women with lower abdominal pain.

B. Patients with acute gynecologic disorders may experience any or all of the following symptoms:
   1. Abdominal pain.
   2. Vaginal bleeding.
   3. Vaginal discharge.
   4. Perineal lesions, often painful.

II. SYMPTOMS.

A. Abdominal pain.
   1. Ectopic pregnancy.
   2. Pelvic inflammatory disease (PID).
   3. Ruptured ovarian cyst.
   4. UTI (see Chapter 19).
   5. Appendicitis (see Chapter 18).
   6. Menstrual cramps.
   7. Endometriosis.
   8. Abruptio placentae (in third trimester).

B. Vaginal bleeding.
   1. Not obviously pregnant.
      a. Ectopic pregnancy.
      b. Ruptured ovarian cyst.
      c. PID.
      d. Dysfunctional bleeding.
      e. Pregnancy with threatened spontaneous abortion.
   2. Obviously pregnant.
      a. Placenta previa.
      b. Abruptio placentae.

      c. Threatened spontaneous abortion.

      d. Heavy bloody show.

C. Vaginal discharge.

  1. Vaginitis.

      a. Fungal *(Candida albicans).*

      b. Protozoal *(Trichomonas vaginalis).*

      c. Bacterial *(Gardnerella vaginalis).*

      d. Viral *(herpes simplex).*

  2. Salpingitis or cervicitis.

      a. Chlamydia.

      b. Gonorrhea.

      c. Other bacteria.

      d. Mixed.

D. Perineal lesions.

  1. Herpes simplex genitalis.

  2. Bartholin's abscess.

  3. Syphilis.

  4. Chancroid and other less common entities such as granuloma inguinale and lymphogranuloma venereum.

III. SPECIFIC DIAGNOSTIC ENTITIES.

A. Ectopic pregnancy.

  1. Symptoms (any of these may be absent).

      a. Menstrual period overdue.

      b. Lower abdominal pain.

      c. Vaginal bleeding.

      d. Weakness or syncope as a result of blood loss.

  2. Findings.

      a. Signs of hypotension if significant intraabdominal or vaginal bleeding has occurred.

      b. Adnexal mass.

      c. Uterus may be slightly enlarged.

      d. Elevated β-subunit of human chorionic gonadotropin (β-HCG) in blood or urine. This assay should detect pregnancy by the time of the missed menstrual period.

      e. If a β-specific HCG pregnancy test is positive, and if the patient is hemodynamically stable, ultrasonography should be performed. Failure to identify an intrauterine pregnancy in a patient with a positive pregnancy test result strongly suggests ectopic pregnancy. Detection of an adnexal mass is not necessary for a presumptive diagnosis. However, in some cases, adnexal mass or blood in the culde-sac may be detected.

      f. Intrauterine pregnancy may not be detectable by ultrasonography before 6 weeks from the last menstrual period (4 weeks after conception). Ultrasonography very early in the course of pregnancy therefore may not be able to distinguish between intrauterine and ectopic pregnancy.

g. In uncertain cases, or when the patient is too unstable to undergo ultrasonography, culdocentesis may be useful by demonstrating nonclotting blood caused by the ruptured ectopic pregnancy.

3. Treatment.

a. Replacement of blood loss as needed with IV fluids and blood (see Chapter 1).

b. Gynecologic consultation and surgery.

c. If ectopic pregnancy is possible but the diagnosis has not been established after evaluation, stable patients with no sign of active bleeding may be discharged from the ED, with reevaluation scheduled within 1 to 2 days. The patient must be cautioned, however, to return to the ED immediately if signs of rupture occur, such as increased abdominal pain, significant vaginal bleeding, or dizziness. A quantitative β-HCG level should be ordered as a baseline for comparison in 1 to 2 days.

B. Spontaneous abortion.

1. Symptoms.

a. Any bleeding in early pregnancy must be considered at least a *threatened abortion.*

b. Cramping is often present.

2. Findings.

a. Blood may be seen at the cervical os.

b. The os may be dilated *(inevitable abortion),* perhaps with tissue extruding.

c. Ultrasonography is very useful for evaluating the intrauterine contents and condition of the fetus.

3. Treatment.

a. There is no adequate treatment for threatened spontaneous abortion. Bed rest is thought by some to decrease the chance of progression from threatened to inevitable abortion.

b. If abortion does occur, the process may conclude spontaneously with extrusion of all the products of conception.

c. If bleeding is prolonged or excessive, dilation and evacuation should be considered by the gynecologist.

d. Blood should be obtained for typing and Rh determination, and anti-Rh factor antibody should be given to Rh-negative women who have vaginal bleeding.

C. PID.

1. *Chlamydia trachomatis* and *Neisseria gonorrhoeae* are the most common causes of PID. However, other pathogens such as GI or GU flora may also be cultured.

2. PID may progress from infection of only the cervix, through extended involvement of the endometrium, myometrium, salpinges, and peritoneum.

3. Symptoms.
    a. Symptoms may range from absent to incapacitating, depending on the acuity and the extent of infection.
    b. Lower abdominal pain is the most common presenting complaint.
    c. Vaginal discharge and sometimes bleeding, along with dysuria and dyspareunia, may also be present.
4. Findings.
    a. Lower abdominal tenderness is the most common finding on palpation of the abdomen.
    b. Cervical motion tenderness is usually present in patients with acute abdominal pain.
    c. Adnexal tenderness indicates infection of the salpinges and is usually bilateral.
    d. An adnexal mass suggests tuboovarian abscess.
    e. A discharge may be seen extruding from the os in many cases.
    f. Fever is often present but may be intermittent.
    g. Leukocytosis is usually present in acute PID, and often an elevated sedimentation rate as well.
5. Treatment.
    a. Swabs of the cervix should be obtained for chlamydial and gonorrheal studies. Testing of serum for syphilis should be considered.
    b. Mild cases with no significant peritoneal signs may be treated with outpatient therapy as long as there is close follow-up.
        (1) Treatment should include coverage of both chlamydial infection and gonorrhea.
        (2) Ceftriaxone, 250 mg IM, or alternatively a combination of cefoxitin, 2 g IM, plus probenecid, 1 g PO, is given in the ED.
        (3) The aforementioned parenteral medication is then followed by a 14-day course of doxycycline, 100 mg bid.
        (4) An alternative regimen to ceftriaxone (or cefoxitin) plus doxycycline, is the following:
            (a) Ofloxacin, 400 mg bid × 14 days, plus:
            (b) A 14-day course of either metronidazole, 500 mg bid *or* clindamycin, 450 mg qid.
        (5) Neither doxycycline nor ofloxacin should be given in pregnancy. Metronidazole is contraindicated during the first trimester and has not been proved safe for the rest of pregnancy.
    c. Patients with significant peritoneal signs or fever should be admitted to the hospital for IV antibiotic therapy.
    d. If a tuboovarian abscess is suspected, laparoscopy should be considered for further evaluation.

D. Ovarian cyst.
1. Symptoms.
   a. An intact ovarian cyst may be asymptomatic.
   b. Menstrual cycles may be irregular; vaginal bleeding may range from absent to heavy.
   c. If the cyst ruptures, pain occurs suddenly as a result of intraabdominal bleeding, which may be only slight and of brief duration, or it may be life-threatening.
2. Findings.
   a. Palpation of the abdomen may reveal unilateral tenderness in patients with intact ovarian cysts. Rupture of the cyst will lead to significant abdominal tenderness, often diffuse and accompanied by peritoneal signs.
   b. Vaginal bleeding may be present or absent, with either an intact or a ruptured ovarian cyst.
   c. An adnexal mass may be palpated with either an intact or a ruptured cyst.
   d. If the cyst has ruptured, there may be signs of hypovolemia.
   e. Ultrasonography may reveal both the cyst and free blood in the cul-de-sac.
3. Treatment.
   a. If there is no acute bleeding, gynecologic consultation should be obtained to consider hormonal manipulation.
   b. If there is significant acute bleeding (vaginal or intraabdominal), immediate evaluation for possible surgery is indicated. Fluid resuscitation should be initiated as required (see Chapter 1).

E. Vaginitis.
1. Symptoms. Vaginal discharge, burning, itching, and sometimes dysuria.
2. Findings.
   a. A vaginal discharge is usually discovered on examination.
   b. Specimens should be obtained for microscopic evaluation. Saline and potassium hydroxide preparations will usually reveal the specific pathogen.
3. Treatment.
   a. Yeast *(C. albicans)*.
      (1) A variety of topical intravaginal preparations are available, some without prescription. Effective agents include miconazole, clotrimazole, butoconazole, terconazole, and tioconazole. Depending on the medication, 3 to 7 days of treatment is sufficient. Single-dose topical treatment is less effective.
      (2) An option to topical intravaginal medication is fluconazole, 150 mg PO in a single dose.
      (3) If there is skin involvement, clotrimazole or miconazole cream can also be applied twice a day.

    b. *Trichomonas.*
      (1) Metronidazole (Flagyl), 2 g in a single dose.
      (2) Teratogenesis has not been found in animal studies, but the manufacturer recommends withholding metronidazole therapy during the first trimester of pregnancy. Many gynecologists withhold it during the second and third trimesters as well. An alternative although less effective regimen is clotrimazole, 100 mg intravaginally at bedtime for 7 days.
      (3) The sexual partner should be treated also to prevent reinfection of the woman, which may occur even if the man is asymptomatic.
    c. Bacterial vaginosis.
      (1) This disorder is caused by the pleomorphic rod *G. vaginalis.*
      (2) Metronidazole gel, 0.75% intravaginally bid × 5 days, or clindamycin 2% cream, intravaginally qhs for 7 days, are both effective.
      (3) Alternative regimens are metronidazole, 500 mg PO bid × 7 days, or clindamycin, 300 mg PO bid × 7 days.
      (4) These drugs should be used with caution in pregnancy.

F. Herpes genitalis.
  1. Symptoms.
    a. Often a prodrome occurring several hours or days before the skin lesion, consisting of hyperesthesia, paresthesia, or itching, in the perineum, buttock, or leg.
    b. Local perineal pain and often dysuria and discharge.
    c. Fever, malaise, and, in severe cases, urinary retention may be present.
  2. Findings.
    a. Exquisitely tender vesicles and/or ulcers are found on the external genitalia. Pain may preclude pelvic examination.
    b. Inguinal lymphadenopathy, fever, and bacterial superinfection of viral lesions may be present.
    c. The acute infection will spontaneously resolve within 1 to 2 weeks, although recurrence is common.
  3. Treatment.
    a. Oral acyclovir (Zovirax), 400 mg tid × 10 days. This drug is moderately effective in shortening the course of initial episodes, and a 5-day course may be somewhat helpful for severe recurrent episodes if started early. IV acyclovir may be required for extremely severe cases.
    b. Local agents such as aluminum acetate (Burow's Solution, Domeboro) may be soothing.
    c. If the viral lesions become superinfected with bacteria, local and sometimes systemic antibiotic therapy will be required.

    d. Urinary retention may result from extreme dysuria or peri-urethral edema. Such patients will require the insertion of an indwelling bladder catheter.

    e. There is some evidence of an increased incidence of cervical carcinoma in women who have a history of herpes genitalis infections. Therefore patients should be encouraged to have periodic pelvic examinations and Papanicolaou smears.

    f. Active genital herpes at the time of vaginal delivery can be catastrophic for the neonate. Patients with a history of genital herpes should be instructed to inform their obstetrician so that serial examination and herpes cultures can be considered during the weeks before delivery. Active infection would indicate cesarean section.

G. Bartholin's abscess.

    1. Symptoms. Pain in the vulvar region.

    2. Findings. Tender, fluctuant mass at the introitus.

    3. Treatment.

        a. Incision and drainage through the mucosal surface of the labia minora.

        b. Irrigation and drain insertion.

        c. Antibiotics and culture if there is fever or adenopathy.

           (1) Doxycycline, 100 mg bid.

           (2) Culture for gonococcal, chlamydial, and gram-negative organisms.

H. Placenta previa. Low implantation of the placenta at or near the cervical os. This may become clinically apparent after the twentieth week, but particularly in the last trimester.

    1. Symptoms.

        a. Vaginal bleeding.

        b. No significant abdominal pain.

    2. Findings. *Caution:* Pelvic and rectal examinations are contraindicated in the ED. They should be performed only by an obstetrician in a delivery room prepared for immediate cesarean section. Accidental dislodging of a placenta previa by the examiner's finger or by a speculum may lead to a fatal hemorrhage.

        a. Bleeding from the vagina.

        b. No significant tenderness on palpation of the abdomen.

        c. Ultrasonography demonstrating a low-lying placenta.

    3. Treatment.

        a. Fatal hemorrhage can result. IV lines should be established, coagulation studies ordered, blood typed and cross-matched, and fluid resuscitation given as needed (see Chapter 1).

        b. Emergency cesarean section may be indicated if bleeding is significant. Obstetric consultation should be obtained.

I. Abruptio placentae. Premature separation in third trimester of a normally located placenta.
1. Symptoms.
   a. Severe abdominal pain.
   b. Vaginal bleeding may or may not be present.
2. Findings.
   a. Uterine rigidity and tenderness on palpation.
   b. Blood may or may not be present at the introitus.
   c. Ultrasonography may reveal the abruption.
3. Treatment.
   a. Preparation should be made for major fluid resuscitation if needed (see Chapter 1).
   b. Initial coagulation studies should be drawn because disseminated intravascular coagulation and amniotic fluid embolism can occur.
   c. Obstetric consultation should be obtained to determine the need for immediate vaginal delivery vs. cesarean section.

J. Eclampsia and preeclampsia.
1. Preeclampsia refers to the symptom complex during pregnancy that includes edema, proteinuria, and hypertension ($>140/>90$ or a rise of 30 mm Hg systolic or 15 diastolic over baseline values).
2. Eclampsia refers to the aforementioned pattern, with the addition of seizures. Hyperactive deep tendon reflexes may indicate an increased risk for seizures.
3. Treatment.
   a. Seizures.
      (1) The acute seizure may be treated with a benzodiazepine such as diazepam (Valium), 2 to 5 mg/min IV to maximum of 20 mg, or lorazepam (Ativan), 1 to 2 mg IV to a maximum of 10 mg.
      (2) Magnesium sulfate is effective for the treatment of acute eclamptic seizures and hypertension, as well as for prophylaxis after seizures.
         (a) A common regimen is 2 to 6 g IV over 5 to 20 minutes (no more than 2 g/5 min), followed by an IV infusion at 1 to 3 g/hr.
         (b) If respiratory suppression or cardiac dysrhythmias occur as a result of excessive magnesium administration, these can often be reversed with IV calcium: a 10% solution of calcium chloride (up to 10 ml) or a 10% solution of calcium gluconate (up to 20 ml). These volumes provide equivalent amounts of calcium ion.
   b. *Acute hypertension.* Diastolic pressure above 110 mm Hg should be treated with hydralazine, 5 to 20 mg IV push every 20 to 30 minutes, to maintain diasystolic BP at about 90 mm Hg. Sudden, severe drops in BP should be avoided.

21

Altered Level of Consciousness, Metabolic Encephalopathy, and Neurologic Emergencies

I. ALTERED LEVEL OF CONSCIOUSNESS AND META-BOLIC ENCEPHALOPATHIES.

A. General considerations.

1. Altered levels of consciousness may range from mild confusion and disorientation to profound coma.
2. Causes.
   a. Drug intoxication or withdrawal.
   b. Alcohol intoxication or withdrawal.
   c. Poisons.
   d. Diabetes: hypoglycemia and hyperglycemia.
   e. Hypoxia.
   f. Sepsis.
   g. CNS pathology.
      (1) Head trauma.
      (2) Stroke.
      (3) Infection: meningitis, encephalitis, or abscess.
      (4) Hypertensive encephalopathy.
      (5) Increased intracranial pressure of any cause.
   h. Metabolic encephalopathies.
      (1) Renal failure.
      (2) Hepatic failure.

(3) Adrenal insufficiency.

(4) Thyrotoxicosis and myxedema.

i. Factitious or hysterical coma.

B. Physical examination.

1. Secure the ABCs as indicated.

2. Perform a physical examination, and in the conscious patient, a mental status examination (see Chapter 29).

3. Serial examination is important. When indicated, the Glasgow Coma Scale or similar scale is useful for documentation of deteriorating or improving level of consciousness (Fig. 21-1).

4. Several specific findings on neurologic examination may provide a clue to the etiology.

   a. *Level of consciousness.* Deep coma is usually due to global impairment such as a metabolic disorder, drug overdose, or severe hypoxia. Less common causes are brain stem hemorrhage or infarction. Thalamic lesions often produce stupor. Deep coma is rarely caused by lesions of the cerebral cortex unless the lesion is bilateral or there is a major mass effect with increased intracranial pressure.

   b. *Pupils.* Metabolic factors or drug ingestion rarely abolish completely the pupillary response to light. An exception is overdose of an anticholinergic agent. Small reactive pupils occur with thalamic lesions. Midposition-fixed pupils indicate dysfunction in the midbrain or medulla. Fixed, pinpoint pupils suggest narcotic effect or a pontine lesion. A single dilated pupil indicates third nerve pressure that is usually due to uncal herniation on the same side or to ocular trauma.

   c. *Doll's eyes.* The normal response (i.e., the presence of doll's eyes) occurs when the head of the supine patient is turned to the side and both eyes remain with fixed gaze toward the ceiling (i.e., they do not turn with the head). Very limited or absent movement is reported as "doll's eyes absent" and indicates a lesion below the upper pons. This test cannot be performed if head or neck trauma is suspected until cervical injury is ruled out by clinical or radiologic evaluation.

   d. *Posturing, reflexes, and muscle tone.* Decorticate (flexor) positioning occurs with bilateral hemispheric insult above the midbrain, whereas decerebrate (extensor) positioning suggests midbrain or upper pontine dysfunction. Abnormal reflexes, especially Babinski's sign, reflect interference with the corticospinal tracts. Increased muscle tone is found with midbrain lesions, less so with pontine lesions, and tone is often flaccid with medullary lesions.

   e. *Respiration.* Deep, hyperpneic breathing suggests acidosis (e.g., ketoacidosis) or dysfunction of the midbrain or

Glasgow Coma Scale

Eyes	Open	Spontaneously	4
		To verbal command	3
		To pain	2
	No response		1
Best motor response	To verbal command	Obeys	6
	To painful stimulus*	Localizes pain	5
		Flexion — withdrawal	4
		Flexion — abnormal (decorticate rigidity)	3
		Extension (decerebrate rigidity)	2
		No response	1
Best verbal response**		Oriented and converses	5
		Disoriented and converses	4
		Inappropriate words	3
		Incomprehensible sounds	2
		No response	1
Total			3-15

The Glasgow Coma Scale, based upon eye opening, verbal, and motor reponses, is a practical means of monitoring changes in level of consciousness. If response on the scale is given a number, the responsiveness of the patient can be expressed by summation of the figures. *Lowest* score is 3; *highest* is 15.

*Apply knuckles to sternum; observe arms.
**Arouse patient with painful stimulus if necessary.

FIG. 21-1 Glasgow Coma Scale.

upper pons. Cheyne-Stokes respiration occurs with metabolic coma or bilateral hemispheric damage. Apneustic or ataxic breathing is caused by lesions of the pons and medulla.

C. Laboratory and radiologic investigations.

1. An approximate serum glucose level can rapidly be determined at the bedside in less than a minute. If hypoglycemia is present, immediately administer 50 ml (25 g) of 50% dextrose IV. If alcohol abuse is suspected, give thiamine, 100 mg IV before the dextrose to preclude precipitation of acute Wernicke's encephalopathy.

2. Other helpful studies may include CBC, electrolytes, creatinine, BUN, calcium, definitive glucose, osmolality, blood gases, carbon monoxide, and urinalysis.

3. If drug intoxication is suspected, toxicology studies of blood, urine, and gastric aspirate may be indicated (see Chapter 28).

4. CT scan of the head and cervical spine radiographs should be obtained when appropriate.

D. Treatment.

1. As discussed in Section I, C, 1, the ABCs are secured as required and hypoglycemia immediately corrected.

2. If narcotic overdose is suspected based on history or pinpoint pupils, administer naloxone (Narcan), 0.8 mg IV.

E. Specific causes of stupor and coma.

1. *Drug intoxication, withdrawal, and poisoning* (see Chapter 28).

2. *Alcohol.*

   a. Several types of acute alcoholic syndromes are seen in the ED.

      (1) *Acute alcoholic intoxication.* Decreased level of consciousness ranging from simple inebriation to coma with airway and ventilatory compromise.

      (2) *Acute withdrawal.* Agitation, tremulousness, and hyperreflexia, ranging from mild symptoms to delirium tremens. The rate of decline of blood alcohol level determines withdrawal symptoms; withdrawal can occur despite a significant blood alcohol level.

      (3) *Delirium tremens.* Severe symptoms of withdrawal, plus confusion, hallucinations (especially tactile), and risk of convulsion and death.

      (4) *Wernicke's encephalopathy.* Confusion, amnesia, confabulation, ataxia, nystagmus, ophthalmoplegia. The blood alcohol level may be low, but the patient has a history of significant malnutrition in addition to chronic alcoholism. There is some evidence that administration of IV dextrose without prior thiamine may precipitate an acute, and possibly permanent, encephalopathy.

b. Treatment.
   (1) All these patients should be evaluated for other causes of stupor and coma in addition to the effects of alcohol, especially for occult trauma.
   (2) A blood or breath alcohol level can be obtained. If the level is not consistent with the clinical state, other causes of altered mental status must be considered. If the alcohol level is sufficient to explain the degree of obtundation, other causes are still possible and must be investigated more thoroughly if the altered level of consciousness declines, or if it does not normalize over a time course consistent with alcohol clearance.
   (3) Intoxication is treated with IV hydration and airway protection as needed. IV thiamine and multivitamins are frequently administered because chronic alcoholics are often malnourished.
   (4) Withdrawal is treated with benzodiazepines: for mild symptoms, diazepam (Valium), 10 to 20 mg PO or chlordiazepoxide (Librium), 25 to 50 mg PO as needed; for significant withdrawal, diazepam, 10 mg IV as needed, with observation for excess sedation. Delirium tremens requires hospital admission for controlled withdrawal.
   (5) Wernicke's encephalopathy is treated with thiamine, 100 mg IV and hospital admission.

3. **Diabetic hypoglycemia.** — LOW BLOOD SUGAR
   a. Diagnosis.
      (1) Hypoglycemia occurs in a diabetic patient with inadequate glucose intake after insulin or oral hypoglycemic medication, or occasionally after excessive exercise.
      (2) It can occur in alcoholic patients without diabetes. In this setting, occult hypoglycemia may present as persistent seizures seemingly as a result of alcohol withdrawal.
      (3) Symptoms range from bizarre behavior or confusion to seizures or coma. Significant diaphoresis is common.
   b. Treatment.
      (1) A bedside test for semiquantitative blood sugar level should be performed immediately and a clot sent to the laboratory for precise glucose measurement.
      (2) The conscious patient able to drink may be given oral fruit juice with added sugar. Most patients, however, will require IV dextrose (D-glucose), 50 ml (25 g) of a 50% solution.
      (3) If IV access is not attainable, glucagon, 1 ml IM, may be effective.

High Blood Sugar

4. **Diabetic hyperglycemia.** (See Chapter 30 for discussion of ketoacidosis in children.)
    a. Diagnosis.
        (1) Diabetic hyperglycemia may occur with or without ketoacidosis. Both disorders can cause massive dehydration, and ketoacidosis is often associated with hyperkalemia despite total body potassium deficit.
        (2) Acute hyperglycemia may occur in a known diabetic patient or may be the presenting syndrome of new-onset diabetes. Nonketotic, hyperosmolar hyperglycemia is particularly common in adult patients with previously undiagnosed type II diabetes. Diabetic ketoacidosis (DKA) may occur at any age.
        (3) Findings may include dehydration, mental status alteration ranging from mild confusion to coma, vomiting, and sometimes abdominal pain. Ketoacidosis is accompanied by hyperventilation (Kussmaul's breathing) and the sweet odor of ketones on the breath.
        (4) Baseline laboratory studies should include urinalysis and a determination of the levels of serum glucose, ketones, osmolality, electrolytes, and in severe cases, ABGs.
    b. Treatment.
        (1) For unconscious patients, treatment should begin before definitive laboratory studies are available and should be based on the bedside serum glucose test result.
        (2) IV fluids.
            (a) One liter of normal saline is given over the first hour (2 liters if hypotensive) until serum electrolyte and BUN levels are available to guide further therapy.
            (b) Because water loss usually exceeds sodium loss, half-normal saline is used after several liters of normal saline.
            (c) Serum osmolality should be measured by the laboratory but may be estimated by using the following formula:

$$2(Na + K) + \frac{blood\ sugar}{18} = serum\ osmolality$$

            (d) Hyperosmolar, nonketotic patients may require large amounts of IV fluid to restore homeostasis. Careful monitoring of fluid balance is essential.
        (3) Insulin.
            (a) A standard regimen consists of an initial bolus of regular insulin, 0.1 U/kg, followed by a continuous IV infusion of 0.1 U/kg/hr.

(b) As the serum glucose level falls below 300 mg/dl, a solution containing 5% dextrose should be administered and the insulin tapered off to prevent the development of iatrogenic hypoglycemia. The goal is to reduce serum glucose by 75 to 100 mg/dl/hr because more rapid reduction can result in cerebral edema.

(c) Nonketotic, hyperosmolar patients are often very sensitive to insulin. Their serum glucose may fall precipitously. Insulin should thus be given carefully, and a smaller amount is usually required compared with that needed for DKA patients. In many such patients, hyperglycemia may be corrected primarily by significant IV fluid hydration, with relatively small amounts of insulin.

(4) Potassium.

(a) Hyperkalemia is usually present if the patient is acidotic because the cells buffer serum hydrogen ion by exchanging it for intracellular potassium. However, potassium is excessively lost in the urine, leading to total body deficit despite hyperkalemia. As acidosis is corrected, the initial hyperkalemia converts to hypokalemia.

(b) Potassium replacement in DKA should begin as the serum potassium falls into the normal range below 5.5 mEq/L. The rate of potassium administration is determined by the frequently measured serum level and is generally 10 to 15 mEq IV/hr. The rate should be somewhat faster if hypokalemia is present, and the potassium should be administered more slowly and very carefully if an elevated serum creatinine reflects renal failure.

(5) Bicarbonate.

(a) Mortality in DKA is more closely associated with the serum pH than the glucose level.

(b) However, administration of sodium bicarbonate is controversial. Particularly in children, its use has been associated with hypokalemia, hypomagnesemia, cerebrospinal fluid (CSF) acidosis, and most important, cerebral edema.

(c) If used, sodium bicarbonate should be reserved for patients with profound acidosis (pH 7.1 or less). Sodium bicarbonate, 2 mEq/kg, can be administered slowly over 1 to 2 hours. Bicarbonate should not be given for more moderate acidosis because treatment with fluids and insulin will result in a return to normal pH.

5. **Hypoxia.** Confusion, obtundation, or coma may be caused by inadequate cerebral oxygenation (see Chapters 3 and 17).
6. **Sepsis.** Overwhelming infection can lead to confusion, obtundation, or coma. This is particularly common in older people with pneumonia (see Chapter 17) or urosepsis (see Chapter 19), and in anyone with CNS infection (as discussed in Section VII).
7. **CNS pathology.**
   a. **Increased intracranial pressure (ICP).** Any disorder leading to elevated ICP can present with altered consciousness. Causes include CNS tumor, hematoma, edema, and infection.
   b. **Head trauma** (see Chapter 7).
   c. **Hypertensive encephalopathy.**
      (1) Diagnosis.
         (a) Sudden severe elevation of blood pressure with development of confusion, which may progress to obtundation and coma. Seizures may occur.
         (b) Underlying disorders may include preexisting hypertension, acute glomerulonephritis, preeclampsia, or rarely pheochromocytoma.
         (c) Clinical findings may include papilledema and focal neurologic signs.
      (2) Treatment.
         (a) Obvious CNS signs indicate the need for rapid evaluation and initiation of therapy. Appropriate studies should be ordered and the blood pressure lowered pharmacologically.
         (b) Nitroprusside (Nipride) is suitable for virtually all hypertensive emergencies. Administration requires constant nursing surveillance and usually an arterial line to monitor its immediate and often profound effect. The dose is 50 mg in 500 ml of D_5W, with the bottle covered with aluminum foil to limit the drug's exposure to light. The infusion rate should start at 0.5 µg/kg/min and be increased based on the response. The average required rate is 3 µg/kg/min. The goal is to reduce pressure by about 30% to 40%.
         (c) Labetalol (Normodyne) is an alternative, 20 mg IV over 2 minutes. Additional doses of 20 to 80 mg may be given q10min as needed to a maximum of 300 mg. Labetalol can be given by continuous infusion rather than bolus, 2 mg/min initially, with adjustment to achieve desired effect. Labetalol has both α- and β-adrenergic blocking properties and should not be used in a patient with CHF, heart block, or bronchospastic disease.

        (d) BP is often elevated in acute stroke and should not necessarily be lowered (see Section VI). Hypertensive encephalopathy therefore must be distinguished from stroke.

  d. **Stroke** (see Section VI).

  e. **CNS infection** (see Section VII).

8. Renal failure.

  a. Diagnosis.

    (1) Gradual onset of coma, usually with a prior history of renal disease.

    (2) Elevated BUN and creatinine levels.

  b. Treatment.

    (1) Hyperkalemia is the immediate concern. Evaluate the T waves of the ECG and measure the serum potassium level. If hyperkalemia is present, treat as described in Chapter 2.

    (2) Arrange for dialysis.

9. Hepatic failure (hepatic encephalopathy).

  a. Diagnosis.

    (1) Progressive deterioration of mental state and history of liver disease.

    (2) Signs of liver failure may include jaundice, ascites, asterixis, fetor hepaticus, and spider nevi.

    (3) The most common precipitating factor is increased nitrogen load from GI bleeding or excess dietary protein. Other precipitants include drugs, fluid and electrolyte disturbance, and infection.

    (4) Liver enzymes are abnormal. Ammonia level is elevated.

  b. Treatment.

    (1) The precipitating cause must be eliminated.

    (2) Protein absorption from the gut can be reduced by administering the osmotic laxative lactulose, 30 ml PO, or via nasogastric (NG) tube to start, and by sterilizing the gut with oral or NG neomycin, 1 g q6h.

    (3) Avoid medications metabolized in the liver if possible.

10. Endocrine conditions.

  a. **Adrenal (addisonian) crisis.**

    (1) Diagnosis.

      (a) Usually occurs in the steroid-dependent patient with infection or major stress, or who has stopped taking steroid medication.

      (b) Can occur in patients with carcinoma or tuberculosis spreading to the adrenal gland.

      (c) Has presenting symptoms of hypotension, confusion, and sometimes a cushingoid appearance.

      (d) Hyponatremia, hyperkalemia, and acidosis may be present.

(2) Treatment.
    (a) Rapid-volume replacement using normal saline.
    (b) Rapid corticosteroid replacement using IV hydrocortisone, 100 mg immediately and q4-6h.

b. **Hypothyroid crisis (myxedema coma).**
  (1) Diagnosis.
    (a) Obtundation can be precipitated by drug ingestion, infection, cold, or trauma.
    (b) Coma may be preceded by the insidious onset of clinical signs and symptoms of myxedema, sometimes in a patient with previous hyperthyroidism treated by pharmacologic thyroid ablation or surgery.
    (c) Examination reveals hypothermia; hypoventilation; bradycardia; and perhaps pericardial and pleural effusion, ascites, and myxedema of the face and skin.
  (2) Treatment.
    (a) Adequate ventilation and careful IV fluid administration.
    (b) Treatment of hypothermia. Passive rewarming is usually sufficient (see Chapter 27).
    (c) L-thyroxine, 0.3 to 0.5 mg IV.
    (d) Hydrocortisone, 100 mg IV to prevent acute adrenal insufficiency sometimes precipitated by thyroxine administration.

c. **Hyperthyroid crisis (thyroid storm).**
  (1) Diagnosis.
    (a) Thyroid storm often occurs in patients with known hyperthyroidism at the beginning of treatment. It can also be precipitated by infection, metabolic disorders, severe illness, or abrupt withdrawal from drugs.
    (b) Signs and symptoms of hyperthyroidism are present and exaggerated. Findings include fever and tachycardia, and often atrial dysrhythmias, vomiting, and dehydration.
    (c) Severe cases may cause high-output heart failure, coma, and death.
  (2) Treatment.
    (a) Treat hypotension with fluids and vasopressors as needed (see Chapters 1 and 2).
    (b) Treat significant fever with acetaminophen, 1 g PO.
    (c) Block peripheral β-adrenergic effects of thyroid hormone with propranolol, 1 mg q5min IV, as needed.
    (d) Draw blood for thyroid studies and then block thyroid hormone production with propylthiouracil, 300 to 400 mg PO or NG q6h.

(e) Block release of thyroid hormone by giving potassium iodide PO or NG (5 drops, 40 mg/drop) or sodium iodide IV (1 to 2 g). Wait 1 to 2 hours after propylthiouracil administration before starting iodide to prevent organification of the iodide.

(f) Stop peripheral conversion of T_4 to T_3 with dexamethasone, 2 mg IV q6h.

(g) Treat the underlying precipitating cause.

II. SYNCOPE.

A. Definition. A sudden, transient loss of consciousness, with or without prodromal symptoms, followed within seconds to minutes by regaining of consciousness to the level of preevent mental status. Confusion may persist for a short time, especially if the causative factor is still present.

B. Evaluation.

1. Take an accurate history of events or symptoms preceding the syncope.

2. Focus the physical examination on the cardiovascular and neurologic systems and exclude inapparent hemorrhage (GI, vaginal, intraperitoneal).

3. The BP and pulse should be measured with the patient supine. If they are not significantly abnormal, orthostatic vital signs can be obtained.

4. A CBC and ECG are usually part of the workup unless a psychogenic vasovagal event is obvious. Additional tests are obtained as indicated.

5. The cause is often not found in the ED, and close follow-up is essential. Admission to the hospital may be necessary for patients in whom life-threatening cardiac or vascular causes are likely.

C. Etiology.

1. Neurologic. Seizure, transient ischemic attack, and stroke can all cause syncope.

2. Cardiac.

  a. Dysrhythmias.

    (1) Significant tachycardia and bradycardia can cause syncope by decreasing cerebral perfusion. A prodrome of light-headedness may precede actual syncope.

    (2) Sudden onset of syncope without prodrome, however, strongly suggests sudden ventricular tachycardia or fibrillation.

  b. Valvular.

    (1) Aortic and mitral valve diseases are common causes of syncope.

    (2) Atrial myxomas and left atrial thrombi can cause syncope through the ball-valve effect or embolization.

(3) Congenital heart disease may cause syncope in children as a result of valve or shunt abnormalities.

(4) Asymmetric hypertrophic cardiomyopathy with subaortic stenosis is an increasingly recognized cause of often fatal syncope precipitated by exercise in young people.

3. Vascular (neurovascular).

a. *Vasovagal syncope.* This is the most common type of syncope and is caused by anxiety. Psychogenic vasovagal syncope is usually preceded by dizziness, tachycardia, and sometimes hyperventilation.

b. *Vasodepressor syndrome.* Essentially a severe form of vasovagal syncope, this condition is generally not caused by anxiety. Patients are susceptible to excessive vagal tone resulting in profound bradycardia and/or vasodilation. There may be a prodrome of dizziness and nausea, or syncope may occur suddenly without much warning. Prophylactic β-blockade or permanent-demand pacemakers are frequently used to prevent acute episodes.

c. *Loss of compensatory venoconstriction.* Certain drugs and several conditions block compensatory venoconstriction when the upright position is assumed. These include antihypertensive drugs, Parkinson's disease, diabetic and alcoholic neuropathies, syphilis, Guillain-Barré and Shy-Drager syndromes, and syringomyelia.

d. *Carotid sinus syndrome.* An abnormally sensitive carotid sinus responds to head and neck movement, coughing, or sneezing, leading to bradycardia and syncope. Some drugs (digitalis and propranolol) may act directly on the sinus.

e. *Micturition syncope.* Syncope occurs during micturition and defecation, when excessive vagal stimulation produces bradycardia and consequent decreased cerebral perfusion.

4. Miscellaneous.

a. *Dehydration.*

b. *Anemia.*

c. *Endocrine:* Hypothyroidism, Addison's disease, pheochromocytoma, and hypoglycemia.

III. DIZZINESS AND VERTIGO.

A. Definition. The term *dizziness* is very nonspecific and is used by different people to describe different symptoms. There are several specific forms.

1. Vertigo.
A feeling of motion, that the person or the surroundings are rotating. This is usually due to a "peripheral" disorder involving the eighth cranial nerve or the inner ear. "Central" vertigo is caused by brain dysfunction, typically

in the portion supplied by the vertebrobasilar arterial system such as the cerebellum and brain stem.

2. *Faintness.* A feeling of weakness and impending loss of consciousness that often precedes syncope.

3. *Dysequilibrium.* A loss of balancing without frank dizziness.

B. Etiology.

1. *Dizziness.* The list of disorders associated with dizziness is endless and includes any cause of weakness, infection, hypotension, dysrhythmia, dehydration, or anxiety.

2. *Peripheral vertigo.* Most patients with vertigo have vestibular/labyrinthine dysfunction. Symptoms are often severe, with nausea and vomiting, and may be intermittent and recurrent. There are several types of peripheral vertigo, but these may be difficult to distinguish in the ED:

   a. *Benign positional vertigo.* Precipitated by rapid head movement; each episode resolves in several minutes. It usually occurs in young people and is often associated with an upper respiratory tract infection.

   b. *Labyrinthitis.* Beginning with the sudden onset of vertigo, often with hearing loss and tinnitus, labyrinthitis does not resolve in minutes but may continue for hours or days. It is often associated with inflammation or infection of the ear or head.

   c. *Vestibular neuronitis.* Occurs in the younger and middle-age groups with sudden severe attacks of vertigo, nausea, and vomiting. Symptoms increase over several hours and then diminish spontaneously over several days, with mild symptoms often persisting for weeks or even months. It is often associated with a recent viral infection.

   d. *Ménière's disease.* Usually occurs in the middle-aged and has presenting symptoms of tinnitus, hearing loss, and vertigo, with pallor, nausea, and vomiting. Attacks last several hours and usually terminate abruptly. They may occur in clusters, with periodic recurrences over many years.

   e. *Other causes.* Drugs, allergy, and infections.

3. *Central vertigo.* The dizziness of central vertigo is less rotational than that of peripheral vertigo, and it may not be intermittent. Nausea and vomiting are often absent.

   a. *Vertebrobasilar artery insufficiency.* Atherosclerotic disease impairs cerebral blood flow to the vestibular centers of the brain stem. Symptoms may be intermittent if caused by transient ischemic attacks. Usually, but not always, vertebrobasilar insufficiency is accompanied by other neurologic symptoms such as ataxia and sensory and motor impairment. It should be suspected in the elderly patient with vertigo.

b. *Cerebellar infarction and hemorrhage.* These serious conditions are characterized by cerebellar findings on examination. Hemorrhage is a neurosurgical emergency; operative decompression may be life-saving. Symptoms begin suddenly and include headache, vertigo, ataxia, and vomiting.

c. *Posterior fossa tumors.* The most common are acoustic neuromas. The symptoms are initially peripheral involving the eighth cranial nerve, typically vertigo, unilateral sensorineural hearing loss, and tinnitus. The tumor may eventually extend centrally to cause signs and symptoms referable to the cerebellopontine angle, such as depressed corneal reflexes and brain stem dysfunction.

d. *Posttraumatic dizziness.* This is very common after head injury and is often associated with headaches.

C. Evaluation.

1. The goal is to distinguish dizziness from vertigo, and in the case of vertigo, peripheral from central etiology.

2. History and physical examination are important, particularly of the neurologic and ophthalmologic systems.

3. Nonneurologic sources of dizziness should be considered, such as inapparent bleeding and anemia.

4. Factors suggesting peripheral vertigo include sudden onset, severe symptoms lasting hours, symptom-free intervals between episodes, unidirectional horizontal nystagmus (never vertical), absence of other neurologic findings, auditory symptoms, and relationship to head movement or position.

5. Factors suggesting central vertigo include a more gradual onset and milder but continuous symptoms, multidirectional nystagmus, presence of other neurologic findings (especially cerebellar), absence of auditory symptoms, and less association with head movement or position.

6. Physical examination may include provocative tests to elicit the symptoms. A positive test suggests peripheral etiology. An example is the Nylen-Barany test:

a. The patient is abruptly brought from a sitting to a lying position, with the head extended to 30 to 45 degrees, held over the edge of the table, and turned to one side.

b. The patient is observed for nystagmus and vertigo.

c. The maneuver is then repeated, with the head turned to the opposite side.

7. Cerebellar examination is important (e.g., finger-to-nose, heel-to-shin, rapid alternating movements, and gait testing if the patient is not too sick to walk). Positive findings point strongly toward central cerebellar dysfunction.

D. Treatment.

1. Symptomatic treatment is often helpful, and most of these diseases are peripheral, self-limiting, and benign. However, additional evaluation is indicated for those patients with

unexplained neurologic findings or in whom a more serious cause is suspected.

2. CT scanning can be helpful, but the posterior fossa is often not well visualized by this technique. MRI and magnetic resonance angiography (MRA) are useful for visualizing the portions of the brain perfused by the posterior vertebrobasilar circulation.

3. Cerebellar hemorrhage may require emergency surgery for decompression. Cerebellar infarction may lead to fatal edema. Both warrant expeditious neurologic or neurosurgical consultation.

4. Peripheral vertigo can be treated symptomatically.
   a. Diazepam (Valium), 2 to 10 mg IV, is very effective.
   b. Antihistamines and phenothiazines with anticholinergic activity are also quite useful.
      (1) Promethazine (Phenergan), 12.5 to 25 mg IV, or 25 to 50 mg PO, IM, or PR, q4-6h.
      (2) Prochlorperazine (Compazine), 5 to 10 mg PO, IM, or IV, q4-6h.
      (3) Meclizine (Antivert), 25 to 50 mg PO q6h to a total of 100 mg/day.
      (4) Diphenhydramine (Benadryl), 50 mg PO q4h.

IV. SEIZURES.
(For seizures in children, see Chapter 30.)
A. General considerations.
1. Seizures may be major motor with tonic-clonic movement, partial with focal motor movement, or nonconvulsive (e.g., petit mal, psychomotor).
2. Patients may present to the ED still seizing in status epilepticus, in a postictal state with altered level of consciousness, or fully recovered.
3. There may be a history of seizure disorder, or this may be a first-time event.

B. Etiology.
1. The differential diagnosis of seizures is quite long. Among ED patients, common causes include the following:
   a. Idiopathic chronic seizure disorder (epilepsy).
   b. Subtherapeutic anticonvulsant medication level, usually from noncompliance with medication regimens.
   c. Alcohol withdrawal.
   d. Hypoglycemic insulin reaction.
   e. Brain trauma.
   f. Hypoxia.
2. More rare causes in the ED include the following:
   a. Alcoholic hypoglycemia.
   b. Meningitis.
   c. Brain tumor.
   d. Metabolic abnormalities such as hyponatremia.

C. Initial evaluation.

1. Ensure the ABCs.
2. Rapidly perform a bedside serum glucose determination and correct hypoglycemia with 50 ml (25 g) IV of 50% dextrose.
3. If the patient has a known seizure disorder and is supposed to be taking anticonvulsant medication, obtain serum levels of those drugs.
4. If there is no prior history of seizure, obtain definitive levels of glucose, electrolytes including calcium and magnesium, and other studies as indicated.

D. Treatment.

1. Active seizing usually stops spontaneously after several minutes. If not, a number of drugs are effective. With any of the IV regimens, however, the patient must be closely watched for possible hypotension, and with the sedative drugs, for respiratory suppression as well.
2. Benzodiazepines are quite effective in stopping seizures. Diazepam acts somewhat more quickly, but lorazepam (Ativan) lasts longer.
   a. Lorazepam, 0.1 mg/kg IV, at a rate of 1 to 2 mg/min to a maximum of 10 mg.
   b. Diazepam, 5 mg IV to start, then titrated slowly to a maximum of 20 mg IV.
3. Phenobarbital may be effective if benzodiazepines are not. A typical regimen is 10 mg/kg IV at 50 mg/min.
4. If the patient will be placed on a phenytoin class drug, a loading dose can be given IV if necessary, or PO in the conscious patient.
   a. The oral route is safest, phenytoin (Dilantin), 15 to 18 mg/kg PO. Although it is generally recommended to divide this into two or three doses over several hours, 1 g is frequently given in a single dose.
   b. The loading dose of IV phenytoin is 18 mg/kg infused at a maximum rate of 50 mg/kg. Fosphenytoin (Cerebyx) can be infused more rapidly than phenytoin, is better tolerated at the IV site, and can be given IM. The loading dose of fosphenytoin is 15 to 20 mg of "phenytoin equivalent" (PE) per kilogram, infused at a rate of 100 to 150 mg PE/min. Because both drugs can cause hypotension and cardiac dysrhythmias, monitoring of cardiac rhythm and blood pressure are necessary.

E. Additional evaluation and treatment.

1. After the acute seizure is stopped, additional evaluation should be considered if there is no prior seizure history.
2. Workup of initial seizure includes metabolic studies mentioned previously, plus CT scan evaluation for blood, tumor, or other structural abnormalities.

3. Lumbar puncture should be considered if meningitis is a possibility, or if the patient does not return to baseline neurologic function and a cause is not apparent.
4. Unstable patients should be admitted to the hospital.
5. The stable patient can often be discharged to the care of responsible friends or family, with arrangements made for further neurologic evaluation.
   a. Generally the patient is placed on phenytoin maintenance, beginning with 300 mg/day in a single dose or divided doses.
   b. The patient should be instructed not to drive motor vehicles. Many states have laws requiring mandatory reporting of seizure disorders.

V. HEADACHE.
A. Etiology.
   1. *Tension headache.* The most common form of headache, tension usually causes a bandlike bilateral frontal or temporal pain or occipital pain, often with neck ache.
   2. *Vascular headache.*
      a. *Common migraine.* 80% of migraine headaches. This form has a nonspecific prodrome with typical migraine symptoms (sometimes bilateral) severe pain, with nausea, vomiting, and photophobia.
      b. *Classic migraine.* 20% of migraine headaches. Pain is preceded by up to an hour of prodrome consisting of visual symptoms such as scintillating scotomata or visual impairment, followed by typical migraine symptoms.
      c. *Cluster headache.* Extremely severe, unilateral retrobulbar pain lasting several minutes to 2 hours, accompanied by nasal congestion and tearing, occurring in clusters each day over several weeks to months.
   3. *Warning leak of a subarachnoid hemorrhage (SAH).* A "sentinel bleed" may precede a major hemorrhagic stroke by several hours, days, or weeks. Diagnosing this warning leak is crucial to prevent the full stroke.
   4. *Stroke.* Ischemic stroke may cause headache, but sudden onset of severe pain is typical with hemorrhagic stroke, either intracerebral or subarachnoid (see Section VI).
   5. Other causes of headache include meningitis, tumor, temporal arteritis, hypertension, and carbon monoxide poisoning.
B. Evaluation.
   1. The most crucial goal is to rule out potentially critical causes. A careful history is important, as is a neurologic examination.
   2. SAH, including sentinel bleed, begins suddenly and maximizes in intensity within 1 to 2 minutes. It is often described as the worst headache of one's life. It may or may not be accompanied by neck pain or meningismus.

a. CT scanning detects significant subarachnoid blood, including 90% to 98% of sentinel bleeds.
b. Lumbar puncture (LP) is more sensitive, detecting blood in virtually all sentinel bleeds.
c. If the history is suggestive of a warning leak, strong consideration should be given to LP if the CT is negative. If the history is significantly suspicious, LP is mandatory.

3. Meningitis causes neck pain increased by flexion, usually with resistance to passive flexion by the examiner (meningismus). LP should be performed if meningitis is suspected.

C. Treatment.

1. Prochlorperazine (Compazine), 5 to 10 mg IV, is quite effective in abolishing both the nausea and pain of many types of headache.
2. Metoclopramide (Reglan), 10 to 20 mg IV, may also be effective.
3. Sumatriptan (Imitrex), 6 mg SC, may abort migraine. This drug should not be used in patients at risk for vasoconstriction (coronary artery disease, hypertension, peripheral neurologic symptoms, etc.).
4. Dihydroergotamine (DHE-45), up to 2 mg (2 ml) IV, may also abort migraine. This drug should not be used in patients at risk for vasoconstriction (coronary artery disease, hypertension, peripheral neurologic symptoms, etc.).
5. Narcotic analgesics and antiemetics may be necessary.

VI. TRANSIENT ISCHEMIC ATTACK AND STROKE.
A. Definition.

1. There are two general types of nontraumatic stroke or cerebral vascular accident (CVA): ischemic and hemorrhagic.
2. **Ischemic stroke** accounts for about 80% to 85% of CVAs.
   a. Nonhemorrhagic stroke may be embolic, thrombotic, or stenotic in origin and may involve large vessels or small vessels in either the extracranial or intracranial circulation.
   b. Atheromatous lesions may thrombose, embolize, or merely impede circulation sufficiently to cause cerebral necrosis.
   c. Common extracranial arterial sites of atheroma are the carotid and vertebrobasilar systems.
   d. Another common source of embolization is the heart, either a fibrillating left atrium, an endocarditic valvular lesion, or a postinfarction left ventricular mural thrombus.
3. **Hemorrhagic stroke** accounts for about 15% to 20% of nontraumatic CVAs.
   a. There are two types of hemorrhagic strokes: intracerebral hemorrhage (ICH), which results from hypertensive disease, and SAH, which results from intracranial (but extracerebral) aneurysm or less commonly arteriovenous malformation (AVM).

  b. ICH and SAH are to be differentiated from traumatic hemorrhage, which is usually more superficial, either epidural or subdural (see Chapter 7).
  4. **Transient ischemic attack** (TIA) is an acute ischemic event that resolves completely and quickly, by definition within 24 hours, but usually within 1 to 2 hours. It is a harbinger of ischemic stroke. The relationship between TIA and ischemic CVA is somewhat analogous to that between angina and MI.

B. Evaluation.

  1. History and neurologic examination are important.
     a. Ischemic stroke causes lateralized neurologic deficits but rarely loss of consciousness unless the brain stem is involved. Headache and nausea are usually relatively mild or absent.
     b. Intracranial hemorrhage typically occurs very suddenly with severe headache and often vomiting. Neurologic function deteriorates quickly, and obtundation and coma are not uncommon. Lateralized deficits are present (if not obscured by deep coma).
     c. Subarachnoid hemorrhage also occurs very suddenly, with severe headache and often vomiting. However, lateralized deficits are not found, with the possible exception of cranial nerve dysfunction. Meningismus is usually, but not always, present.

       A young person with stroke, or the sudden onset of the worst headache of one's life, is strongly suspicious for SAH because ICH and ischemic stroke are usually the results of long-standing hypertensive and atheromatous disease in the elderly.
     d. Posterior circulation (vertebrobasilar) strokes, whether ischemic or hemorrhagic, may cause cerebellar findings such as ataxia and vertigo.
     e. Differential diagnosis.
       (1) Bell's palsy causes unilateral paresis of the seventh cranial nerve without other neurologic findings (although fifth nerve sensory symptoms may occur).
         (a) Unlike the muscles of the lower face, those of the forehead are innervated by seventh nerve fibers from both sides, which join in the ganglion to form the peripheral nerve. Because Bell's palsy is a lower motor neuron disorder, the patient is unable to wrinkle the forehead.
         (b) In contrast, stroke affecting the seventh cranial nerve involves the upper motor neuron, but innervation to the forehead is overlapping and thus preserved by fibers from the other side. The forehead can thus be wrinkled in the stroke patient with a facial droop but not in the patient with Bell's palsy.

    (2) Migraine syndrome can sometimes cause hemipare-
    sis, even without headache. A prior history is helpful
    in differentiating this from stroke, as is the presence
    of a visual aura if that occurred.

 2. Noncontrast CT is the most important study. (Contrast
  may obscure blood.) Its purpose is to rule out acute hemorrhage.

  a. Ischemic stroke generally is not detectable by CT during the first 24 to 48 hours. The CT ordered from the
   ED is thus negative for acute pathology in ischemic
   stroke.

  b. Acute hemorrhage greater than 1 cm in diameter is reli-
   ably detected by CT. However, smaller subarachnoid
   bleeds may be missed (approximately 5% of sentinel
   bleeds). See Section V, B for discussion of CT vs. LP in
   the diagnosis of SAH.

 3. The carotid arteries can be evaluated noninvasively with
  color Doppler ultrasonography. The study should be
  obtained on an emergent or semiemergent basis in the patient with anterior circulation TIA because expeditious
  carotid endarterectomy may be effective in preventing
  stroke.

 4. CT is less sensitive than MRI for evaluation of the posterior
  fossa. MRA may provide even better evaluation of the posterior circulation. However, MR may not be available on a
  stat. basis in many hospitals.

 5. Other modalities include angiography and transcranial
  Doppler ultrasonography, but these are generally not ordered during the ED phase of care.

C. Treatment.

 1. The ABCs must be secured.

 2. Patients with stroke often present with elevated BP. This
  should not be lowered in most patients because increased
  perfusion pressure is believed to be a beneficial compensatory mechanism in stroke. Sustained hypertension (>220
  mm Hg systolic or >120 mm Hg diastolic) may be gradually lowered with nitroprusside or labetalol.

 3. TIA is often treated with aspirin or ticlopidine to try to prevent further clotting. As discussed previously, consideration
  should be given to carotid studies to evaluate the utility of
  expeditious endarterectomy to prevent stroke.

 4. Ischemic stroke has recently been shown to be responsive
  to thrombolytic therapy in a subset of patients.

  a. Current indications for t-PA (Activase) are an ischemic
   stroke less than 3 hours from the onset of symptoms, of
   moderate intensity and not improving, with no hemorrhage or major signs of early infarct on CT, and with
   blood pressure less than 185 mm Hg systolic and less
   than 110 mm Hg diastolic without aggressive treatment.

      b. However, thrombolytic therapy of ischemic stroke is a rapidly evolving area of research, and the physician should be familiar with the latest indications and contraindications before using a thrombolytic drug.

      c. The dose of t-PA is 0.9 mg/kg, not to exceed 90 kg, 10% of the total dose given over 1 minute, the remainder over 60 minutes.

      d. At this time, aspirin and heparin are not used concurrently with t-PA for stroke (as opposed to thrombolytic therapy of MI; see Chapter 15).

  5. Heparinization is used in some patients with ischemic stroke, especially that caused by carotid artery dissection. Neurologic consultation should be obtained before anticoagulation.

  6. Hemorrhagic stroke may be amenable to emergency surgery, but often it is not. An exception is cerebellar hemorrhage (and some cases of cerebral infarction with significant edema), for which surgical decompression may be life-saving.

  7. Prophylactic surgery or endovascular occlusion to prevent further bleeding from an aneurysm or AVM should strongly be considered in patients with SAH.

  8. The major determinant of neurologic impairment in SAH may be delayed vasospasm rather than the bleeding itself. This secondary ischemia occurs several days to weeks after the hemorrhage. Prophylactic calcium blockade with nimodipine, 60 mg PO q6h can be effective. This is generally not started in the ED.

  9. Increased ICP from cerebral edema after stroke may occur but not usually during the ED phase of care. Treatment involves hyperventilation and osmotic agents.

VII. MENINGITIS.

(See Chapter 30 for discussion of meningitis in children.)

A. General considerations.

  1. Meningitis may be viral, bacterial, fungal, or protozoal.

  2. Fulminant meningitis may cause rapid deterioration. If strongly suspected, antibiotics can be started before CT or LP.

  3. Common bacterial pathogens in older children and adults include *Neisseria meningidites* and *Streptococcus pneumoniae.* In older patients and alcoholics, *Haemophilus influenzae* and *Enterobacter* can also be found.

  4. Meningococcemia causes a petechial rash and may occur without meningitis.

B. Evaluation.

  1. Symptoms typically include headache and stiff neck. Fever, altered mental status, seizures, and focal neurologic deficits can occur, particularly with bacterial meningitis.

   2. Examination usually reveals meningismus.
   3. LP should be performed. The CSF contains WBCs, lymphocytes with viral mengingitis, and polymorphonuclear cells with bacterial (or early viral) meningitis.
   4. Other CSF findings suggestive of bacterial meningitis include turbidity, organisms on Gram's stain, CSF glucose less than 70% of the serum level, and elevated protein.
   5. CT should be performed before LP if there is any question of increased ICP, as might occur with an abscess.

C. Treatment.
   1. Antibiotic therapy should be started before CT, and even before LP if that will be delayed, in the critically ill patient strongly suspected of having bacterial meningitis.
   2. Empiric therapy of suspected or proven bacterial meningitis should be started in the ED. Several IV regimens are commonly used in adults and older children.
      a. Penicillin, 5 million units, or ampicillin, 2 g.
      b. Ceftriaxone, 2 g, or cefotaxime, 2 g.
      c. Combination of both penicillin or ampicillin plus ceftriaxone or cefotaxime.
      d. In penicillin-allergic patients, chloramphenicol can be substituted.
      e. In geographic regions with significant pneumococcal resistance to penicillin, vancomycin can be added to the cephalosporin instead of a penicillin.
   3. Continuing therapy should be determined by CSF C&S results.
   4. Antibiotic prophylaxis of contacts.
      a. Prophylaxis is generally unnecessary for ED staff unless there has been close contact, such as mouth-to-mouth resuscitation or perhaps endotracheal intubation.
      b. Prophylaxis of household or other close contacts is recommended.
         (1) For meningococcus: rifampin, 600 mg PO bid, for 4 doses (5 mg/kg/dose in children).
         (2) For *Haemophilus:* rifampin, 600 mg PO, in a single dose qd for 4 doses (20 mg/kg/dose in children).

22

Head and Neck Emergencies

I. ACUTE AIRWAY OBSTRUCTION.

A. Obstruction caused by a foreign body. If the patient cannot talk or is cyanotic, in respiratory distress, or obviously not ventilating, the following measures can be taken.

1. Foreign bodies in the airway can sometimes be dislodged by forceful percussion over the upper part of the back.

2. An abdominal thrust (Heimlich maneuver) may also be successful. The examiner's hands are interlocked and placed over the epigastrium of the supine patient. Forceful pressure is then applied. A patient who is seated or standing may be grasped from behind. Back blows and abdominal thrusts are most applicable in the nonmedical setting when no equipment is available.

3. The patient's pharynx may be swept with the examiner's fingers, with a bite block (or in the nonmedical setting, an improvised object such as a wallet) first placed between the teeth to prevent biting.

4. If the equipment is available, direct laryngoscopy may be used.

5. If the patient cannot be ventilated around the foreign object, intubation should be attempted.

6. If the rapid use of some or all of the aforementioned measures is unsuccessful, an emergency cricothyrotomy should be performed (see Chapter 4).

B. Obstruction caused by laryngospasm. Laryngospasm may occlude the airway and require cricothyrotomy. If time permits, however, intubation may be possible, with care taken not to traumatize the vocal cords. Sometimes anesthetic spray (e.g., benzocaine [Cetacaine]) directed at the cords may break the laryngospasm and allow intubation. Lidocaine, 75 to 100 mg IV, may also be successful.

II. FOREIGN BODY IN AIRWAY OR ESOPHAGUS.

A. A patent airway must be ensured as the initial step (see Section I).

B. Etiology.

1. Certain foreign bodies are common in particular age-groups: safety pins, coins, grapes, and peanuts in children; and dentures, food, and bones in adults.

2. Fish bones are most often found in the faucial tonsil or at the base of the tongue in the lingual tonsil. Safety pins, coins, and dentures often lodge in the cricopharyngeal area, and smaller objects such as tacks and peanuts are frequently found in the trachea or bronchi.

3. Predisposing risk factors include esophageal webs or strictures.

C. Symptoms and signs.

1. A foreign body in the airway may cause pain, cough, hoarseness, hematemesis, agitation, inspiratory stridor, respiratory distress, and possibly cyanosis.

2. A foreign body in the esophagus may cause drooling, localized pain, referred pain (especially to the jugulosternal notch), odynophagia, inability to swallow, and regurgitation.

D. Physical examination.

1. Examine the mouth, pharynx, larynx, neck, and chest. Search for signs of obstruction, hemorrhage, or perforation.

2. Laryngoscopy should be performed as needed. The pharynx is anesthetized with benzocaine spray or lidocaine gargle (Viscous Xylocaine). Indirect mirror laryngoscopy with the patient in a sitting position may reveal the foreign body. Direct laryngoscopy can be performed with the patient supine. If available, fiberoptic laryngoscopy can be extremely useful.

E. Radiographs.

1. Radiographs of the neck, chest, or abdomen may reveal a radioopaque foreign body. For suspected nonradioopaque foreign body aspirated into the lungs, inspiratory and expiratory films of the chest in frontal and lateral projections may reveal characteristic areas of hyperaeration and/or hypoaeration.

2. Radiographic contrast studies such as barium swallow may be useful for esophageal obstruction. Consultation before obtaining such studies is advisable, since some endoscopists prefer to proceed directly to esophagoscopy.

F. Treatment.

1. Foreign bodies visible in the upper airway can sometimes be easily removed.

2. Foreign bodies of the lower airway usually require removal via bronchoscopy.

3. Esophageal foreign bodies.

   a. Meat impacted in the esophagus can be softened by drinking small amounts of meat tenderizer (papain) in water.

    b. Glucagon, 1 ml IV, or diazepam, 5 to 10 mg IV, may relax esophageal smooth muscle and allow passage into the stomach. Alternatively, glucagon may induce vomiting and regurgitation of the impacted food.

    c. Endoscopic removal may be required if the preceding measures fail.

III. FOREIGN BODY IN THE NOSE OR EAR CANAL.

A. Any object small enough to pass into the nostril or external auditory meatus may be found lodged in these areas. Such objects are frequently wedged in because of unskilled attempts at removal. A child's reluctance or inability to cooperate may complicate the problem.

B. Signs and symptoms.

1. Nose. Pain, sneezing, or unilateral nasal obstruction may be present. Later, findings may include bleeding accompanied by fetor and a foul discharge.

2. Ear. Later signs in the ear may resemble those of external otitis or chronic otitis media.

C. Treatment.

Shrinking the nasal mucosa with a vasoconstricting nose spray or drops (e.g., NeoSynephrine) may be helpful. Forceps or an ear curette may be used to extract the foreign body from the nose or ear canal. A small suction catheter may sometimes be effective as well.

IV. INGESTION OF CAUSTICS.

The most common offenders are acids and alkali used in household cleaning, such as lye, ammonia, potassium permanganate, and sulfuric acid. (See Chapter 28 for a discussion of poisoning.)

A. History. Ascertain the time of ingestion, the quantity and nature of the material ingested, and whether the ingestion was accidental or on purpose.

B. Physical examination.

1. Examination of the oral cavity, pharynx, and larynx may reveal marked reddening of the mucosa, denuded areas, or a coagulum of the caustic agent. This examination should be performed gently to avoid inadvertent vomiting of the offending agent back into the esophagus and pharynx.

2. Vital signs and vital organ function should be evaluated. Airway maintenance is essential, and tracheotomy eventually may be required.

C. Diagnostic evaluation.

1. Radiographs of the chest and cervical soft tissues should be considered in any significant case to look for signs of esophagogastric perforation such as free air.

2. Early endoscopy should be performed by an experienced endoscopist. Contrast studies should be obtained only after endoscopic consultation because contrast material can obscure the findings on endoscopy.

D. Treatment.
1. Antibiotics (e.g., penicillin, 1 million units IV q6h) should be given early to cover the gram-positive oral flora.
2. No attempt should be made to induce vomiting because this may reexpose the esophagus to the caustic agent.
3. Extended in-hospital treatment including surgery is often necessary. Early surgical or gastroenterologic consultation is important.

V. EPISTAXIS.
A. Etiology.
1. The most common site of bleeding is the anterior portion of the nasal mucosa along the septum.
2. Underlying causes of epistaxis include hypertension, anticoagulant medication or other coagulopathies, digital trauma or foreign body in children, blunt trauma to the nose, and upper respiratory tract infection.

B. Management.
1. BP control.
   a. In cases of major blood loss, draw blood for hemoglobin, hematocrit, platelet count, clotting parameters, and type and crossmatching as indicated. Administer IV fluids and blood as required (see Chapter 1).
   b. If the patient is significantly hypertensive, often reassurance and control of active bleeding will result in lowering the BP. If necessary, administer appropriate agents such as nifedipine, 10 mg PO.
2. Hemostasis.
   a. Prepare the necessary equipment, including a head mirror and adequate light, suction apparatus and nasal aspirating tips, cotton, bayonet forceps, silver nitrate sticks, and topical anesthetic such as tetracaine (Pontocaine) or cocaine 4%.
   b. Position the patient appropriately, seated but slightly reclined. Give the patient a basin into which blood and secretions may be expectorated.
   c. Protect yourself and the patient with aprons or gowns, gloves, and facial shield.
   d. Aspirate all clots and debris from the nose.
   e. Check the pharynx for bleeding posteriorly.
   f. Pack the nose with a large cotton pledget dampened lightly with the topical anesthetic. These agents also provide vasoconstriction and may decrease bleeding.
   g. If the bleeding has stopped and the site has not been identified, light abrasion of the anterior septum with a cotton applicator may cause renewed bleeding and allow identification of the site.
   h. When the bleeding point is identified, chemical cautery may be used with the application of silver nitrate. This

will stop most nosebleeds. Occasionally electrocautery will be required. Injection of the mucosa with lidocaine beforehand is advisable.

i. If the bleeding is stopped, emphasize that the patient should not manipulate the nose or engage in exceptional activity for several days.

j. If the patient is still bleeding after the aforementioned procedure, an anterior pack can be placed with lubricated gauze stripping, layered from the floor to the roof of the nose. The patient is reevaluated in 1 to 2 days.

k. If the patient is still bleeding, or if the examination demonstrates that the bleeding is in the posterior portion of the nose, insert a posterior nasopharyngeal pack and pack anteriorly against it through the nose.

   (1) Commercially available epistaxis balloons are excellent. If not available, a 30-ml Foley catheter can be used (nos. 14 to 16 for adults, no. 12 for children).

   (2) Anesthetize the pharynx and soft palate with anesthetic spray (e.g., Cetacaine). Use a cotton pledget dampened with anesthetic (e.g., 4% cocaine) to anesthetize the nose.

   (3) Lubricate the catheter with antibiotic ointment and pass it through the anterior nares until it is visible in the oropharynx.

   (4) Inject 8 ml of air, and withdraw the catheter until it is engaged in the choanae. Then inflate another 2 to 4 ml of air.

   (5) While an assistant maintains gentle traction on the catheter, firmly pack petrolatum gauze into the nose anteriorly against the Foley balloon.

   (6) Protect the nostril and columella with soft gauze or cotton, and anchor the catheter.

   (7) A significant incidence of hypoxia can occur in patients with posterior packs. Hospitalization with close observation should be considered, especially for the elderly patient.

VI. INFECTION.

A. Pharyngitis.

1. Viral infections account for most sore throats.

2. Bacterial infections of the pharynx and tonsils can be caused by a number of organisms, but group A β-hemolytic *Streptococcus* and *Gonococcus* are the only types that require antibiotics. Untreated streptococcal infections can be associated with the later development of rheumatic fever or glomerulonephritis.

3. Diagnosis.

   a. Both viral and streptococcal infections can cause pharyngeal erythema, mucosal petechiae, tonsillar exudate, and cervical adenopathy. The greater the number of the afore-mentioned findings, the greater the possibility of strepto-coccal infection. However, pharyngitis in mononucleosis is often associated with all these signs. A frequent additional finding in mononucleosis is posterior cervical adenopathy.

b. Definitive diagnosis is made by culture. Full C&S of the throat is unnecessarily expensive. A culture to rule out *Streptococcus* infection is preferred. Rapid streptococcal screens give fairly accurate results in less than 1 hour. If gonorrhea is suspected by history, swabbing for gonorrheal studies is suggested.

4. Treatment.

a. For streptococcal pharyngitis, use one of the following regimens.

(1) Benzathine penicillin, 1.2 million units IM, or:

(2) Penicillin VK (phenoxymethyl), 250 mg qid for 10 days; or:

(3) If the patient is allergic to penicillin, alternatives are erythromycin, 250 mg qid for 10 days, or azithromycin, 500 mg on the first day, followed by 250 mg daily for another 4 days.

b. For gonococcal pharyngitis, one of the following regimens may be used.

(1) Ceftriaxone, 125 mg IM, or:

(2) Cefixime 400 mg PO, or ciprofloxacin 500 mg PO, or ofloxacin, 400 mg PO.

B. Peritonsillar abscess.

1. *Symptoms.* Prominent complaints are severe sore throat, worse on one side, with severe pain on swallowing (odynophagia). Weakness, chills, fever, and trismus are common. Trismus may prevent the patient from opening the mouth to allow adequate inspection.

2. *Findings.* The patient is toxic and febrile; also noted are muffled speech, drooling, trismus, and contralateral displacement of the edematous uvula. There is fullness at the juncture of the soft palate and the lateral margin of the palatine tonsil, and asymmetry is usually noticeable. Cervical adenopathy frequently is present. Respiratory obstruction may occur.

3. Treatment consists of aspiration, incision and drainage, and parenteral antibiotics. Ear, nose, and throat consultation is strongly suggested.

C. Croup and epiglottitis. (See Chapter 30).

D. Otitis.

1. Classification, terminology, definitions, and even the need for antibiotic therapy of ear infections are areas of controversy.

a. By common definition, serous otitis is a viral infection, and otitis media with effusion is bacterial. However, clinical impression is not always confirmed by culturing of middle ear fluid.

b. Most bacterial infections are self-limited, but treatment may shorten the course and lessen the chance of progression to mastoiditis.

c. The discussion below includes the traditional definitions and therapy.

2. Serous otitis.

a. *Symptoms.* The ears feel occluded and there is a sensation of "fullness." Hearing may be decreased. Discomfort may be present but is not usually severe.

b. *Findings.* The TM may at first be retracted with alteration of the light reflex. As fluid accumulates in the middle ear, the TM becomes dull. Bubbles may occasionally be seen in the fluid behind the TM.

c. *Treatment.* The goal is to decrease swelling around the eustachian tube to allow the fluid to drain. Oral and/or nasal decongestants are used. Because the infection is thought to be viral, antibiotics are not usually prescribed.

3. Bacterial otitis media (otitis media with effusion).

a. Symptoms.

(1) All the symptoms of serous otitis described in the last section may be experienced, but otalgia is the prominent complaint. Fever is common.

(2) In young children who cannot verbalize the complaint of ear pain, fever and vomiting may be the only obvious symptoms.

b. Findings.

(1) Early in the course, the eardrum may exhibit only dilated vessels.

(2) Eventually the entire drum becomes red with altered landmarks. The light reflex is lost, and the drum may bulge.

(3) Pneumatic otoscopy reveals an immobile TM.

c. Treatment.

(1) Although no definitive study has proven decongestants to be effective, they are often prescribed with the hope of easing the pressure sensation of otitis.

(2) Otitis media with effusion is by definition a bacterial infection and therefore is usually treated with antibiotics.

(a) Amoxicillin, 250 mg tid for 10 days (in children 40 mg/kg/day in 3 divided doses), is most commonly prescribed.

(b) Alternative regimens include erythromycin, trimethoprim-sulfamethoxazole (Septra, Bactrim), amoxicillin-clavulanate (Augmentin), erythromycin-sulfisoxazole (Pediazole), and various cephalosporins.

4. Otitis externa.

a. *Etiology.* A bacterial infection of the external auditory canal, this disorder is often induced by foreign material such as water from swimming, or a cotton-tipped applicator used to clean the ear.

b. *Symptoms.* At first only itching may be present, but eventually pain develops, especially with chewing. A sense of fullness and hearing loss may also occur.

c. Findings.

(1) Manipulation of the auricle causes pain, and periauricular tenderness and adenopathy may be present.

(2) Although the external auditory canal may at first be only red, swelling is usually found, often with pus, which may occlude the canal.

d. Treatment.

(1) Gently wipe or aspirate the discharge.

(2) If there is significant swelling, a ¼-inch gauze wick should gently be inserted into the canal.

(3) Antibiotic drops should be prescribed (e.g., Cortisporin 4 drops qid).

(4) Systemic antibiotics should be used if there is fever, significant periauricular adenopathy, or accompanying otitis media.

E. Acute sinusitis.

1. *History.* Onset often follows an upper respiratory tract infection, facial trauma, or a tooth extraction.

2. *Symptoms.* Nasal blockage, pain over the involved sinus, fever, chills, malaise, and orbital discomfort are common; symptoms may be unilateral or bilateral.

3. *Findings.* Tenderness to percussion over the involved sinus is usually present. Facial swelling, warmth, and erythema may occur as well. The infected sinus may fail to transilluminate. Intranasal examination may reveal injected swollen turbinates and mucous membranes. The teeth may be sensitive to percussion. Check for a dental focus of infection, especially if toothache is an early symptom.

4. If the diagnosis is not obvious from history and physical examination, radiographs can be helpful by revealing clouding of the sinus and thickening of the sinus mucosa. CT scanning is diagnostic.

5. *Treatment.* Antibiotic therapy may include amoxicillin, trimethoprim-sulfa, amoxicillin-clavulanate, or a cephalosporin. Also suggested are systemic and local nasal decongestants, high fluid intake, and humidification of the environment. Ten days of antibiotic therapy may be sufficient for acute sinusitis, but chronic infection may require 2 to 3 weeks of treatment. Surgical drainage and irrigation of the sinus are occasionally required.

VII. ORAL AND DENTAL INFECTIONS.

A. Patients with *dental caries* commonly present to the ED with toothache. Analgesics may be given and the patient referred to a dentist.

B. A *dental abscess* may be suggested by the presence of fever, swelling, acute submandibular adenopathy, or tenderness to percussion of the tooth. Penicillin should be prescribed (250 mg four times a day) and the patient referred to a dentist for drainage. If there is evidence of facial cellulitis, especially if pointing toward the orbit, IV antibiotics may be required.

C. *Stomatitis* presents with ulceration of the gums or tongue.

   1. Etiologic agents may include herpes simplex, the coxsackieviruses, or *Candida* (thrush).

   2. Findings. Herpes simplex usually causes one or more localized ulcers or vesicles. Coxsackievirus generally causes more widespread ulceration or vesiculation. In thrush, the oral mucosa or tongue displays erythema or a white coating.

   3. Local application or rinsing with viscous lidocaine may be helpful. Severe herpes infections may respond to acyclovir (Zovirax), 200 mg five times a day. Thrush is treated with clotrimazole troche, 10 mg five times a day for 10 to 14 days.

VIII. TEMPOROMANDIBULAR JOINT (TMJ) DISORDERS.

A. Inflammation may be chronic or acute and typically causes pain on jaw motion and chewing. Pain may be referred to the ear. Nonsteroidal antiinflammatory drugs may help temporarily, and referral to a specialist is suggested.

B. Dislocation of the TMJ is caused by displacement of the mandible in an anterior direction. The patient is unable to close the mouth. Reduction is achieved by downward and backward traction on the jaw. Parenteral analgesic and muscle relaxant may be required (see Chapter 12).

23

Ophthalmologic
Emergencies

I. GENERAL CONSIDERATIONS.

A. In all patients with eye problems except those for whom intervention must be initiated without delay, visual acuity should be tested before diagnostic or therapeutic manipulation. Each eye should be tested separately and the results noted in the medical record. If the patient wears glasses, the acuity may be recorded with the glasses in place and the notation "corrected" made.

B. The standard Snellen eye chart should be used whenever possible and the smallest line discernible by the patient recorded. A pinhole can be used for patients who did not bring their corrective lenses. If the patient is unable to read even the largest figures on the chart, he or she should be asked to count the number of fingers the examiner holds, to detect finger movement, and to perceive light, in that order.

C. Examination of the eye should usually include a funduscopic examination. Examination with the slit lamp (if available) should be used in appropriate cases. Tonometry should be performed if increased intraocular pressure is suspected. This is easily done with the Schiøtz tonometer, applanation or air-puff tonometers, or the TonoPen. Normal intraocular pressure is 12 to 20 mm Hg.

D. The use of topical corticosteroid preparations for the emergency patient can be dangerous because of the ophthalmologic complications these drugs may produce. Therefore these medications should be used only with specific indications and with the assurance of prompt ophthalmologic follow-up.

II. CONJUNCTIVITIS AND KERATITIS.

A. **Bacterial conjunctivitis.** The patient has conjunctival injection, copious mucopurulent discharge, and may give a history of the lids sticking together. Staining of the discharge reveals polymorphonuclear leukocytes and bacteria. The discharge may be cultured and broad-spectrum antibiotic drops administered, such as bacitracin, neomycin, gentamicin, or sulfacetamide.

B. Epidemic keratoconjunctivitis. This is caused by an adenovirus and is highly communicable. Signs include conjunctival and lid edema with mild hyperemia and scanty, watery discharge. There may be swelling and tenderness of the preauricular lymph nodes. The most important consideration is preventing the spread of the disease by carefully sterilizing ophthalmic instruments and warning the patient of the infectious nature of the process. The condition usually resolves in 2 to 3 weeks without treatment.

C. Other viral conjunctivitis. This may have accompanying upper respiratory tract infection. The eye is injected and uncomfortable, and there may be some discharge. A Gram's stain of this reveals monocytes. Although a topical decongestant such as naphazoline (Vasocon) may be administered, these disorders improve without therapy.

D. Herpes simplex keratitis. Patients generally complain of unilateral eye irritation, photophobia, and occasionally blurred vision. There may be corneal hypesthesia. The most characteristic finding is irregular dendritic ulcers on the cornea that take fluorescein stain. Topical corticosteroid therapy may result in corneal perforation and should be avoided. Viricidal preparations such as trifluridine (Viroptic) are used, and ophthalmologic consultation should be obtained.

III. ACUTE LOSS OF VISION.

A. Some common causes of acute visual loss are listed in Box 23-1. Several of the more important ones are discussed in sections IV and V.

B. Some of these entities may display characteristic abnormalities on funduscopic examination.

BOX 23-1
Common Causes of Acute Visual Loss

Acute angle-closure glaucoma
Central retinal artery occlusion
Central retinal vein occlusion
Vitreous hemorrhage
Macular hemorrhage
Retinal detachment
Ischemic optic neuropathy
Functional

C. Patients with acute retinal detachment may experience total unilateral visual loss or a decreased visual field. This may be preceded by floaters or flashes of light. The patient may complain of a curtain descending across a portion of the visual field. Although the edge of some detachments may be seen on direct ophthalmoscopy, more peripheral involvement requires the use of indirect ophthalmoscopy.

D. The most important cause of ischemic optic neuropathy is temporal arteritis. This is characteristically seen in older patients and may be accompanied by temporal headache, muscular pains, and other constitutional symptoms. A markedly elevated erythrocyte sedimentation rate is characteristically present. If this diagnosis is made, treatment with high-dose corticosteroids should be initiated.

1. Methylprednisolone, 80 to 100 mg IV, as an initial dose.
2. Prednisone, 40 mg/day, which may ultimately be tapered by the consulting physician.

IV. OCCLUSION OF THE CENTRAL RETINAL ARTERY.

A. The history is a sudden painless loss of unilateral vision. The objective findings are an absence of the direct reaction of the pupil to light, diffuse gray edema of the retina, and poor filling of the retinal vascular tree (compared with that of the other eye). The prognosis with regard to the return of vision depends on the duration and the degree of retinal anoxia. Permanent damage is likely to occur if the duration of visual loss exceeds 2 hours.

B. Initial treatment consists of measures aimed at vasodilation in the area supplied by the carotid arteries. Having the patient breathe into a paper bag is a widely used form of therapy. Alternatively, a commercially available mixture of 95% oxygen and 5% carbon dioxide may be used for 5 minutes of each hour. Because this may cause systemic vasodilation, the BP should be closely monitored during such treatment. Intermittent manual massage of the globe may dislodge an arterial clot. Other measures such as anterior chamber paracentesis may be performed by those practiced in the procedure.

V. ACUTE ANGLE-CLOSURE GLAUCOMA.

A. Acute angle-closure glaucoma is an emergency that must be recognized and treated without delay.

B. The patient usually complains of severe pain in the eye. This may be accompanied by blurred vision, nausea, and vomiting. Rarely, headache and nausea may be the only symptoms.

C. Physical examination reveals the following:

1. Conjunctival infection, especially around the limbus.
2. Clouding of the cornea.
3. Shallowness of the anterior chamber.
4. Midsized pupils.
5. High intraocular pressure on tonometry.

D. Treatment.
   1. Initial treatment should consist of the instillation of a topical miotic such as 2% or 4% pilocarpine drops every 15 minutes.
   2. Topical β-blockers, such as timolol, should be instilled to reduce aqueous humor. Care should be taken in patients with cardiac or bronchospastic disease, since systemic absorption occurs.
   3. Acetazolamide (Diamox), 500 mg, should be given IV to reduce aqueous production.
   4. An osmotherapeutic agent (such as mannitol, 1.5 to 2.0 g/kg administered IV over 30 to 60 minutes). This will draw fluid from the globe by osmotic mechanisms. Care should be taken in elderly patients because osmotic agents may produce vascular overload.
   5. Ophthalmologic consultation should be sought and the patient admitted to the hospital.

VI. ACUTE ANTERIOR UVEITIS (IRITIS, IRIDOCYCLITIS).

A. A number of illnesses may predispose, including collagen-vascular disorders, ulcerative colitis, tuberculosis, and various viral infections.
B. The patient usually experiences pain in the eye, blurred vision, and significant photophobia. The eye is red, with particular dilation of the vessels around the limbus. The pupil is miotic and may be irregular. Slit-lamp examination reveals flare and cells in the anterior chamber, as well as cellular deposits on the endothelial surface of the cornea.
C. Treatment consists of pupillary dilation and cycloplegia with 1% homatropine drops and referral of the patient to an ophthalmologist for topical corticosteroid therapy.

VII. HORDEOLUM AND CHALAZION.

A. A hordeolum (sty) is a staphylococcal abscess of a meibomian gland of the eyelid. It is a tender, erythematous lesion that may be accompanied by significant lid edema. Treatment is the application of hot compresses and the instillation of topical antibiotics four times daily.
B. A chalazion is a lipogranulomatous reaction in an obstructed meibomian gland. It is a nontender localized swelling of the lid. Treatment is hot compresses and referral for elective surgical excision.

24

AIDS and Oncologic and Hematologic Emergencies

I. AIDS.

A. Definitions.

1. AIDS is the result of infection with HIV type 1, which in turn causes a progressive loss of CD4 lymphocytes, leading to the development of opportunistic infections and malignancies.

2. The clinical staging system instituted by the Centers for Disease Control and Prevention (CDC) in 1993 for classification of HIV disease on the basis of CD4 counts includes overt infection, category B (formerly AIDS-related complex), and AIDS-defining conditions.

   a. HIV-positive patients with CD4 counts above 500 cells/μl are likely to have few symptoms, although lymphadenopathy, seborrheic dermatitis, and oral leukoplakia or aphthous ulcerations may be seen.

   b. With CD4 counts below 500 cells/μl, the patient may have presenting symptoms of recurrent herpes simplex or varicella zoster infections, oral or vaginal candidiasis, or bacterial infections (e.g., sinusitis, bronchitis, community-acquired pneumonia, tuberculosis).

   c. At CD4 counts less than 200 cells/μl, opportunistic infections and malignancies are common. These include *Pneumocystis carinii* pneumonia, CNS toxoplasmosis, disseminated or esophageal candidiasis, lymphoma, and Kaposi's sarcoma.

   d. Advanced disease is associated with severe immunosuppression (CD4 counts are below 50 cells/μl). Such patients may exhibit cryptococcal meningitis, disseminated *Mycobacterium avium* complex disease, or other opportunistic infection.

B. Presentations to the emergency department.

1. Fever.

   a. In patients with known AIDS, fever is common. A diagnostic workup would be initiated when the fever pattern changes or new systemic or localized symptoms develop (Table 24-1).

   b. Because fever can represent a presentation with a variety of bacterial, viral, fungal, and protozoal organisms, a thorough history and physical examination should be performed in each instance. Special emphasis should be placed on the respiratory tract, CNS, and the abdomen.

2. Skin eruption.

   a. Cutaneous lesions are common in patients with HIV infection and may represent an array of underlying infectious processes, although noninfectious lesions are also seen.

   b. Infectious skin lesions.

      (1) Viral: herpes simplex, varicella zoster, molluscum contagiosum.

         (a) Herpes simplex infection may be extensive and disseminated, involving the oral mucosa and gastrointestinal tract.

         (b) Treatment for herpes simplex infection is acyclovir, 200 mg five times daily, for 10 days for mucocutaneous lesions. Extensive cutaneous involvement or gastrointestinal or CNS involvement requires a higher dose or IV acyclovir.

         (c) Varicella zoster infection may represent the initial manifestation of HIV infection.

TABLE 24-1
Fever in Patients With AIDS

Abnormality	Cause of fever
Severe oral candidiasis	*Candida* esophagitis
Neurologic deficits	Toxoplasmosis or cryptococcal meningitis
Exanthem	Disseminated herpes, disseminated cryptococcal disease or drug fever (especially trimethoprim-sulfamethoxazole)
Deteriorating visual acuity	Disseminated cytomegalovirus
Progressive anemia with or without liver function abnormalities	*Mycobacterium avium-intracellulare*
Increasing lymphadenopathy	Lymphoma or mycobacterial disease

From Hollander H: Practical management of common AIDS-related medical problems, *West J Med* 146:237-240, 1987.

       (d) Treatment of dermatomal varicella zoster is acyclovir, 800 mg five times daily, or famciclovir, 500 mg three times daily. Disseminated infection requires treatment with IV acyclovir.

   (2) Bacterial skin infections include folliculitis, cellulitis, and impetigo.

   (3) Fungal infection may produce dermatophyte or *Candida* skin involvement, or skin lesions may represent disseminated cryptococcosis or histoplasmosis.

  c. Noninfectious skin lesions: these include Kaposi's sarcoma, seborrhea, and psoriasis.

3. Oral lesions.

  a. Oral lesions commonly represent candidiasis, herpes simplex infection, hairy leukoplakia, or aphthous stomatitis.

  b. Kaposi's sarcoma can occur on the palate without involvement elsewhere.

  c. Dysphagia or odynophagia may be the result of esophagitis caused by *Candida,* herpes simplex virus, cytomegalovirus, or lymphoma.

4. Neurologic signs and symptoms (e.g., altered mental status, seizures, headache).

  a. CNS infection is the most common cause of neurologic presentations. Fever is usually present. Lumbar puncture should be performed if meningitis is suspected. Cryptococcal infection is common, although meningitis may also be viral, bacterial, or tuberculous. Focal encephalitis is most commonly due to *Toxoplasma.*

  b. Other neurologic syndromes associated with AIDS include AIDS dementia complex and peripheral neuropathy.

5. Respiratory system: shortness of breath, cough.

  a. Pulmonary complaints are very frequent among patients with HIV infection.

  b. The most common cause of shortness of breath is *Pneumocystis carinii* pneumonia. Dyspnea, nonproductive cough, and diffuse interstitial infiltrates on chest radiograph are characteristic.

  c. Other causes of pneumonia are bacteria, viruses (especially cytomegalovirus), fungi and mycobacteria (e.g., tuberculosis and *M. avium*).

6. Gastrointestinal tract: dysphagia (see 3, c), abdominal pain, vomiting, diarrhea.

  a. Diarrhea is the most common gastrointestinal complaint and should suggest an infectious cause.

  b. The most common agent of infectious diarrhea in these patients is *Cryptosporidium.* Others include *Candida, M. avium,* cytomegalovirus, herpes simplex virus, *Campylobacter, Shigella, Salmonella,* and *Giardia.*

  c. Evaluation should include stool culture for bacteria and parasites, and staining for fecal leukocytes, cryptosporidium, and acid-fast bacilli.

C. Precautions for health care workers.
1. The major risk to health care workers is associated with percutaneous exposure to blood or blood-containing body fluids of patients with HIV infection. Other types of exposure carry significantly less risk.
2. Adhere to CDC guidelines to minimize the risk of disease transmission.
3. Observe universal precautions with respect to blood and blood-containing body fluids.
4. Follow needle, fluid, and soiled object disposal policies.
5. In general, reserve respiratory precautions (e.g., mask and physical isolation) for patients with known or suspected tuberculosis. *Pneumocystis carinii* pneumonia is not contagious.
6. Institutional policies should be developed for the management of occupational exposure. The advisability of postexposure prophylactic antiviral therapy is controversial but usually recommended for primary exposure to blood known to be or strongly suspected of carrying HIV. However, side effects of prophylactic therapy are common.

II. ONCOLOGIC EMERGENCIES.
A. General considerations.
1. Emergencies in cancer patients present to the emergency physician in four major ways.
   a. A patient not known to have cancer has initial symptoms.
   b. An emergency arises during the course of a patient's cancer therapy.
   c. An emergency arises in a terminal patient.
   d. The emergency is unrelated to the patient's cancer.
2. The event must be assessed in the context of the patient and the specific disease. The following questions should be answered if possible before initiating therapy:
   a. Is the emergency related to the patient's malignant disease?
   b. What is the tumor cell type, stage, and present extent?
   c. What surgery, radiation, or chemotherapy has the patient already undergone?
   d. Does there remain an effective therapy likely to produce a good remission?
   e. What is the realistic probability of cure or long-term control?
   f. What is the patient's quality of life and, if appropriate, have decisions been discussed or finalized regarding the intensity of therapeutic efforts to be undertaken should life-threatening situations occur?
B. Neurologic emergencies. Treatment for the following conditions should be instituted as soon as the diagnosis is suspected.
1. Cerebral herniation.
   a. *ICP.* ICP is a nonlinear function of brain, CSF, and cerebral blood volume. A small increase in ICP may produce a sudden major deterioration in clinical condition. Simi-

larly, a small reduction in ICP after therapy may significantly alleviate the patient's condition.

b. Causes.
   (1) Primary or metastatic tumors.
   (2) Cerebral hemorrhage.
   (3) Subdural hematomas.
   (4) Cerebral abscess.
   (5) Acute hydrocephalus.
   (6) Radiation-induced cerebral necrosis.

c. Presentation (see Chapter 21).
   (1) Headache.
   (2) Herniation syndromes.
   (3) Altered mental status.
   (4) Seizures, focal or generalized.
   (5) Focal neurologic signs similar to stroke.

d. Treatment.
   (1) Institute endotracheal intubation for significant elevation. Pretreat with lidocaine, 1 to 2 mg/kg IV, to protect against a raised ICP.
   (2) Initiate hyperventilation to reduce the $PaCO_2$ to 25 to 30 mm Hg.
   (3) Consider giving mannitol, 1 to 2 mg/kg IV.
   (4) Consider dexamethasone, 20 to 100 mg IV: its onset of effect is slower than that of intubation or mannitol.
   (5) Surgical decompression based on CT scan findings may be needed.

2. **Seizures.**
   a. Causes.
      (1) Seizure is common as a presenting symptom of neurologic involvement in the cancer patient.
      (2) A seizure may be due to a primary tumor or from metastatic, metabolic, infectious, or vascular causes.
   b. Treatment (see Chapter 21).

3. **Spinal cord compression.** This condition requires prompt diagnosis and initiation of treatment to preserve function. It may be the presenting syndrome of cancer or occur in a patient with known malignancy.
   a. Causes.
      (1) Breast, lung, renal and prostate tumors, lymphoma, and multiple myeloma are the most common causes.
      (2) Epidural spinal cord compression is typically the result of metastatic disease to the spine.
   b. Presentation.
      (1) Local or radicular pain occurs in 95% of epidural metastases and precedes other symptoms by weeks or months.
      (2) In cervical spine metastases, a classic presentation is unilateral high neck pain aggravated by turning, with radiation to the shoulder or occiput.

      (3) Pain is accentuated by percussion, Valsalva maneuver (such as coughing or sneezing), neck flexion, and straight leg raising.

      (4) Motor weakness or ataxia progressing to paralysis.

      (5) Sensory loss (paresthesias, hypoesthesia, or dysesthesia.)

      (6) Autonomic findings (incontinence, urinary retention).

  c. Diagnosis.

      (1) Spinal radiographs are essential in any cancer patient complaining of new, persistent, or worsening back or neck pain. These may show osteolytic or osteoblastic lesions, pedicle erosion, or vertebral body collapse.

      (2) Further evaluation may include CT, MRI, or myelography.

  d. Treatment.

      (1) Obtain early consultation with an oncologist or radiation therapist and a neurosurgeon.

      (2) Early initiation of radiation is the mainstay of treatment.

      (3) Surgical decompression may be indicated in certain circumstances.

4. CNS infections.

  a. Causes.

      (1) Cancer patients are compromised hosts with impaired immune systems resulting from one or more of the following:

        (a) Underlying disease.

        (b) Corticosteroid therapy.

        (c) Chemotherapy.

        (d) Splenectomy.

        (e) Radiation.

      (2) Most CNS infections occur in leukemia, lymphoma, or head and neck cancer. The latter patients are susceptible as a result of fistulas and direct invasion, which allow organisms access to the CNS.

  b. Major types.

      (1) Meningitis.

        (a) *Presentation.* Headache, fever, and an altered level of consciousness are common. Delay in diagnosis may occur as a result of assigning fever to a systemic source, headache to metastases, and the altered mental status to a metabolic or toxic encephalopathy.

        (b) Diagnosis.

          (i) Lumbar puncture should be done after checking coagulation studies including the platelet count. It may be necessary to replenish the coagulation system with fresh frozen plasma and platelets before the procedure (see Section II, G, 5).

(ii) A CT scan should precede the lumbar puncture if there is any suggestion of a mass lesion.

(c) Treatment (see also Chapter 21).

(i) Combination therapy is preferred until the
culture results are available. The choice of antibiotics is based on the peripheral WBC, and
the results of Gram's staining (Table 24-2).

(ii) Ampicillin, 2 g IV every 4 hours, should be
added when *Listeria monocytogenes* is suspected.

(iii) When gram-negative rods and neutropenia
are present, initial therapy should include an
aminoglycoside (loading dose, 2 mg/kg) plus
a third-generation cephalosporin (cefotaxime,
2 g IV every 4 hours) or a semisynthetic penicillin (carbenicillin, 400 to 500 mg/kg/day
given every 4 hours).

(2) *Cerebral abscess.* This usually presents to the ED as a
herniation syndrome (see Chapter 21).

(3) *Encephalitis.* This is very unusual but difficult to diagnose. The CT scan shows cerebral edema, and the
spinal tap shows pleocytosis and an elevated protein
concentration without any organisms. Herpes zoster
and *Toxoplasma gondii* are the most common causes.
Patients should be admitted when the diagnosis is suspected.

TABLE 24-2
**Organisms Commonly Causing Meningitis in Different
Neoplastic Diseases**

Primary tumor	Organism	
	WBC >2700/mm^3	WBC <2700/mm^3
Lymphoma	*Listeria monocytogenes* *Diplococcus pneumoniae* *Cryptococcus neoformans*	Gram-negative rods
Leukemia		
Acute	—	Gram-negative rods, especially *Pseudomonas aeruginosa*
Chronic Head/spine	*Cryptococcus neoformans* *Staphylococcus aureus* Gram-negative rods	
Others	*Listeria monocytogenes* *Diplococcus pneumoniae*	Gram-negative rods

From Yarbro JW, Bornstein RS: *Oncologic emergencies,* Philadelphia, 1981,
Grune & Stratton.

C. Vascular disorders.

1. *Causes.* A poorly defined state of hypercoagulability in cancer patients produces three conditions of importance:

   a. *Disseminated intravascular coagulation.* Agitation, lethargy, seizures, and stupor are common, as are focal deficits such as focal seizures, hemiparesis, aphasia, and cortical blindness. The neurologic effects may be seen before laboratory results become abnormal. When laboratory tests are abnormal, these show thrombocytopenia, prolongation of prothrombin and partial thromboplastin times, elevation of fibrin degradation products, and reduction of fibrinogen level.

   b. *Marantic endocarditis.* Bronchiolar carcinoma, or adenocarcinoma of the lung, is the most common primary source, and cerebral infarction is the most common cause of death in these patients.

   c. Sagittal sinus thrombosis occurs with sinus compression or invasion by leukemic or solid-tumor infiltration of the dura, or as a nonmetastatic remote effect of the cancer. It can present with acute neurologic effects (especially sixth cranial nerve palsy, producing diplopia) or a slow progression of obtundation. It is difficult to diagnose and may require MRI or high-resolution arteriography with a review of the venous and arterial phases.

D. Toxic and metabolic abnormalities.

1. *Causes.* Cancer patients are susceptible because the underlying disease can cause organ failure, electrolyte and nutrition disturbances, and drug reactions. Also, impaired liver function and retarded metabolism cause drug side effects.

2. *Presentation.*

   a. Common presentations include acute or subacute changes in mental status, aberrant behavior, confusion, fever, and headache.

   b. Consider hypoglycemia and unintentional narcotic overdose as causes.

   c. First rule out a mass lesion or infection and check the levels of electrolytes, BUN, glucose, calcium, ABGs, and liver function tests.

3. *Treatment.* Manage as indicated, depending on the identified metabolic abnormality. These patients usually require hospital admission for management.

4. *Specific metabolic states.* The following are the most common metabolic abnormalities:

   a. Hypercalcemia (see Chapter 2).

   b. Acute adrenal insufficiency (Addisonian crisis; see Chapter 21).

   c. SIADH. ADH (arginine vasopressin), stored in the posterior pituitary gland, is secreted in response to extracellular fluid (ECF) osmolality changes. Secretion increases as osmolality increases. Renal mechanisms then retain water, and the osmolality decreases. SIADH results from continued ADH release, which causes continued water retention and dilutional hyponatremia. The usual feedback loop is not functional.

(1) Causes.

   (a) Ectopic ADH production, most common in oat cell carcinoma, primary and metastatic brain tumors, non–small-cell lung carcinoma, and rarely pancreatic carcinoma.

   (b) *Chemotherapy.* The mechanism is unclear. It occurs with cyclophosphamide, vincristine, and vinblastine.

   (c) After the administration of narcotics, antidepressants, and phenothiazines, commonly used drugs in cancer patients.

   (d) Pneumonia and CNS disorders may cause SIADH, and these conditions are fairly common in cancer patients.

(2) *Presentation.* This is primarily dependent on the rate of hyponatremia development. Moderate symptoms occur below 125 mEq/L, and below 115 mEq/L they are severe. Nausea, anorexia, and weakness are common early symptoms, progressing to vomiting, lethargy, seizures, and coma.

(3) Diagnostic criteria.

   (a) Hyponatremia with no evidence of volume depletion and edema.

   (b) Normal thyroid, renal, and adrenal function.

   (c) No diuretic therapy.

   (d) Inappropriately high urine sodium concentration.

   (e) Decreased plasma osmolality when the urine sodium concentration is high.

(4) Treatment.

   (a) *Mild hyponatremia.* Water restriction of 500 to 750 ml/24 hr.

   (b) *Severe hyponatremia, especially with seizures.* Rapid correction of hyponatremia with furosemide, 1 mg/kg IV, and a saline infusion to replace urine losses. Check electrolyte levels frequently, and replace as indicated. If necessary, 3% saline may be used. This requires monitoring of central venous pressure and urine output. Assess serum sodium every 1 to 2 hours. Correct the serum level to no more than halfway to normal over the first 8 hours.

E. Effects of radiation and chemotherapy.

1. Radiation therapy.

   a. Irradiation of the pelvis and abdomen produces anorexia, vomiting, cramps, and loose stools, which are treated with a low-residue diet. Occasionally these patients require opiate-type drugs to control the diarrhea. Sometimes it is necessary to stop radiation treatment, and severe cases may require hospitalization.

b. More severe gastrointestinal problems include strictures, fistulas, and intestinal obstruction. Perforation may occur.

c. Hematuria, if mild, may respond to the removal of stimulants from the diet (tea, coffee, alcohol, and spices). Severe hematuria requires admission for Foley irrigation and cystoscopy.

d. Pulmonary syndromes.

   (1) Acute radiation pneumonitis occurs 2 to 3 months after treatment, with the insidious onset of exertional dyspnea, low-grade fever, nonproductive cough, and progressive radiographic pulmonary interstitial findings confined to lung treatment portals.

   (2) Restrictive lung disease occurs 9 to 12 months after treatment. It presents with pulmonary fibrosis.

   (3) Lobular or lobar radiologic patterns, pleural effusion, or mediastinal lymphadenopathy are uncommonly due to radiation, and other causes, usually infectious, should be sought.

2. Chemotherapy.

   a. *GI toxicity.* This is very common with certain agents. Treatment with antiemetics may require careful combinations of different agents, and side effects may occur (Box 24-1).

   b. *Pulmonary toxicity* (Box 24-2). The difficulty is in differentiating drug toxicity from infection and tumor, and a biopsy may be required to make the diagnosis.

BOX 24-1
Commonly Used Antiemetic Medications

Phenothiazines
   Prochlorperazine (Compazine)
   Thiethylperazine malate (Torecan)
   Chlorpromazine (Thorazine)
Butyrophenones
   Haloperidol (Haldol)
   Droperidol (Inapsine)
Miscellaneous
   Metocopramide hydrochloride (Reglan)
   Dexamethasone (Decandron)
   Trimethobenzamide hydrochloride (Tigan)
   Ondansetron (Zofran)

BOX 24-2
Chemotherapeutic Agents Causing
Pulmonary Damage

CYTOTOXIC
Busulfan (Myleran)
Cyclophosphamide (Cytoxan)
Bleomycin sulfate
Nitrosoureas (carmustine, lomustine, semustine)
Chlorambucil (Leukeran)
Mitomycin C
Hydroxyurea
Procarbazine hydrochloride

NONCYTOTOXIC
Methotrexate
Procarbazine hydrochloride
Bleomycin sulfate
Cyclophosphamide

---

   c. *Cardiac toxicity.* The most common causes are anthracy-clines (doxorubicin and daunorubicin) and cyclophos-phamide. Anthracyclines produce dysrhythmias, conduction defects, and cardiomyopathy.

   d. *Neurotoxicity.* Virtually any deficit may occur, as may meningeal irritation after the intrathecal administration of chemotherapeutic agents.

   e. Allergic reactions. These range from skin rashes, fevers, and chills to exfoliative dermatitis and frank anaphylaxis. Fevers respond to acetaminophen and antihistamines. Anaphylaxis, though rare, may occur after prolonged exposure to certain specific drugs.

F. Cardiopulmonary conditions.
  1. Cardiac.
    a. Dysrhythmias and cardiac failure occur from the effects of antineoplastic drugs (see Section E, 2, c). However, cardiac effects of pericardial effusion and pulmonary embolism are more frequent, as are dysrhythmias resulting from electrolyte disturbances.

    b. Superior vena cava obstruction presents with shortness of breath; cyanotic swelling of the face, neck, and shoulders; and distended neck veins. It is the result of invasion or extrinsic compression of the superior vena cava by tumor.

The onset is usually gradual. Administer oxygen and elevate the head of the bed. Obtain oncology and thoracic surgical consultation.

2. Pulmonary.
   a. Chemotherapy effect (see Section E, 2).
   b. Respiratory failure occasionally occurs unexpectedly in cancer patients who have received blood transfusions or undergone surgery.
   c. Life-threatening pulmonary infections caused by immunosuppression from chemotherapy or radiation therapy occur very rapidly.
      (1) Sepsis may present with fever or hypothermia.
      (2) Tachycardia and unexplained hypocapnia without radiologic changes may be the first signs of respiratory failure. Early aggressive treatment with antibiotics and intubation as indicated are essential.

G. Oncologic hematologic emergencies (see Section III for general discussion of hematologic emergencies).
   1. *Erythrocytosis.* This condition is usually secondary, and the most common tumor is a hypernephroma. Hyperviscosity causes dizziness, headaches, angina, and TIAs. The signs are retinal vein engorgement and facial redness. If the situation is urgent, phlebotomize 1 unit to reduce the red cell mass.
   2. *Leukocytosis.* In the blastic crisis of chronic granulomatous leukemia, the count may be 100,000 cells/cm^3, which produces leukostasis, thrombosis, vasospasm, and hypoxia. Immediate chemotherapy is indicated.
   3. *Thrombosis and hemorrhage.* Solid tumors are associated with a significant incidence of these events, up to 10%. Thromboembolic events occur with GI tract adenocarcinomas and tumors of the pancreas, ovary, and breast. Compensated disseminated intravascular coagulopathy (DIC) is common in these patients, with increased fibrinogen, fibrin, and platelets. When these levels fall, uncompensated DIC is occurring and requires urgent treatment.
   4. *Thrombocytosis.* Usually not problematic in cancer patients.
   5. *Thrombocytopenia.* In the cancer patient, this may be due to decreased platelet production by marrow infiltration as a result of leukemia, lymphoma, or carcinoma, or the effects of chemotherapeutic drugs (especially cytosine arabinoside). Thrombocytopenic patients seldom bleed until the platelet level is below 25,000/cm^3. Consider platelet transfusion if the condition is urgent (e.g., active bleeding with severe thrombocytopenia). One unit of random-donor platelets will raise the platelet count by 10,000/cm^3. Give 4 to 6 units, and assess the platelet count after 1 hour.

H. Infections.

1. Important predisposing factors.
   a. The malignancy itself and its effects.
   b. Surgery, chemotherapy, and radiation alter the anatomic barriers to infection.
   c. Radiation and chemotherapy impair the immune system and the inflammatory response.
   d. Neutropenia is a very important single factor.
2. Evaluation.
   a. Perform a thorough physical examination to ascertain any source of infection.
   b. Obtain a CBC, urinalysis, chest radiograph, and other diagnostic tests as indicated. Before initiation of therapy, culture blood, urine, throat, and any area suggestive of infection for aerobic and anaerobic organisms and atypical pathogens.
   c. Fever is very important. If present, it mandates a full workup. If the temperature is above 101°F without a history of recent blood product administration, there is an 80% chance of infection if the patient has advanced malignancy and neutropenia.
3. *Treatment.* This may include oncology or infectious disease consultation, broad-spectrum antibiotics, and close surveillance in the hospital.

III. HEMATOLOGIC AND COAGULATION EMERGENCIES.

(See Section II, G for discussion of oncologic hematologic emergencies.)

A. Hematologic emergencies.

1. Emergent anemia.
   a. Causes.
      (1) Blood loss is the most common cause and presents with signs of shock. Beware of subtle signs in infants and the elderly, who may decompensate rapidly.
      (2) Check the history for bleeding diathesis, drugs, and underlying diseases.
   b. Evaluation.
      (1) Examine the patient for bruising and petechiae (include the palate and conjunctiva). Perform a stool guaiac test, and check the urine for hematuria. Look for vaginal blood, and do a full pelvic and rectal examination.
      (2) Type and crossmatch the blood; check the CBC and smear, prothrombin time (PT) and PTT, electrolytes, glucose, creatinine; and save serum for later studies.
   c. Treatment (see Chapter 1).
2. Red cell destruction anemias (Box 24-3).
   a. Causes. These occur rarely in emergency medicine but require immediate intervention.
      (1) For a classification and common drugs causing hemolytic anemia, see Box 24-4.

BOX 24-3
Classification of Hemolytic Anemias

Intrinsic
  Enzyme defects
    Glucose-6-phosphate dehydrogenase deficiency
    Pyruvate kinase
  Membrane abnormality
    Spherocytosis
    Elliptostomatocytosis
    Paroxysmal nocturnal hemoglobinuria
    Spur cell anemia
  Hemoglobin abnormality
    Hemoglobinopathies
    Thalassemias (discussed with microcytic anemias)
    Unstable hemoglobin
    Hemoglobin M
Extrinsic
  Immunologic
    Alloantibodies
    Autoantibodies
  Mechanical
    Microangiopathic hemolytic anemia
    Cardiovascular such as prosthetic heart valve disease
  Environmental
    Drugs
    Toxins
    Infections
    Thermal
  Abnormal sequestrations as in hypersplenism

From Rosen P, et al: *Emergency medicine,* ed 3, St Louis, 1992, Mosby.

BOX 24-4
Drugs Associated With Hemolysis in G-6-PD Deficiency

Analgesics and antipyretics: acetanilid, aspirin, phenacetin
Antimalarials: primaquine, quinacrine, quinine
Nitrofurans
Sulfa drugs: sulfamethoxazole, sulfacetamide
Sulfones
Miscellaneous: napthalene, fava beans, methylene blue, phenhydrazine, nalidixic acid

From Rosen P, et al: *Emergency medicine,* ed 3, St Louis, 1992, Mosby.

(2) *Sickle cell disease.* In the United States, this is the most common type seen in the ED, although it is dependent on the population served. Sickle C disease and thalassemia also produce sickling.

(a) In sickle trait, only one parent has an abnormal gene.

(b) In sickle cell disease, all the hemoglobin is abnormal because both parents contribute the abnormal gene.

(c) The trait occurs in 10% of African-Americans. It is rarely symptomatic, although it can cause renal-concentrating problems, spontaneous hematuria, and at high altitude, splenic infarction.

(d) Sickle cell disease crisis presents with severe abdominal, bone, or joint pain, commonly in the back, ribs, and long bones, and often is precipitated by cold, stress, and infection. It mimics embolism, infection, and colic.

(e) Sickle cell disease patients have an increased susceptibility to infection, especially to *Pneumococcus, Salmonella, Staphylococcus,* and *Haemophilus.* Bone and splenic infarction are also common (Table 24-3).

(f) If no infection or other complication is present, treatment of sickle cell crisis is symptomatic and supportive: IV fluids, oxygen, and pain relief.

TABLE 24-3
Organ Damage Seen in Hemoglobin Sickle Cell Disease

Organ or system	Injury
Skin	Stasis ulcer
Central nervous system	Cerebrovascular accident
Eye	Retinal hemorrhage
Cardiac	Congestive heart failure
Pulmonary	Intrapulmonary shunting, embolism, infarct, infection
Vascular	Occlusive phenomenon at any site
Liver	Hepatic infarct, hepatitis secondary to transfusion
Gallbladder	Increased incidence of gallstones caused by bilirubin
Urinary	Hyposthenuria, hematuria
Genital	Decreased fertility, impotence, priapism
Skeletal	Bone infarcts, osteomyelitis, aseptic necrosis of the hip
Leukocytes	Relative immunodeficiency
Erythrocytes	Chronic hemolysis

From Rosen P, et al: *Emergency medicine,* ed 3, St. Louis, 1992, Mosby.

(g) Proper disposition and close supportive follow-up are crucial to the successful management of this disabling disease.

B. Coagulation disorders. The coagulation cascade is shown in Fig. 24-1.

1. Evaluation.

   a. The clinical presentation of patients with coagulopathies may include frank hemorrhage (either internal or external) or dermatologic findings such as ecchymosis or petechiae.

   b. The useful laboratory tests include the CBC and peripheral smear, PT and PTT, platelet count, and bleeding time. Consider fibrinogen levels, thrombin time, clot solubility, and factor levels. Also evaluate the need for selected tests of liver and renal function.

2. Specific disorders.

   a. *Vascular disorders.* Capillary fragility disorders may be idiopathic (thrombotic thrombocytopenic purpura), infectious (meningococcemia), or allergic (drug reaction). The vasculitis may be complicated by thrombocytopenia.

   b. *Platelet disorders.* Usually occurring in women, with mild to moderate bleeding. Epistaxis, menorrhagia, and GI loss are common. The bleeding time is prolonged, and the platelet count can be low, normal, or high.

   c. *Thrombocytopenia* (see also section II, G, 5). Causes include platelet loss (e.g., through massive transfusion), sequestration (e.g., hypersplenism), decreased production resulting from congenital condition or acquired factors (e.g., alcohol, thiazide diuretics), or increased destruction (e.g., idiopathic thrombocytopenic purpura [ITP]).

   d. Coagulation pathway disorders.

      (1) Usually they present as soft-tissue or intramuscular hemorrhage.

      (2) Congenital forms usually appear in men.

      (3) Hematuria and hemarthrosis are more common.

      (4) The bleeding time is normal except in von Willebrand's disease.

      (5) *Evaluation.* The PT and PTT are the basic tests for evaluation of these disorders.

         (a) If the PT is abnormal and the other test results are normal, there is an extrinsic pathway abnormality via factor VII deficiency. The most common causes are liver disease, coumarin use, and vitamin K deficiency.

         (b) If the PTT is abnormal and the other test results are normal, this reflects heparin use or inherited clotting disorder. The factor VIII assay is most important. Two forms of factor VIII deficiency are as follows:

            (i) *Hemophilia A.* This is the result of decreased factor VIII activity. Most of these cases result

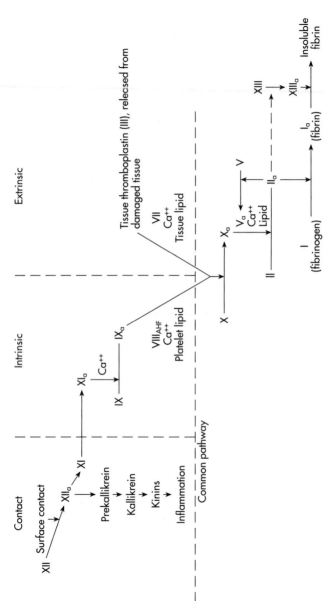

FIG. 24-1 Coagulation pathway. (From Rosen P, et al: *Emergency medicine*, ed 3, St Louis, 1992, Mosby.)

from the sex-linked recessive form, and the remainder appear to be spontaneous. The most common bleeding sites are in deep muscle, joints, the urinary tract, and the CNS. For therapy, see Box 24-5 and Table 24-4. An allergy to cryoprecipitate may require diphenhydramine, 25 to 50 mg IV.

(ii) *Hemophilia B (Christmas disease).* It is clinically indistinguishable from hemophilia A, but much rarer. It is diagnosed by a factor IX assay and treated with a special plasma prothrombin complex (Proplex) using a similar schedule to that for hemophilia A.

(iii) *von Willebrand's disease.* The absence of a specific type of factor VIII activity affects platelet function. It is milder than hemophilia A and usually presents with mucosal and cutaneous bleeding. Factor VIII (antihemophilic factor [AHF]) levels are in the 50% to 60% range. Treatment is with cryoprecipitate or desmopressin.

BOX 24-5
Sample Protocol for Cryoprecipitate Therapy*

OBTAINING CRYOPRECIPITATE

One bag of cryoprecipitate equals 80 units of factor VIII.

Fill out the form as for blood (order in bags), and record the weight of the patient in pounds.

If patient's blood type is known to the blood center, no blood sample is needed. If the blood type is not known, a 10-ml red-topped tube is sent for typing.

If possible, ABO type-specific cryoprecipitate is used. Full crossmatching is not necessary.

After cryoprecipitate has been thawed and pooled, it has an expiration time of 4 hours and must be transfused within this time.

ADMINISTRATION OF CRYOPRECIPITATE

Cryoprecipitate must be administered through a blood filter. If preferred, a platelet concentration infusion set may be used instead of the regular blood filter. This set allows for administration by an intravenous push.

The details for nursing and physician roles in administration may be detailed in this protocol.

From Rosen P, et al: Emergency medicine, ed 3, St Louis, 1992, Mosby.
*Similar protocols may be made for the use of fresh frozen plasma or single-donor plasma.

TABLE 24-4
Dosage of Factor VIII$_{AHF}$

Bleeding risk	Desired factor VIII level (%)	Initial dose (units/kg)
Mild	5–10	12.5
Moderate	20–30	25
Severe	50 or greater	50

Standard calculation

1. Patient's plasma volume (50ml/kg × weight in kg) × (Desired level of factor VIII in percent) − (Present level of factor VIII in percent) = Number of units for initial dose
2. In emergency therapy, the present level of factor VIII is assumed to be zero
3. One unit is the activity of the coagulation factor present in 1ml of normal human male plasma
4. Because the half-life of factor VIII is 8 to 12 hours, the desired level is maintained by giving half the initial dose every 8 to 12 hours
5. Cryoprecipitate is assumed to have 70 to 80 units of factor VIII per bag; factor VIII concentrates list the units per bottle on the label

From Rosen P, et al: *Emergency medicine,* ed 3, St. Louis, 1992, Mosby.

    (c) If the PT and PTT are both abnormal, this reflects a deficiency of the common coagulation pathway. The most frequent cause is DIC, diagnosis of which is based on tests shown in Table 24-5. Treatment depends on whether hemorrhage or coagulation dominates the clinical picture.

        (i) For hemorrhage, administer platelets, fresh frozen plasma, and blood.

        (ii) For coagulation (i.e., fibrin deposition), consider heparin, although its effectiveness varies with the cause. Prompt hematology consultation is advised.

TABLE 24-5
Laboratory Diagnosis of Disseminated Intravascular Coagulation

Test	Finding	Pathophysiology
Peripheral smear	Low platelets, schistocytes, red blood cell fragments	Red blood cell fragmentation on fibrin strands; schistocytes not always seen
Platelet count	Low (usually < 100,000/mm^3)	Consumed in clotting; lower numbers are reflected in bleeding time
Prothrombin time	Prolonged	Factors II and IV consumed
Partial thromboplastin time	Prolonged	Factors II, V, and VIII consumed
Thrombin time	Prolonged	Decrease in factor II and fibrin degradation products
Fibrinogen level	Low	Factor II consumed; may be difficult to interpret because this is an acute-phase reactant
Fibrin degradation products	Zero to large	Dependent on the amount of secondary fibrinolysis
Serum creatinine or urinalysis	May be abnormal	Functional assessment of organ most commonly injured by fibrin deposition

From Rosen P, et al: *Emergency medicine*, ed 3, St Louis, 1992, Mosby.

25

Emergencies in the Patient With Prior Organ Transplant

I. GENERAL CONSIDERATIONS.

A. The immunosuppressed patient is seen with increasing frequency in community EDs. Many have undergone organ transplantations performed at major centers and then return home to their local communities. Emergency physicians need to be familiar with the problems specific to these patients.

B. In general, complications of organ transplantation are of three interrelated types causing similar symptoms: infection, drug toxicity, and rejection.

C. Immunosuppression impairs the ability to fight not only infection but also malignancy. Lymphoma is particularly common, as are cancers of the skin, lip, and cervix.

D. This chapter discusses first the specific immunosuppressive agents, then the broad category of infections encountered because of these agents, and finally specific considerations for the various transplanted organs.

II. IMMUNOSUPPRESSIVE AGENTS.

A. All immunosuppressive drugs increase the risk of infection. Immunosuppression also reduces the inflammatory response, thus often masking the physical signs of infection.

B. **Azathioprine.**
   1. Inhibits both deoxyribonucleic acid (DNA) and ribonucleic acid (RNA) synthesis.
   2. Decreases both humoral and cell-mediated immunity.
   3. Complications: mucositis and malignancy, especially lymphomas.

C. **Steroids (glucocorticoids).**
   1. Inhibit release of interleukins.
   2. Decrease both humoral and cellular immunity.

   3. Complications: GI hemorrhage, osteoporosis, avascular hip necrosis, impaired wound healing, diabetes, cataracts.

D. Cyclosporine.
   1. Inhibits interleukin production by helper-inducer (CD4) cells.
   2. Decreases cellular immunity.
   3. Complications: renal toxicity and malignancies (especially lymphomas).

E. Methotrexate.
   1. Interferes with folic acid metabolism and thus DNA synthesis and repair.
   2. Inhibits lymphocyte proliferation.
   3. Complications: GI, hepatic, renal, pulmonary, and cerebral toxicity.

F. Antilymphocyte antibodies (antithymocyte globulin [ATG] and OKT3).
   1. Prepared in animals, these globulins attack the patient's lymphocytes.
   2. Inhibit cellular immunity.
   3. Complications: fever, chills, headache, hypotension.

III. INFECTIONS IN THE TRANSPLANTED PATIENT.

A. General considerations.
   1. Transplant recipients are susceptible to the same overall types of infections.
   2. More than 80% of transplant recipients develop clinical infection during the first year, especially during the immediate postoperative period, and during episodes of rejection when immunosuppressive treatment is intensified.
   3. As in any immunosuppressed patient, signs and symptoms of infection are often subtle. Fever and leukocytosis may be absent, with fatigue and malaise the only symptoms.
   4. Suppression of humoral immunity leads to acute bacterial infection with extracellular bacteria and some protozoa.
   5. Suppression of cell-mediated immunity causes infection with opportunistic organisms such as intracellular bacteria, fungi, protozoa, worms, and viruses.

B. Organisms.
   1. Bacteria.
     a. Gram-positive: staphylococcus, streptococcus, pneumococcus, meningococcus.
     b. Gram-negative: *Haemophilus, Escherichia coli, Pseudomonas.*
     c. Opportunistic: tuberculosis and other mycobacteria, *Nocardia, Listeria.*
   2. Fungi. *Candida, Aspergillus, Cryptococcus, Histoplasma.*
   3. Viruses. Herpes simplex and herpes zoster, Epstein-Barr, hepatitis B and C, cytomegalovirus.
   4. Protozoa. *Pneumocystis, Toxoplasma, Giardia.*
   5. Worms. *Strongyloides.*

C. Organs infected.
  1. The transplanted organ is of course at risk for infection, particularly postoperatively.
  2. Regardless of which organ is transplanted, the following organs are frequently infected because of immunosuppression: lungs, kidney, liver, and CNS.

IV. SPECIFIC ORGAN TRANSPLANTS.
A. Kidney.
  1. The most commonly transplanted organ. Death is rare because the rejected or infected transplant can be removed, dialysis initiated, and a repeat transplant performed.
  2. Rejection.
     a. Acute: fever, tenderness over graft, renal failure.
     b. Chronic: nephrosclerosis leading to hypertension and renal failure.
  3. Specific considerations.
     a. Cyclosporine is renal toxic and suppresses signs of rejection. Distinguishing rejection from drug toxicity as a cause of renal failure may be difficult.
     b. Hypertension is common in renal failure patients even after transplantation.
     c. Cardiac and cerebral arteriosclerotic vascular disease is accelerated in renal failure patients even after transplantation.

B. Heart.
  1. Cyclosporine has revolutionized cardiac transplantation. Current 1- and 5-year survival rates are 95% and 70%, respectively.
  2. Although more than 2500 cardiac transplantations were performed annually throughout the world by 1989, there are more than 20,000 potential recipients in the United States, with only 2000 potential donors.
  3. Rejection.
     a. Immunosuppression involves lifetime triple therapy with cyclosporine, azathioprine, and prednisone, with OKT3 and ATG often added during the early phase.
     b. Acute: heart failure, dysrhythmias, and elevated lymphocyte count may be clues. Echocardiography may reveal prolongation of isovolume relaxation time, but percutaneous endocardial biopsy is diagnostic.
     c. Chronic: a major long-term survival risk is accelerated coronary artery atheroma resulting from fibrointimal hyperplasia caused by chronic rejection.
  4. Physiology of the transplanted heart.
     a. The transplanted heart is denervated, but the posterior wall and sinus node of the recipient heart are still in place.
     b. The ECG thus reveals two independent atria: a recipient P wave dissociated from the QRS and a donor P wave linked to the QRS, which reflects donor ventricular activity.

    c. The donor heart rate is generally about 100, but both rate and contractility can increase because of circulating catecholamines. Total cardiac output can thus reach about 70% of normal.

  5. Specific considerations.

    a. Lymphoma is common because of cyclosporine.

    b. Heart failure and dysrhythmias may reflect either rejection or MI, which is often a sequela of chronic rejection.

    c. Although partial renervation sometimes occurs, the transplanted heart is denervated—*infarction usually does not hurt.*

C. Lung.

  1. Single lung transplantation is most common, but double lung and heart-lung transplantations are not uncommon.

  2. Arterial circulation through the bronchial arteries is not reestablished during surgery. The lung is supplied by the pulmonary circulation until collaterals develop.

  3. One- and 2-year survival rates are 68% and 60%, respectively, but are rising.

  4. Rejection.

    a. Acute: cough, fever, dyspnea, adventitial lung sounds.

    b. Chronic: bronchitis-type symptoms.

  5. Infection.

    a. Pneumonia is a major risk because of impaired host defenses: diminished cough reflex because the lung is denervated, decreased ciliary action and alveolar macrophage function, and colonization during prolonged postoperative intubation.

    b. Gram-negative bacterial infection is most common, but staphylococcal, community-acquired, nosocomial, and opportunistic pneumonias are also frequent.

  6. Specific considerations. Rejection presents like infection and may be impossible to distinguish in the ED.

D. Liver.

  1. Liver transplantation is now routine; thousands are performed annually in the United States.

  2. One-year survival ranges from 50% for those critically ill at the time of surgery, to 85% in the healthiest recipients. Survival for repeat transplantations is about 50%.

  3. Rejection.

    a. Fever, pain over graft site, increasing bilirubin and liver enzymes, and often leukocytosis.

    b. The same findings may occur with failure to engraft, biliary or vascular obstruction, hepatitis, drug toxicity, or recurrence of original hepatic disease.

    c. Liver biopsy is diagnostic.

  4. Specific considerations. Metabolic derangement may be massive. It is impossible to distinguish the etiology of transplanted liver failure in the ED.

E. Bone marrow.

1. Bone marrow transplantation is performed for one of two reasons.
   a. Replacement of deficient marrow (e.g., aplastic anemia).
   b. Replacement of marrow destroyed by aggressive cancer chemotherapy (e.g., leukemia, lymphoma, breast).

2. Before transplantation, cyclophosphamide is used to totally destroy host marrow to prevent rejection. Donor marrow is then infused intravenously.

3. Rejection. Because recipient marrow is destroyed pretransplantation, immunosuppressive medication is unnecessary unless graft rejection or graft-versus-host disease (GVHD) occurs (see Section IV, E, 5).

4. Infection is a major risk, even more so than with other transplantations.
   a. The recipient marrow has been destroyed, and resistance to infection is totally dependent on successful engraftment of the donor marrow. Rejection therefore causes infection.
   b. Failure to engraft is characterized by failure of new donor cells to appear in the peripheral blood. With rejection, donor cells appear but then disappear. Rejection is usually due to inadequate preoperative recipient marrow obliteration.
   c. After the first year, complete immune competence has usually been reestablished. Because immunosuppressive medication is not used (unlike with other transplanted organs), there is no longer a risk for infection.

5. GVHD.
   a. If the patient survives the initial infection risk, the major complication of bone marrow transplantation is GVHD. Donor lymphocytes attack host tissue throughout the body, particularly skin, GI tract, and liver.
   b. Symptoms: rash, diarrhea, abdominal pain, ileus, and liver dysfunction.
   c. Treatment is immunosuppression as with other transplantations.
   d. Mortality is about one in three for victims of moderate-to-severe GVHD, either from infection or organ failure.

6. Specific considerations.
   a. Infection is the cause of most ED visits by bone marrow recipients.
   b. After the first year, infection may reflect GVHD.

V. IMPLICATIONS FOR EMERGENCY PHYSICIANS.

A. Even seemingly minor infections may be related to immunosuppression and imply a life-threatening potential.

B. Infection, rejection, and drug toxicity may be impossible to distinguish in the ED. A multispecialty team approach is often required.

26

Dermatologic Disorders

I. DRUG ERUPTION.

A. Drugs may cause virtually any type of dermatitis. Skin lesions may even appear after treatment with a drug that has been discontinued if it or its metabolites persist in the system.

B. Treatment begins with discontinuation of therapy with the inciting agent. Itching can be controlled by the application of a drying antipruritic lotion such as calamine or the administration of antihistamines. If the condition is severe, systemic corticosteroid therapy should be instituted such as 40 to 60 mg of prednisone daily until improvement is noted, followed by tapering of the dose. This is most likely to be necessary for severe erythema multiforme, drug-induced toxic epidermal necrolysis, or vasculitis.

II. FEBRILE ILLNESS WITH RASH (Table 26-1).

A. Gonococcal dermatitis.

1. *Appearance.* Lesions, often multiple with a predilection for periarticular regions of the distal extremities, begin as erythematous or hemorrhagic papules that evolve into pustules and vesicles with an erythematous halo and may have a gray or hemorrhagic center.

2. *Management.* Hospitalization is usually recommended.

3. *Treatment regimens.*

   a. Ceftriaxone, 1 g IM or IV every 24 hours, to be continued for 24 to 48 hours after improvement begins. Oral therapy should then be given with one of the following to complete 7 days of therapy:

      (1) Cefixime, 400 mg BID.

      (2) Ciprofloxacin, 500 mg BID (contraindicated in patients under 17 years of age and pregnant or lactating women).

   b. Patients allergic to penicillin or cephalosporins. Spectinomycin, 2 g IM q12h, instead of ceftriaxone.

B. Hand-foot-and-mouth disease. Coxsackievirus infection produces a distinctive syndrome of stomatitis and exanthem involving the hands and feet. The rash is maculopapular, begins

TABLE 26-1
Features of Various Eruptions of Febrile Illness

Eruption	Area of initial involvement	Direction of spread	Other features
Hand-foot-and-mouth disease	Face or trunk	Extremities	Oral lesions
Measles	Forehead or neck	Trunk, extremities	Koplik's spots
Roseola	Trunk	Neck and extremities	High fever
Rubella	Face	Neck, trunk, and extremities	Lymphadenopathy
Scarlet fever	Chest	Head and extremities	Desquamation

on the face or trunk, and spreads to the extremities. Oral lesions are bullae that evolve into erosions. All lesions are painful. Treatment is symptomatic.

C. Lyme disease. Lyme disease is the most common tick-borne disease in the United States, most common in the Northeast, upper Midwest, and Pacific Coast. The infection begins with the rash of erythema migrans (EM; see below) and flulike symptoms, which may progress after days to weeks to a disseminated stage and in months to years to a late stage, which may include cardiac, articular, and neurologic involvement.

1. The diagnosis is best made on clinical and epidemiologic grounds. The most distinctive clinical feature of early disease is EM, seen in 60% to 80% of cases. Usually appearing after 8 to 9 days (range 2 to 28 days) at the site of an infected tick bite, EM begins as a nonpainful, nonpruritic erythematous macule. The lesion expands over days to weeks to attain a well-demarcated annular appearance, with central clearing that produces a target configuration. Lesions are usually larger than 5 cm in diameter, sometimes attaining 50 to 60 cm. They typically resolve 3 to 5 weeks after their appearance but may persist for longer periods. Atypical lesions may be crusted, vesicular, oval, or triangular. Multiple lesions may occur.

2. Treatment of early Lyme disease characterized by EM without neurologic manifestations or carditis should be with doxycycline, 100 mg bid; amoxicillin, 500 mg qid; or cefuroxime, 500 mg bid for 10 to 30 days. Doxycycline should not be administered to children.

D. Measles. Measles (variola) has an onset with fever and malaise. Cough, coryza, and conjunctivitis begin within 24 hours. Koplik's spots (irregular, small, red spots with bluish-white centers appearing on the buccal mucosa) are pathognomonic of the disease. Maculopapular erythematous lesions involve the forehead and upper part of the neck and spread to the trunk, arms, legs, and feet. Koplik's spots begin to disappear coincidentally with the appearance of the rash. Treatment of measles is symptomatic only.

E. Meningococcemia.

1. The severity varies from a mild illness to an acute, fulminant, sometimes fatal infection. Its onset is usually sudden, with fever, chills, myalgias, and arthralgias. A rash develops in three fourths of cases and initially consists of macular nonpruritic erythematous lesions that appear on the trunk or extremities, are 2 to 15 mm in diameter, and blanch on pressure. Petechiae may be present and may coalesce into the large intracutaneous hemorrhages of purpura.

2. Early treatment is imperative. Penicillin G is the drug of choice. Adults should receive 24 million units daily in divided IV doses, and children should receive 250,000 U/kg/day. Chloramphenicol should be administered to patients with penicillin allergy.

3. Household contacts and medical personnel who have had close contact with the patient's secretions should receive treatment with rifampin, 300 mg twice daily for 4 days.

F. Roseola infantum.
A benign illness with a high fever, skin eruption, and a paucity of other physical findings, usually in children 6 months to 3 years of age. The fever typically has an abrupt onset and rises rapidly to 39 to 41° C. The rash usually appears after 2 to 3 days of fever. Lesions are pink macules or maculopapules 2 to 3 mm in diameter and blanch on pressure. The infant may not appear particularly ill despite the high fever. The cause of the illness is infection with human herpesvirus 6. The prognosis is excellent, although febrile convulsions may occur.

G. Rubella.
Rubella (German measles) is characterized by fever, skin eruption, and generalized lymphadenopathy. A day prodrome of headache, malaise, sore throat, coryza, and a low-grade fever antedates the rash, which appears on the face and spreads rapidly to the neck, trunk, and extremities. The appearance is pink-to-red maculopapules that disappear in 3 days. The most severe complication is fetal damage when the illness occurs during pregnancy.

H. Scarlet fever.

1. Caused by a group A β-hemolytic streptococcal infection, the illness has an abrupt onset with fever, chills, malaise, sore throat, and rash. This consists of a generalized papular eruption overlying a hyperemic base that may spare the perioral area. The skin has a rough "sandpaper" texture. There may be erythematous lesions or petechiae on the palate. Desquamation of the involved areas follows resolu-

tion. Late complications include rheumatic fever and acute glomerulonephritis.

2. Penicillin is the drug of choice. For children younger than 10 years old, use 600,000 units of benzathine penicillin and 600,000 units of aqueous procaine penicillin intramuscularly. For older children and adults, the dose of benzathine penicillin is 900,000 units. Patients allergic to penicillin should receive erythromycin, 250 mg four times daily for 10 days.

I. Toxic shock syndrome. Toxic shock syndrome is an acute febrile illness characterized by a rash that is typically a diffuse, blanching, macular erythroderma. The redness may involve the palms and soles and be accompanied by generalized nonpitting edema. The rash may rarely be vesicular or petechial. Accompanying mucous membrane inflammation is common. Pharyngitis (sometimes with strawberry tongue), conjunctivitis, or vaginitis may be seen. As a rule, the rash fades within 3 days of its appearance. This is followed by a full-thickness desquamation, most commonly involving the hands and feet.

1. The syndrome most often occurs in young women using tampons but may also occur in men and children. It has frequently been linked to culture of exotoxin-producing *Staphylococcus aureus.*

2. In addition to rash, toxic shock syndrome is composed of high fever, hypotension, and constitutional symptoms. The onset and progression are strikingly rapid. Criteria require the presence of (1) fever of at least 38.9° C; (2) hypotension with a systolic blood pressure of 90 mm Hg or less, (3) skin rash, and (4) involvement of at least three organ systems. Hypotension is the result of decreased vasomotor tone and leakage of fluid from the intravascular to the interstitial space.

Systemic involvement may produce myalgias, arthralgias, adult respiratory distress syndrome, encephalopathy, renal failure, anemia, disseminated intravascular coagulation, or hepatic or gastrointestinal dysfunction. Headache, muscle or joint pain, alteration of consciousness, vomiting, or diarrhea may be present.

3. Treatment includes IV fluid administration (and vasoactive agents if needed) to maintain BP and urine output. Removal of tampons or treatment of other sources of infection should be undertaken. Antistaphylococcal antibiotic administration is frequently used. Appropriate antibiotics include nafcillin, 2 g IV q4h, or vancomycin, 30 mg/kg/24 hr.

J. Varicella. Varicella (chickenpox) begins with a low-grade fever, headache, and malaise. Skin lesions rapidly progress from macules to papules to vesicles to crusting. Vesicles are 2 to 3 mm in diameter and surrounded by an erythematous border. The hallmark of varicella is the appearance of lesions in all stages of development in one region of the body. The illness is self-limited, and treatment is symptomatic only. The disease is contagious until all vesicles are crusted and dried. Aspirin should be avoided in these patients, since there is evidence for an increased incidence of Reye's syndrome when aspirin is used in the presence of varicella.

III. ERYTHEMA MULTIFORME.

  A. Definition. An acute, usually self-limiting eruption precipitated by a variety of factors (most common factors are drug exposure and herpes simplex infection) and characterized by the sudden appearance of erythematous macules, papules, vesicles, or bullae.

  B. Appearance. The distribution is symmetric, most commonly on the palms, soles, backs of the hands or feet, and extensor surfaces of the extremities. The hallmark is the target lesion (a papule or vesicle that is surrounded by a zone of normal skin and then by a halo of erythema), commonly seen on the hand or wrist.

  C. Stevens-Johnson syndrome. A severe form is occasionally fatal and characterized by bullae, mucous membrane lesions, and multisystem involvement.

  D. Management. Search for an underlying cause. Mild forms resolve spontaneously. Severe cases, including Stevens-Johnson syndrome, require hospital admission for IV hydration and systemic corticosteroid therapy (equivalent of 80 to 120 mg of prednisone daily).

IV. URTICARIA.

  A. A result of immune system activation, urticaria appears as circumscribed raised wheals ("hives") that may be slightly erythematous or display central clearing.

  B. Urticaria can be caused by skin contact, but more often it is a reaction to an ingested or unknown antigen. Almost any drug may produce urticaria, with penicillin and aspirin being the most common. A variety of food and other allergies may also produce urticaria.

  C. The treatment of urticaria involves removal of the inciting factor (when applicable) and the administration of antihistamines and often other agents with antiinflammatory activity.

    1. Histamine$_1$ blockers are the major form of treatment, for example, diphenhydramine (Benadryl), 50 mg IM, followed by 25 to 50 mg q4h or hydroxyzine (Atarax, Vistaril), 50 mg q4h.

    2. Histamine$_2$ blockers are also useful and may be added for severe cases. Cimetidine (Tagamet), ranitidine (Zantac), or similar agents may be used.

    3. Epinephrine, 0.3 mg of 1:1,000 dilution SC, is rapidly effective.

    4. Corticosteroids may be added for significant cases, parenterally in the emergency department, followed by a short course of oral prednisone (e.g., 60 mg for 3 days).

V. FUNGAL INFECTION.

The dermatophytoses ("ringworm") are fungal infections limited to the skin and are characterized by scaling and pruritus. They may involve the scalp, arms, legs, or trunk and classically produce a sharply marginated annular lesion with raised or vesicular margins and central clearing. Lesions should be scraped and examined under the microscope in a potassium hydroxide preparation. Involvement of the intertriginous areas between the toes ("athlete's foot") is common. A number of effective topical antifungal preparations are available (including clotrimazole, haloprogin, miconazole, and tolnaftate), and these should be applied 2 to 3 times daily.

VI. HERPESVIRUS INFECTION.

A. Herpes simplex.

1. Two serotypes of herpes simplex virus (HSV) cause cutaneous infection. HSV-1 affects predominantly nongenital sites (classically the mouth or lips). HSV-2 lesions appear mainly in the genital area. The hallmark is grouped vesicles on an erythematous base. Tender regional lymphadenopathy may be present. Children are more frequently affected with HSV-1 infection than are adults.

2. Genital lesions in the male usually appear on the penile shaft or glans or in the perianal region. In primary cases, fever, malaise, and headache are common. Tender inguinal lymphadenopathy occurs in about half of patients. During recurrences, constitutional symptoms are minimal or absent.

3. The infection is much more severe in the female and may involve the introitus, cervix, or vagina and produce severe pelvic pain, dysuria, vaginal discharge, or urinary retention. Hospitalization may be necessary.

4. Treatment of an initial episode of genital herpes is with acyclovir (Zovirax), 200 mg five times a day for 10 days. Such treatment does not prevent the development of recurrent lesions. Treatment of subsequent recurrence is less effective, but a 5-day course of acyclovir is sometimes helpful if started early.

B. Herpes zoster.

1. Herpes zoster (shingles) occurs exclusively in individuals who have previously had chickenpox and is caused by a reactivation of latent varicella-zoster virus that has been dormant since the initial infection. Pain in a dermatomal distribution may precede the eruption by 1 to 10 days. The rash consists of grouped vesicles on an erythematous base that involves one or several thoracic, abdominal, or facial dermatomes. Although an association with Hodgkin's lymphoma and other malignancies is well known, most cases occur in healthy individuals.

2. Treatment is largely symptomatic, including the administration of codeine-containing analgesics. The administration

of acyclovir, 800 mg 5 times daily for 10 days, is recommended in immunocompromised patients and may be useful in others. Pain that persists after the lesions have healed occurs more commonly in elderly and immunosuppressed patients, may last a number of months, and is often resistant to treatment with analgesic medications. The use of corticosteroids to treat this postherpetic neuralgia is controversial. Prednisone, 40 mg daily for 10 days with tapering, may be administered.

VII. IMPETIGO.

A. A pustular eruption commonly caused by group A streptococci, impetigo begins as 1- to 2-mm vesicles with erythematous margins. When these break, they leave erosions covered with a golden-yellow crust. Postpyodermal glomerulonephritis is a recognized complication.

B. Bullous impetigo is caused by phage group 2 staphylococci. The initial skin lesions are thin-walled, 1- to 2-cm bullae. When these rupture, they leave a thin serous crust.

C. Treatment of localized impetigo should be with application of mupirocin (Bactroban) ointment three times a day. Alternative treatment may include erythromycin, 50 mg/kg/day, dicloxacillin, 12.5 mg/kg/day, or cephalexin, 25 to 50 mg/kg/day. Oral therapy should be used for extensive involvement.

VIII. INFESTATIONS.

A. **Pediculosis.** The diagnosis is made by the identification of louse eggs in the pubic hair. These attach to the bases of the hair shafts and appear as white dots. The patient usually presents with severe itching. Treatment should be with gamma benzene hexachloride (Kwell) or pyrethrum/piperonyl butoxide (RID) shampoo.

B. **Scabies.**

1. Scabies is characterized by severe itching that is usually worse at night. The areas of the body most commonly involved are the interdigital web spaces, wrists, axillae, buttocks, lower back, penis, scrotum, and breasts. Typical lesions are reddish papules or vesicles surrounded by an erythematous border. Secondary infection is common. Close personal contact is involved in transmission.

2. Treatment forms are gamma benzene hexachloride (Kwell) and crotamiton (Eurax) lotion, cream, or shampoo. Clothing and bedding should be treated with boiling or hot water washing.

IX. PEMPHIGUS VULGARIS.

A. An uncommon but potentially fatal disorder of unknown cause, it is a bullous disease most common in men 40 to 60 years old. The typical skin lesions are small flaccid bullae that break easily and form superficial erosions. Any area of the body may be involved. Blisters may characteristically be extended or new bullae formed by applying firm tangential pressure to the intact epidermis.

B. Oral mucous membrane lesions typically antedate cutaneous lesions by several months.

C. Patients with suspected pemphigus should be hospitalized. Treatment with oral corticosteroids in doses of 100 to 300 mg of prednisone or the equivalent should be initiated.

X. SYPHILIS.

A. The chancre is the manifestation of primary syphilis. Chancres usually appear as single lesions but may be multiple. They usually appear on the genital mucous membranes. The chancre is characteristically a painless ulcer about 1 cm in diameter with a clean base and raised borders.

B. There are various cutaneous manifestations of secondary syphilis. Lesions may be erythematous or pink macules or papules, usually with a symmetric, generalized distribution. Pigmented macules and papules classically appear on the palms and soles. Generalized lymphadenopathy accompanies the lesions.

C. The diagnosis of primary syphilis is made by the identification of spirochetes with dark-field microscopy. Serologic tests for syphilis are invariably positive in secondary syphilis but may be negative in the primary stage.

D. Primary and secondary syphilis should be treated with benzathine penicillin, 2.4 million units, by IM injection. Patients with penicillin allergy should be treated with tetracycline, 500 mg four times daily for 15 days.

XI. TOXIC EPIDERMAL NECROLYSIS.

A. There are two forms of toxic epidermal necrolysis (TEN). Both are characterized by the acute loosening of large sheets of epidermis from underlying dermis.

1. One form is associated with *S. aureus* infections (staphylococcal scalded skin syndrome [SSSS]) and is generally seen in children under 6 years old and has an excellent prognosis.

2. The other form is related to the use of medications, infection, or medical illness or is idiopathic. It is associated with a substantial mortality rate.

3. The two conditions are distinguishable by skin biopsy.

B. Treatment of SSSS is with penicillinase-resistant penicillins. IV therapy is with nafcillin, 50 mg/kg daily. If the patient can take oral medications, cloxacillin, 50 mg/kg daily, may be administered.

C. Treatment of nonstaphylococcal TEN includes fluid replacement and the administration of systemic corticosteroids (prednisone in a dosage of 100 to 300 mg daily or its equivalent).

XII. ATOPIC DERMATITIS.

A. Atopic dermatitis is a recurrent condition frequently associated with allergic diseases such as asthma and allergic rhinitis.

B. The skin is dry and lesions scaly, with itching and excoriations prominent.

C. Lichenification (hyperpigmentation, skin thickening, and accentuation of skin furrows) is typical of chronic involvement.

D. The course of the disorder typically involves remissions and exacerbations.

E. Treatment. Dryness is treated by the application of lubricating ointments such as Vaseline, antihistamines, and similar agents for reducing pruritus. Topical corticosteroids (Table 26-2) are the

TABLE 26-2
Medications Commonly Used in Treating Dermatologic Problems

Agent	Adult dosage	Pediatric dosage (mg/kg/day)
Antibiotics		
Dicloxacillin	125-250 mg q6h	12.5-25
Erythromycin estolate	250 mg q6h	30-50
Erythromycin ethylsuccinate	400 mg q6h or 800 mg q12h	30-50
Penicillin V	125-250 q6h	15-50
Tetracycline*	250-500 q6h	25-50†

Agent	Concentration	Applications/day
Topical antifungal agents		
Clotrimazole (Lotrimin)	1%	2
Econazole (Spectazole)	1%	2
Nystatin (Mycostatin)	100,000 U/g	2
Topical corticosteroids		
Betamethasone valerate (Valisone)	0.1%	1-3
Desonide (Tridesilon)	0.05%	2-4
Desoximetasone (Topicort)	0.25%	3-4
Flucinolone acetonide‡ (Fluonid, Synalar)	0.025% and 0.1%	2-4
Fluocinonide‡ (Lidex)	0.05%	2-4
Triamcinolone acetonide (Aristocort, Kenalog)	0.025% and 0.1%	3-4

*Do not use in pregnant women.
†To be used in children over the age of 8 only.
‡Fluorinated agents.

cornerstone of therapy, the ointment form being preferred. Use a fluorinated preparation when involvement is severe (but avoid the use of these on the face).

XIII. CONTACT DERMATITIS.

A. Contact dermatitis is an inflammatory reaction of the skin to physical, chemical, or biologic agents, either irritant or allergic.

B. Treatment.

   1. *Mild dermatitis.* Topical application of antipruritic lotions or cool compresses of aluminum acetate (Burow's Solution).

   2. *Moderate-to-severe dermatitis.* Administration of systemic corticosteroids. Oral prednisone, 60 mg/day for severe cases, and 40 to 60 mg/day for moderately severe cases, should be administered, with tapering begun after 3 to 5 days. Therapy should be continued for 2 to 3 weeks.

   3. Poison oak and poison ivy are particularly common forms of allergic contact dermatitis. In addition to corticosteroids for moderate-to-severe cases, antihistamines are quite helpful, for example, diphenhydramine (Benadryl) or hydroxyzine (Atarax, Vistaril), 50 mg q4h. Topical rather than systemic corticosteroids may be used for milder cases with localized rash.

C. Treatment for acute inflammation.

The application of normal saline or aluminum acetate compresses for 20 minutes every 3 to 4 hours is indicated. Corticosteroid creams may be alternated with wet dressings once the acute inflammatory stage subsides. Reduction of edema is important (diuretics, bed rest, and elevation of the extremity should be used).

27

Environmental
Emergencies

I. THERMAL BURNS.

A. General principles.

1. Burn injuries range from relatively trivial to exceedingly complex.
2. It is important to decide which patient requires hospitalization, what therapy can safely be instituted in the ED, and which patient requires initial procedures before being admitted to the inpatient service or transferred to a burn center.
3. Rigid asepsis (e.g., cap, mask, gown, gloves) should be maintained when treating the patient with a major thermal injury. These wounds are open and subject to contamination.
4. The history should include all details of the accident.
   a. Time and duration of contact.
   b. Location—closed or open space (greater chance of pulmonary injury in a closed space).
   c. Heat source—flame (often deep burn), hot water (less often full-thickness), etc.
   d. Presence of noxious substances—gases, plastics, etc.
   e. Possibility of associated injuries—explosion with shrapnel or glass, motor vehicle accident, etc.
5. The history should also include potentially crucial factors such as preexisting diseases or medications.
6. A complete physical examination is mandatory. Special emphasis should be given to ruling out other injuries.
7. Tetanus prophylaxis should be given if indicated (see Chapter 14).

B. Extent of injury.

1. A rough estimation of the extent and depth of the burn helps determine whether the patient requires hospitalization and IV fluid therapy. Table 27-1 represents a standard technique for estimating the extent of the burn.

TABLE 27-1
How to Estimate the Percentage of Burn

Area	Percentage		
	Infant	Child	Adult
Head and neck	20	15	9
Arms			
Right	10	10	9
Left	10	10	9
Legs			
Right	10	15	18
Left	10	15	18
Trunk			
Front	20	20	18
Back	20	20	18
Perineum	—	—	1
Total	100	105	100

2. The depth of the burn is often difficult to determine. Subsequent infection can convert a partial-thickness wound to a full-thickness one.
3. Superficial burns usually heal with little if any permanent scarring.
   a. First-degree burns involve only the epidermis and are characterized by erythema.
   b. Second-degree burns involve the epidermis and some of the dermis. Blistering and superficial denudation are prominent.
4. Deep burns heal with permanent scarring.
   a. Deep second-degree burns involve most of the dermis. The burned skin may be inelastic and red.
   b. Third-degree burns are full thickness. All layers of skin are destroyed, and scarring is significant. The burned skin is tough, inelastic, and discolored (white or charred). It does not blanch and is anesthetic because blood vessels and nerves are destroyed.

C. Criteria for admission.
   1. If there is any doubt, admit the patient to the hospital. Critical cases should be transferred to a burn center, but only after several IV lines have been established and adequate fluid resuscitation begun.
   2. Outpatient care is appropriate for superficial burns that involve less than 15% of the body surface area in adults and 10% in children.

3. Outpatient care of full-thickness burns less than 2% is reasonable. Patients with deep burns greater than 10% are usually admitted.

4. Other factors that favor admission are extremes of age or involvement of the hands, feet, face, or perineum.

5. Inhalation injuries and electric burns require careful evaluation for admission.

D. Minor burns.

1. Early immersion of the burned area in cool water or the application of cold packs will relieve pain and decrease swelling. Ice should not be applied directly to the skin.

2. The burn should be gently cleaned and debrided of nonviable tissue such as the nonadherent epidermis of already ruptured blisters.

3. Intact blisters generally should not be debrided. Because they are likely to rupture, large tense bullae over joints may be considered for sterile aspiration.

4. First-degree burns can be treated with antibiotic cream. Bandaging is unnecessary.

5. Second-degree burns should be treated with a topical antibiotic and a closed dressing. One common regimen involves neomycin-polymyxin-bacitracin (Neosporin) applied to the burn, with antibiotic-impregnated gauze (Xeroform) over this. The wound should be inspected and the dressings completely changed at 1- to 2-day intervals. Ideally, the patient might apply the topical antibiotic several times a day, although this may be impractical in outpatient therapy.

E. Severe burns.

1. Airway maintenance is vital. Significant burns of the upper airway may require immediate intubation and perhaps eventual tracheostomy to prevent upper airway obstruction from secondary edema.

2. "Pulmonary burns" are thought to be due to chemical injury caused by the inhalation of toxic chemicals. Water vapor in the upper and lower airways usually cools the inhaled gases so that actual thermal injury to the lower airway (lungs) probably does not occur. (A possible exception is steam inhalation, which can cause thermal injury to at least the larger airways of the lung.)

   a. Inhalation injury is suggested by singed nasal hair, soot in the nose or mouth, perinasal and perioral burns, or rhonchi heard on auscultation of the chest.

   b. Inhalation injury may lead to thermal injury to the upper airway or chemical injury to the lower airway, which may eventually cause ARDS.

3. Escharotomy of the chest may be necessary if a dense third-degree eschar restricts ventilation (Fig 27-1).

4. Escharotomy of the extremities may occasionally be required to restore impeded arterial circulation.

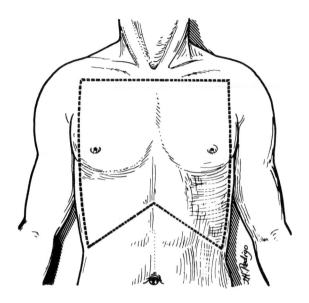

FIG. 27-1 Chest escharotomy.

5. The fluid requirements in a significantly burned patient are enormous. IV lines should be inserted early and resuscitation begun in the ED.
6. Formulas may be used to estimate fluid replacement. It must be emphasized that these are only rough guidelines and care must be individualized.
7. Evidence has demonstrated significant capillary permeability to colloid during the first 24 hours. Initial fluid replacement therefore should be with crystalloid solution. The Parkland (Baxter) formula is recommended.
    a. First 24 hours—Lactated Ringer's solution, 4 ml/kg/percent burn. (Burns greater than 50% are considered 50%.)
        (1) Half the volume over the first 8 hours.
        (2) Half over the next 16 hours.
    b. Such formulas should be used as guidelines only, and patients in shock with unstable vital signs should be resuscitated more aggressively. Maintain a urine output between 30 and 50 ml/hr.
8. Inpatient wound care involves topical antibiotics and periodic debridement.

9. If the patient must be transferred to a burn center, adequate IV fluid resuscitation and airway support (if necessary) should be initiated before transfer.

II. ELECTRIC SHOCK.

A. Injury can result from several mechanisms:
   1. Passage of electric current through tissues.
   2. Electrothermal heat conduction. Most injury is due to this factor.
   3. Massive tetany of the musculature that leads to bone fractures.
   4. Myonecrosis and myoglobinuria from the aforementioned mechanisms.
   5. Ventricular fibrillation or asystole from current passing through the heart.
   6. Asystole secondary to apnea (caused by suppression of the cerebral respiratory center from a current traversing the brain).

B. The skin burn can appear deceptively minor, with massive necrosis of deeper structures initially not apparent. Therefore patients with anything beyond a minor electric burn should be considered for hospital admission.

C. Electrical burns of the mouth in children are usually due to biting an electrical cord or plug. Although such injuries may initially seem trivial, they can quickly progress to massive swelling and airway compromise. Hospitalization should be strongly considered in such injury.

D. The skin burn is treated like any other thermal burn.

E. Underlying injuries must be discovered and treated.

F. If myonecrosis is suspected, the urine should be alkalinized (by administration of IV sodium bicarbonate to maintain urine pH > 8.0) and its volume maintained to reduce the chance of myoglobinuric renal failure (e.g., IV normal saline solution to maintain a urine output of 50 to 100 ml/hr). Osmotic diuretics may be helpful (e.g., mannitol, 0.5 mg/kg 20% solution IV).

G. Lightning causes an electric burn that may produce massive injury or surprisingly little damage.
   1. Because the duration of lightning current is exceedingly brief, lightning often "flashes over" the victim and causes extensive skin damage but relatively little internal injury. Common internal targets, however, are tympanic membranes, eyes, heart, and brain.
   2. Lightning causes death by halting cardiac and brain activity, which leads to cardiac and respiratory arrest. Surprisingly, only one in four patients struck by lightning is killed.
   3. Skin burns from lightning are treated like other electric or thermal burns.
   4. Associated injuries should be sought.

III. HYPERTHERMIC STATES.

A. Hyperthermic disorders fall into four categories: heat cramps, heat syncope, heat exhaustion, and heat stroke. The syndromes may overlap.

B. Heat cramps are due to spasm of the voluntary musculature caused by depletion of electrolytes.

   1. Both salt and water are lost in sweat. The patient with heat cramps has usually replaced the water loss by drinking but has not replaced the salt loss.

   2. Treatment.

      a. Place the patient in a cool place.

      b. Replace NaCl orally with drinks that are high in salt content or IV with normal saline.

C. Heat syncope is caused by vasodilation, often with dehydration as a contributing factor. Orthostatic hypotension is treated with recumbency, cooling, and fluid replacement as needed.

D. Heat exhaustion is a loss of both salt and water; either loss may predominate.

   1. Symptoms include headache, nausea, dizziness, and visual disturbance.

   2. The patient may be moderately febrile.

   3. Use laboratory values to guide the replacement of salt with isotonic fluids or water with hypotonic fluids.

   4. Cool the patient as needed by exposure, fanning, and other methods. If untreated, heat exhaustion may progress to heat stroke.

E. Heat stroke is severe hyperthermia (above 41° C or 106° F) with a loss of heat regulation. The hallmark of heat stroke is CNS impairment. Sweating may be present or absent.

   1. Symptoms include confusion, coma, and seizures.

   2. Fatigue of hypothalamic and sweat gland regulation leads to loss of heat dissipation without dehydration.

   3. Fluid and salt loss varies in severity.

   4. The elderly and infants are particularly at risk. Other predisposing factors are obesity, hyperthyroidism, and drugs such as β-blockers, anticholinergic agents, and diuretics.

   5. Complications may include hyperthermic damage to the brain, liver, kidney, heart, and other tissues.

   6. Treatment is to lower the body temperature rapidly.

      a. Ice packs should be applied to the skin, especially to the axilla, groin, and scalp. Cold water should be splashed on the skin and then evaporated by fanning. A cooling blanket may be helpful.

      b. Iced gastric lavage, cold fluid enemas, and peritoneal dialysis at 10 to 20° C are all effective if logistic concerns can be met.

      c. Immersion in a cold-water bath is generally impractical and interferes with proper monitoring and care.

      d. Shivering must be avoided because it will raise the body temperature. Chlorpromazine, 50 mg IV, may be used to control shivering but may cause hypotension or lower the seizure threshold.

e. Complications may follow, including rhabdomyolysis and myoglobinuria or disseminated intravascular coagulation.

f. Monitor temperature continuously. Discontinue active cooling measures when the core temperature falls to 101 to 102° F.

IV. HYPOTHERMIC STATES.

A. Cold injury may be localized to a peripheral area as in frostbite, or it may be generalized as in hypothermia.

B. Frostbite.

1. Symptoms include numbness, tingling, pain, and burning, which are particularly apparent with rewarming.

2. Examination reveals discoloration, with eventual blistering in severe cases.

3. Treatment consists of rapid rewarming in an agitated water bath at 104 to 108° F (40 to 42° C).

4. It is absolutely crucial to avoid refreezing. If there is any danger of this, it is better to postpone rewarming until a suitable environment can be reached.

5. Wounds should be treated open, with initial debridement of only previously ruptured blisters. Frostbitten tissue is quite fragile and must be handled with great care. Massage is contraindicated. Frostbitten toes and fingers should be gently separated with sterile cotton.

6. Tetanus prophylaxis should be given if indicated (see Chapter 14).

7. In-hospital treatment may include vasodilating medication. Doppler studies may be helpful in assessing deep tissue viability.

C. Hypothermia.

1. Symptoms include progressive shivering, loss of fine motor control, confusion, and coma.

2. Illnesses that predispose to hypothermia include hypothyroidism, hypoglycemia, sepsis, head and spinal cord injury, and acute alcoholic intoxication.

3. Complications can involve dysrhythmias, electrolyte disturbances, pulmonary edema, and paradoxical vasodilation and shock on rewarming.

4. The ECG may show J or Osborne waves, a notching at the end of the QRS segment that is pathognomonic of hypothermia (Fig. 27-2).

5. Treatment consists of controlled rewarming of the central core.

a. Active rewarming of the extremities should be avoided to conserve vasoconstriction until the core temperature is raised.

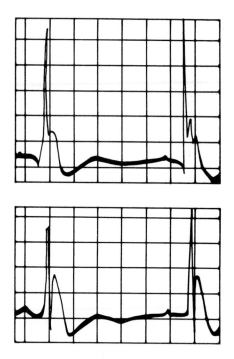

FIG. 27-2 J or Osborne wave in hypothermia.

b. Rapid warming can cause sudden shifts in electrolyte balance and should be avoided (as opposed to frostbite, for which rapid warming is indicated).

c. In mild cases, warmed or electric blankets, heated inspired O_2, and warmed IV solutions may suffice.

d. In severe hypothermia, additional modalities may include gastric lavage, enemas with warm fluid, or peritoneal lavage with isotonic peritoneal dialysate (previously heated through a blood-warming coil to 100° F) at a rate of 2 liters every 20 to 30 minutes. For very severe cases, extracorporeal blood rewarming with a heat exchanger at 40° C may be necessary.

e. A rectal temperature probe is essential for severe cases.

f. After the rectal temperature has reached 86° F (30° C), rewarming should be slowed to a rate not exceeding 2° F (1° C) per hour. A warm-water bath or hydraulic water pad can be used.

g. Dysrhythmias and electrolyte disturbances may occur during rewarming and should be treated as necessary. Ventricular fibrillation or asystole may be refractory to the usual regimens. In such cases, emergency thoracotomy and direct warming of the heart in warm saline may allow successful conversion to a viable rhythm.

h. Severely hypothermic patients may appear dead, with cardiac output and respiration so minimal that BP, pulse, and even heart sounds may not be detected. Because of hypothermic suppression of metabolism, however, many such patients actually recover with little residual deficit. There is wisdom in the old axiom that hypothermic patients should not be considered dead until they are warm and dead.

i. The apparently dead hypothermic victim may thus be alive. The cold heart is extremely susceptible to ventricular fibrillation because of mechanical irritation. Therefore it is often recommended that cardiopulmonary resuscitation not be used in such patients if there are any signs of life unless cardiac monitoring reveals ventricular fibrillation or asystole.

V. DECOMPRESSION ILLNESS (BAROTRAUMA).

A. A rapid decrease in atmospheric or water pressure can lead to inert gases (principally nitrogen) vaporizing out of solution in various parts of the body.

B. Any decrease in ambient pressure can cause decompression illness, including rapid ascent while scuba diving, high-altitude flying with inadequate cabin pressure, or excessively rapid ascent in tunnel workers (caisson disease).

C. Damage may occur in any organ but is particularly common in the lungs, brain, spinal cord, skin, and heart.

1. Nitrogen bubbles may form in the blood and lead to vascular occlusion of any organ.

2. Nitrogen expanding from the dissolved to the gaseous phase may distend cells sufficiently to cause cellular rupture. Fat cells are particularly liable to such damage, which leads to the release of fat into the blood and a subsequent fat embolus to the pulmonary circulation.

3. A similar process may disrupt lung cells, causing pneumothorax or systemic arterial air embolus.

D. Symptoms and signs depend on the organ affected and may range from pruritus and joint pain ("bends") to cough and dyspnea ("chokes") to paralysis and death.

E. Treatment consists of repressurization in a hyperbaric chamber.

1. Care should be taken not to decompress the patient even further during transport. Ground transport is preferred over air transport, if feasible. If air evacuation is necessary, the flight should involve low altitudes in a pressurized aircraft.

2. The patient should be kept at total rest and given high-flow oxygen at 100%.
3. The left lateral, head-down position will reduce the chance of gas bubbles obstructing blood flow through the heart.
4. Specific measures may be required, for example, treatment of dysrhythmias or pneumothorax.

VI. IMMERSION INJURY: DROWNING AND NEAR DROWNING.

A. Hypoxia is the initial, as well as the ultimate, risk from water aspiration.
  1. The immediate response to aspiration is laryngospasm, followed by swallowing of water into the stomach.
  2. Whereas some victims experience continued hypoxia and die from asphyxia, most aspirate additional water as the initial laryngospasm relaxes due to hypoxia and hypercapnia. Stomach contents may also be aspirated into the lungs.
B. Salt water is hypertonic compared with blood, causing additional fluid shift into the alveoli, thereby impairing gas exchange.
C. Fresh water is hypotonic and is rapidly absorbed from the alveoli into the circulation. However, hypotonic water interferes with pulmonary surfactant, causing alveolar collapse and impaired gas exchange.
D. Contrary to formerly held theories, significant hemodilution and hemolysis do not usually occur after absorption of hypotonic water because the amount of aspirated water is relatively small compared with total blood volume.
E. The result of either salt or fresh water aspiration is impaired oxygenation.
F. Additional sequelae may include ARDS, acidosis, dysrhythmias, renal failure, disseminated intravascular coagulation, and hypoxic cerebral damage.
G. ED treatment consists of ensuring adequate oxygenation, with positive airway pressure and endotracheal intubation if necessary.

28

Poisoning, Overdose,
and Envenomation

I. GENERAL CONSIDERATIONS.

A. Poisonings and drug abuse constitute a significant portion of the medical emergencies faced by physicians. About 75% of the cases in the United States occur in children under 5, but 95% of the fatalities are in adults. Poisoning is also common in retarded older children. Suicide and homicidal attempts also result in large numbers of poisonings. Occasional accidental ingestions occur in adults.

B. Household products such as bleaches, polishing fluids, and pesticides are responsible for much of the poisoning in children. The medicine chest and kitchen cabinets are common sources of poison. Studies of poison control centers throughout the United States have shown that more than 1000 different household products have been responsible.

C. In many cases the diagnosis of poisoning or overdose is obvious, and a history of ingestion is easily elicited. In other cases, it is difficult to elicit a history of ingestion or pica. In occasional cases a history of ingestion is never obtained despite clinical and laboratory evidence for poisoning. In puzzling clinical problems for which the cause of the symptoms is not apparent, the possibility of poisoning or overdose should always be considered.

D. Telephone consultation with the regional poison control center may be of assistance in handling toxicologic emergencies.

II. SIGNS AND SYMPTOMS.

A. A large number of symptoms may develop as a result of poisoning, including vomiting, pallor, convulsions, coma, somnolence, burning in the mouth, fever, hyperexcitability, and diarrhea.

B. Physical findings suggestive of poisoning include disturbed states of consciousness, constricted pupils, dilated pupils, cyanosis, abnormal odor of tissues, and increased sweating. The urine may be discolored and the skin stained. The specific symptoms and physical findings often suggest the type of poison ingested.

C. Various clinical syndromes may be helpful in identifying the drug or poison involved.
1. Comatose patients with dry skin, dilated pupils, tachycardia or other dysrhythmias, hyperreflexia, hypotension, and convulsions suggest anticholinergic drug ingestion. Comatose patients with miotic pupils and cardiopulmonary depression suggest narcotic toxicity.
2. Patients with cholinergic poisoning show salivation, lacrimation, sweating, pulmonary edema, bronchoconstriction, bradycardia, miosis, muscular weakness, fasciculation, seizures, and coma.
3. Acute cyanosis and hypotension secondary to methemoglobinemia may be due to nitrate, nitrite, nitrophenol, or nitrobenzene poisoning.
4. Metabolic acidosis with an anion gap may be due to salicylates, methanol, ethanol, ethylene glycol, and isoniazid.
5. Cardiac dysrhythmias may result from cyclic antidepressants (CAs), phenothiazines, cocaine, amphetamines, and cardiac drugs.
6. Nystagmus may occur with sedative-hypnotic drugs and phenytoin. Horizontal or vertical nystagmus is characteristic of phencyclidine (PCP) toxicity.

III. IDENTIFICATION.

A. Although the general nature of the poison may be indicated by symptoms and physical findings, definite identification of the agent is desirable. Examination of the original container for the product is frequently helpful. Containers of most dangerous household chemicals are labeled with a list of ingredients.
B. Often the poisoning substance may not be in its original container. Examination of the remainder of the tablets or pills from the container will often lead to identification of the poisoning compound.
C. A history of peeling lead paint or plaster or other environmental hazards in the home, the industrial plant, or a recreation site should be elicited.
D. Toxicology laboratory.
1. Facilities for clinical toxicologic examination to provide immediate results for certain substances should be present in every hospital dealing with emergencies.
2. Routine urine or serum toxicologic studies should be ordered when appropriate but may be of limited value during the initial ED phase of care. They may take 6 to 8 hours to complete and may not detect the specific ingested agent, that is, a negative result does not rule out intoxication.
3. Determining the salicylate and acetaminophen levels in most possible overdose patients is worthwhile because of the widespread availability.
4. If ingestion of a specific drug is known or suspected, the laboratory may be able to determine not only its presence but also

its serum level. This should be specifically ordered. Among those agents that may be quantified are the following:

Acetaminophen
Salicylates
Carbon monoxide
Digitalis
Ethanol
Iron
Lithium
Theophylline

E. In cases of poisoning, appropriate tests of blood, urine, stomach contents, or vomitus are useful. Direct communication with the toxicology laboratory is helpful with regard to the test required and the urgency of the determination. If a specimen cannot be sent to the laboratory immediately, it should be refrigerated. Preservatives should not be added.

F. A radiograph of the abdomen may show oblong masses (heroin or cocaine in condoms), radioopaque pills, concretions, or liquids. The mnemonic useful for this finding is CHIPES. A negative x-ray does not rule out ingestion of these substances.

C = Chloral hydrate, carbon tetrachloride
H = Heavy metals
I = Iron, iodides
P = Psychotropics (phenothiazines)
E = Enteric coated (salicylates, KCl)
S = Solvents ($CHCl_3$, CCl_4)

G. Examinations such as hemoglobin and hematocrit tests for anemia, determinations for methemoglobinemia, and urine for myoglobin and coproporphyrin may be of value in assessing certain cases of poisoning.

IV. ATTEMPTED SUICIDE (also Chapter 29).

A. Suicide attempts involving ingestion of poisonous substances or excessive doses of medications are common. There is a high frequency of this in adolescents, as well as in older depressed persons. About 50% of adult ingestions are the result of attempts at suicide.

B. In addition to treatment of the poisoning, attention must be given to the psychiatric problems underlying the suicide attempt. Hospitalization is desirable in many such cases. Psychiatric evaluation is essential after the patient has recovered from the immediate effects of the ingestion. If there is suspicion of a homicidal attempt, appropriate legal authorities must be notified. The possibility of child or elder abuse must also be considered.

V. PRINCIPLES OF MANAGEMENT.

A. In the management of poisoning, there are three main principles:
1. The poison may be evacuated and its absorption inhibited if these can be done safely.

2. Supportive and symptomatic therapy should be instituted promptly, including the administration of IV fluids and maintenance of an adequate airway.

3. Any patient with an altered state of consciousness should have a rapid determination of serum glucose, followed by 50 ml of 50% dextrose if hypoglycemia is present. Miotic pupils should prompt administration of naloxone, 0.8 to 2.0 mg, to reverse possible narcotic overdose.

4. If there is a specific antidote for the poison ingested, it should be administered. However, for only a small percentage of poisonings are specific antidotes known (Table 28-1). The availability of a specific antidote does not obviate the need for general supportive measures.

B. Early in the evaluation of each case, a decision must be made about the necessity for hospitalization. Not all cases of ingestion require hospitalization. In doubtful cases, however, hospitalization is the safest choice. Patients with a suicidal risk should be evaluated psychiatrically.

C. A prime consideration is whether evacuation of the stomach is indicated either by the induction of vomiting or by gastric lavage. Evacuation of the stomach is contraindicated in poisonings caused by corrosives such as lye or strong acids. Evacuation is also contraindicated if aspiration of small amounts of the poisonous substance is likely to cause severe aspiration pneumonia. The hydrocarbons are the major groups involved, and recent research has resulted in a more rational approach about when to evacuate the stomach in cases of hydrocarbon ingestion (Boxes 28-1 and 28-2).

D. Many toxicologists think that emptying the stomach is rarely indicated and that instillation of activated charcoal is actually more effective. However, if a decision is made to empty the stomach, the following information may be useful:

1. In most cases of poisoning, the induction of vomiting for emptying the stomach is more efficacious and faster than gastric lavage. For certain drugs (see Section V, E), it may be useful to give charcoal first and then initiate lavage. Vomiting should not be induced, however, in unconscious, stuporous, or seizing individuals or in patients with deteriorating mental status.

2. The initial dose of syrup of ipecac is 30 ml in adults, 15 ml in children, and 10 ml in infants 6 months to 1 year old. The medication should be followed by the ingestion of about 200 ml of water or clear fluids. Vomiting usually occurs within 20 minutes. If vomiting does not occur, the dose may be repeated once. However, the oral administration of additional water is usually more effectual. Syrup of ipecac is relatively ineffective after phenothiazine poisonings because of the antiemetic properties of these compounds.

3. Gastric lavage can be used in unconscious or stuporous patients or if induction of vomiting with syrup of ipecac is not

TABLE 28-1
Effective Antidotes for Specific Intoxications*

Specific agent	Symptoms requiring treatment	Antidote
Acetaminophen (Tylenol; Nebs)	Hepatotoxicity (hepatocellular necrosis)	*N*-acetylcysteine
Anticholinergic agents	Central and/or peripheral anticholinergic symptoms and at least one of the following: Hypertension Hallucinations Convulsions Coma Arrhythmias	
Benzodiazepines	Coma	Flumazenil
Cholinergic agents Physostigmine Neostigmine Pyridostigmine Pilocarpine Bethanechol Methacholine	Cholinergic crisis Diaphoresis Lacrimation Bronchial secretions Excessive urination and defecation Convulsions Fasciculations	Atropine sulfate
Cyanide (potassium cyanide, hydrocyanic acid, laetrile, nitroprusside sodium)	Cyanosis Cardiopulmonary arrest Convulsions Coma	Sodium nitrite Sodium thiosulfate
Digoxin	Major dysrhythmias	Digitalis-specific antibody fragments
Ethylene glycol	Acidosis Oxalate crystals in urine	Ethanol

*See text for dosages.

Continued

TABLE 28-1
Effective Antidotes for Specific Intoxications—cont'd

Specific agent	Symptoms requiring treatment	Antidote
Haloperidol (Haldol) Loxapine succinate (Loxitane) Molindone (Moban) Phenothiazines Chlorpromazine (Thorazine) Thioridazine (Mellaril) Fluphenazine (Prolixin)	Extrapyramidal symptoms: Dystonia Dyskinesia Oculogyric crisis Parkinsonian symptoms	Diphenhydramine Benztropine
Iron salts (ferrous sulfate, ferrous gluconate)	Hypotension Shock Coma (free serum iron present)	Deferoxamine
Methanol	Acidosis Methanol blood level exceeding 20 mg/dl	Ethanol
Methemoglobin-producing agents: Nitrates/nitrites Phenazopyridine Phenacetin	Methemoglobinemia (>30%)	Methylene blue
Narcotic analgesics and related agents (pentazocine [Talwin], propoxyphene [Darvon], diphenoxylate [Lomotil])	Respiratory depression Hypotension Coma	Naloxone
Organophosphate insecticides Malathion Parathion	Cholinergic crisis: Diaphoresis Lacrimation Bronchial secretions Excessive urination and defecation Convulsions Fasciculations Profound weakness Muscular twitching	Atropine sulfate Pralidoxime

---

BOX 28-1

Hydrocarbons: General Indications for Induced Emesis

EMESIS MAY BE INDICATED

1. Ingestion of a large amount of highly toxic hydrocarbon if spontaneous vomiting has not occurred
2. Ingestion of hydrocarbons that contain very toxic additives:
   Halogenated hydrocarbons (e.g., carbon tetrachloride), aromatic hydrocarbons, heavy metals, pesticides

EMESIS NOT GENERALLY INDICATED

1. Low-viscosity compounds for which emesis is of little benefit or increases the risk of aspiration:
   Accidental ingestion of small volumes of gasoline, kerosene, petroleum ether (benzine), petroleum naphtha, naphtha paint thinner, mineral seal oil, mineral spirits, charcoal lighter fluid, furniture polish, oil polish, turpentine
2. High-viscosity compounds unlikely to produce systemic toxicity:
   Asphalt, tar, heavy greases, motor oil, cutting oil, transmission oil, fuel oil, diesel oil, mineral oil, baby oil, petroleum jelly, paraffin wax
3. Ingestion of small amounts of solutions containing 2% to 5% benzene (e.g., gasoline, kerosene)
4. Ingestion of hydrocarbons containing trace quantities of lead

---

Adapted from Rumack BH, editor: *Poisindex,* Englewood, Colo, 1997, Micromedex, Inc.

successful or not indicated. Lavage may be used in semiconscious patients if the gag reflex is present; the patient should be turned onto his or her side. In unconscious patients with no gag reflex, tracheal intubation must precede gastric lavage. Gastric lavage is contraindicated after the ingestion of caustics, ammonia, strychnine, and some petroleum products (see Box 28-1). A lubricated large-bore catheter (larger than 28 French) should be used. Oral gastric intubation in the cooperative or unconscious patient is more effective. Saline can be used for lavage, with instillation and subsequent aspiration of 200-ml amounts of the fluid many times until between 2 and 4 L have been used. In the awake uncooperative patient, a nasogastric tube can be passed nasally and ipecac administered. This tube is inadequate for lavage.

E. Activated charcoal.

    1. Activated charcoal is useful in most types of poisoning. It adsorbs many poisonous compounds and reduces absorption.

Activated charcoal should not be given simultaneously with syrup of ipecac, since it adsorbs the latter. However, the charcoal may be given after vomiting has been induced.

2. Activated charcoal is of no value for binding ethyl alcohol, methyl alcohol, caustic alkalis, mineral acids, organic phosphates, iron, or lithium.

3. The dose of activated charcoal is 1 g per kg body weight. Repeated doses every few hours are recommended for a number of drugs, such as theophylline and drugs that undergo enterohepatic circulation.

F. Catharsis. Cathartics are often recommended, such as magnesium sulfate, 250 mg/kg orally or by gastric tube. Sorbitol is also effective and is often mixed with activated charcoal in a commercial preparation. Repeated doses of cathartic may lead to major dehydration, especially in small children. If activated charcoal is to be repeated, doses after the first should not be mixed with sorbitol.

G. Diuresis and dialysis. Urine output is a good indicator of kidney function, but it may not correlate with the excretion of a drug. In general, drug elimination by renal excretion is independent of urine flow rates. Forced diuresis, often with alteration of urine pH, is useful in certain situations (Box 28-2 and Table 28-2). Dialysis effectiveness depends on a number of factors, including volume of distribution, protein binding, molecule size, and metabolism. Dialysis is indicated for certain drugs (Box 28-3). The value of charcoal hemoperfusion is now clear in certain situations (Box 28-4).

VI. SPECIFIC POISONS AND DRUGS.
A. Salicylates.

1. Salicylate poisoning is common in both adults and children. Salicylates are eliminated primarily by conjugation with glycine to form salicyluric acid. Relative excretion tends to slow as the total amount of salicylates in the body increases. When liver metabolism is saturated, renal excretion becomes the primary route.

2. Symptoms and signs of salicylate poisoning include tinnitus, anorexia, fever, vomiting, sweating, flushed appearance, hyperventilation, delirium, coma, and convulsions. The Phenistix test of urine is useful, as is the ferric chloride test (a purple color after a few drops of 10% $FeCl_3$ are added). The plasma sodium level is usually normal, but the plasma bicarbonate level is usually reduced as a result of hyperventilation. Ketonuria is common.

3. A single serum salicylate level may be misleading, since the level may continue to increase for 6 hours after ingestion. Ideally, a level at 6 hours should be obtained, or at least two samples drawn 1 to 2 hours apart to ensure that the level is not rising.

BOX 28-2
Forced Diuresis

DIURESIS

Hypertonic or pharmacologic diuretics should be given along with adequate fluids. Usual urine flow is 0.5 to 2 ml/kg/hr and with forced diuresis should be 3 to 6 ml/kg/hr. Alkaline or acid diuresis should be chosen on the basis of the drug's pKa so that ionized drug is trapped in the tubular lumen and not reabsorbed. Monitoring urine pH is required.

ALKALINE DIURESIS

This can usually be accomplished with sodium bicarbonate, 1 to 2 mEq/kg IV, and observing for potassium depletion. Administration of potassium chloride may also be indicated. Serum electrolytes and pH must be assessed.

ACID DIURESIS

This may be accomplished with ascorbic acid or ammonium chloride, IV or PO. Serum and urine pH must be followed. Ascorbic acid may be given in doses of 500 mg to 2 g IV or PO as needed to obtain an acid urine (pH of 5.5). PO is less effective than is IV. Ammonium chloride may be used IV or PO at a total dose of 2 to 6 g/day or 75 mg/kg/day in four divided doses. Caution is advised for patients with renal or liver disease.

From Watanabe A, Rumack B, Peterson R: Enhancement of elimination in poisonings, *Topics in Emergency Medicine* 1(3):19-26, 1979, Aspen Systems Corp.

TABLE 28-2
Some Drugs Helped by Forced Diuresis

Toxicant	Type of diuresis
Alcohol	? Effectiveness
Amphetamines	Acid
Bromides	Saline
Isoniazid	Alkaline
Meprobamate	? Effectiveness
Phencyclidine*	Acid
Phenobarbital	Alkaline
Salicylates	Alkaline
Quinine/quinidine	Acid

From Watanabe A, Rumack B, Peterson R: Enhancement of elimination in poisonings, *Topics in Emergency Medicine* 1(3):19-26, 1979, Aspen Systems Corp.
*May precipitate or aggravate myoglobinuria.

BOX 28-3
Dialysis Indications

Immediate dialysis indicated regardless of condition:
    Ethylene glycol and methanol
        If acidotic, start ethanol, then dialyze
Dialysis indicated on basis of condition:

Alcohols	Chloral hydrate	Quinidine
Amphetamines*	Isoniazid	Quinine
Antibiotics	Meprobamate	Salicylates
Barbiturates (long)†	Paraldehyde	Strychnine
Bromides	Potassium	Theophylline

Dialysis not indicated except for support (therapy is intensive supportive care)

Antidepressants (tricyclic and MAO inhibitors also)	Hallucinogens
	Methaqualone
Antihistamines	Methyprylon
Benzodiazepines	Narcotics
Digitalis and related compounds	Propoxyphene
Diphenoxylate	Phenothiazines
Ethchlorvynol	Synthetic anticholinergics and
Glutethimide	belladonna compounds

From Watanabe A, Rumack B, Peterson G: Enhancement of elimination in poisonings, *Topics in Emergency Medicine* 1(3):19-26, 1979, Aspen Systems Corp. MAO, monoamine oxidase.
*Amphetamines respond better to acid diuresis, but if not responding, consider dialysis for severe toxicity.
†While the long-acting (renal cleared) barbiturates are more readily dialyzable than the short (hepatic cleared), dialysis may be helpful if the patient has criteria for supportive dialysis needs (i.e., renal failure, electrolyte imbalance, and hyperthermia).

BOX 28-4
Poisonings Reported Treated With Hemoperfusion

Amanita muscaria	Methsuximide
Barbiturates	Salicylate
Long acting: phenobarbital	Phenytoin
Short acting: secobarbital	Theophylline
Ethchlorvynol	Tricyclic antidepressants

Modified from Watanabe A, Rumack B, Peterson G: Enhancement of elimination in poisonings, *Topics in Emergency Medicine* 1(3):19-26, 1979, Aspen Systems Corp.

4. Serum pH should be determined if the salicylate level is in the toxic range. Metabolic acidosis may be seen, but there may be compensation for this through respiratory alkalosis.

5. Determining the blood salicylate level 6 hours after ingestion and the blood pH is suggested. Levels above 35 mg/100 ml are considered toxic, although there is no good correlation between salicylate levels and symptoms. The level must be evaluated by considering the time elapsed since the ingestion (Fig. 28-1). Toxic doses have much longer half-lives than do therapeutic doses, rising from 4 to 20 hours. Geriatric patients receiving chronic therapy can become poisoned easily when increased doses overload the detoxifying pathways.

6. Treatment.
   a. Vomiting should be induced by syrup of ipecac if ingestion has been relatively recent (e.g., less than 1 hour).

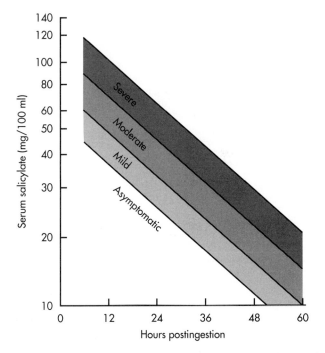

FIG. 28-1 Nomogram relating serum salicylate concentration and expected severity of intoxication at varying intervals after the ingestion of a single dose of salicylate.
(From Done AK: Salicylate intoxication, *Pediatrics* 26:800, 1960.)

b. In significant cases, IV fluids should be started. Elevation of the urine pH to above 7.5 is important, since the reabsorption of salicylate from urine is markedly reduced and excretion of salicylate is greatly enhanced at an alkaline pH.

   (1) IV sodium bicarbonate, 20 to 50 mEq, is given over a period of 5 minutes. If after 10 minutes the urine is not alkaline, an additional 15 mEq is given and repeated every 10 minutes until the urine is alkaline.

   (2) After the urine is alkaline, 10 mEq of sodium bicarbonate per 100 ml of 5% dextrose in half-normal saline is given as a drip at 1.5 to 3.0 ml/min. After a good urinary flow is obtained, serum potassium levels should be monitored and 30 mEq added as needed to each liter of IV fluid.

   (3) Alkalinization of the urine may be difficult to achieve or maintain if insufficient renal tubular potassium leads to preferential reabsorption of hydrogen ion instead of potassium.

   (4) The urine pH should be checked every 30 minutes, and if it is less than 7.5, another 15 to 25 mEq of sodium bicarbonate should be given over a 5-minute period. An indwelling catheter is useful.

   (5) After 2 to 5 hours of treatment, maintenance fluids may be started. In rare cases in which renal failure occurs, hemodialysis or peritoneal dialysis may be considered.

B. Acetaminophen (Tylenol).

1. Overdose with this drug has become more common. It causes severe liver damage because it depletes the glutathione supply. It seldom causes significant symptoms less than 24 hours after ingestion.

2. Clinical course.

   a. Evidence of hepatotoxicity becomes apparent after 2 to 3 days, including right upper quadrant pain, hepatomegaly, and bleeding.

   b. Either uneventful recovery or progressive liver failure ensues, with coma, severe metabolic disturbances, and occasionally death.

3. Treatment.

   a. Obtain a serum acetaminophen level initially and at least 4 hours after ingestion.

   b. If the level is above the diagonal line on the nomogram in Fig. 28-2, start *N*-acetylcysteine administration; load with 140 mg/kg, followed by 70 mg/kg every 4 hours for 18 doses given orally as a 5% solution.

   c. If a significant overdose is suspected and a serum level is not rapidly obtainable, start administering *N*-acetylcysteine

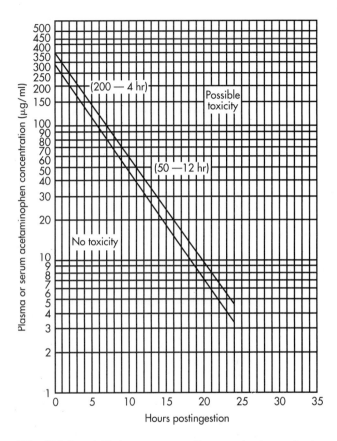

FIG. 28-2 Rumack-Matthew nomogram for acetaminophen poisoning.
Semilogarithmic plot of plasma acetaminophen levels vs. time. *Cautions for use of
the graph:* (1) the time coordinates refer to time of ingestion; (2) serum levels drawn
before 4 hours may not represent peak levels; (3) the graph should be used only in
relation to a single acute ingestion; (4) the lower solid line 25% below the standard
nomogram is included to allow for possible errors in acetaminophen plasma assays
and estimated time from ingestion of an overdose. (Adapted from Rumack BH,
Matthew H: Acetaminophen poisoning and toxicity, *Pediatrics* 55:871, 1975.)

until the level is available. The maximal effect is obtained if
it is given within 10 hours of ingestion.

    d. Give activated charcoal with *N*-acetylcysteine.

C. Psychotropic drugs. Psychotropic drug poisoning is particularly prevalent among adolescents and young adults. In

general, the clinical manifestations are somewhat similar, and treatment is essentially the same, with some specific exceptions. Some of the more common psychotropic drug overdoses are discussed.

1. Barbiturates.
   a. A short-acting barbiturate (e.g., secobarbital, pentobarbital) overdose is most common, and single doses of 2 to 3 g can be life-threatening or fatal. Long-acting barbiturates (e.g., phenobarbital) have a wider margin of safety; single doses of 5 g or more are generally fatal (serum level higher than 120 μg/ml).
   b. The clinical presentation in mild cases includes drowsiness, nystagmus, ataxia, and dysarthria. In more severe cases, profound CNS depression may occur with deep coma, areflexia, hypotonia, apnea, hypotension, and hypothermia.
   c. Treatment.
      (1) The principles of management given in Section V should be followed, with special attention paid to the recognition of rapid deterioration in the level of consciousness and ventilation. Hypotension requires aggressive treatment with fluids and vasopressors if necessary.
      (2) Short-acting barbiturates are poorly dialyzable, and forced diuresis is of little value. Supportive care is important, with dialysis indicated if there is renal failure.
      (3) Phenobarbital is effectively excreted with forced alkaline diuresis (see Box 28-3 and Table 28-2). Hemodialysis is effective for long-acting barbiturate overdoses.
2. Glutethimide (Doriden).
   a. The lipid solubility of this drug makes measurement of serum concentration of almost no value.
   b. The clinical presentation is similar to that of barbiturates, with the additional anticholinergic effects of tachycardia, paralytic ileus, and mydriasis.
   c. Treatment.
      (1) See Section V, and monitor for sudden changes in consciousness and ventilation.
      (2) Hemodialysis is of little or no value.
3. Major tranquilizers.
   a. Clinical presentation.
      (1) Aliphatic and piperidine phenothiazines (chlorpromazine [Thorazine], thioridazine [Mellaril], mesoridazine [Serentil]) produce CNS depression with coma and seizures after the ingestion of large amounts. Hypothermia or hyperthermia can result.

Tachycardia, hypotension, paralytic ileus, urinary tract retention, and cardiac dysrhythmias including ventricular tachycardia can occur.

(2) Piperazine phenothiazines (fluphenazine [Prolixin], trifluoperazine [Stelazine], perphenazine [Trilafon]), haloperidol (Haldol), and thioxanthines (thiothixene [Navane] can produce CNS excitation with agitation, delirium, muscular rigidity, spasm, twitching, hyperreflexia, tremor, and seizures. Other manifestations include impaired temperature regulation, autonomic nervous system dysfunction, and cardiac dysrhythmias. Frank extrapyramidal signs can occur with excessive intake or as a side effect with normal doses.

b. Treatment.

(1) Induced emesis may not be effective because almost all phenothiazines have antiemetic properties. Gastric lavage should be instituted immediately and activated charcoal administered.

(2) Patient assessment must include cardiac monitoring for dysrhythmias.

(3) Hypotension should be treated with volume expansion and, if necessary, α-adrenergic stimulators (metaraminol, norepinephrine). The use of β-adrenergic drugs may cause further hypotension.

(4) Dystonic reactions are treated with IV diphenhydramine, up to 50 mg slowly, or IV benztropine (Cogentin), 2 mg.

(5) Forced diuresis and dialysis are of little value.

4. Lithium carbonate.

a. Toxicity correlates with serum lithium concentrations; levels higher than 2 mEq/L are toxic. Toxicity can follow an acute overdose or chronic use with poor monitoring of serum levels, coadministration of diuretics, restricted sodium intake, or dehydration.

b. Clinical presentation.

(1) Early signs are nausea, tremor, drowsiness, thirst, and muscle irritability.

(2) Severe poisoning produces muscle fasciculation, twitching, rigidity, clonus, hyperreflexia, seizures, hypothermia, obtundation, and coma. The electrocardiogram shows a prolonged Q-T interval and inverted T waves.

c. *Treatment.* Forced saline diuresis with alkalinization of the urine is the most effective therapy in mild cases. In the event of any serious clinical signs, neuropsychiatric abnormality, or a level of 4.0 mEq/L or more at 6 hours, hemodialysis should be considered, even if the patient is asymptomatic.

5. Cyclic antidepressants.
   a. Tricyclic (TCAs): Amitriptyline (Elavil), desipramine (Norpramin), imipramine (Tofranil), nortriptyline (Pamelor).
   b. Tetracyclic: maprotiline (Ludiomil).
   c. Overdose with CAs can present as an anticholinergic syndrome.
   d. After rapid oral absorption, TCAs are widely distributed in body tissues and are highly protein bound, with less than 1% in the plasma even after an overdose. Toxicity is due to the blocked reuptake of norepinephrine, an atropine-like anticholinergic effect, and a direct myocardial depressant effect.
   e. Clinical presentation.
      (1) Primarily with the tricyclic agents, cardiotoxicity is a major cause of mortality and produces myocardial depression, prolongation of His-Purkinje conduction, and dysrhythmias from anticholinergic activity. The latter includes supraventricular tachydysrhythmias.
      (2) The following can also occur: respiratory depression, grand mal seizures, hypotension, hypertension, shock, abnormal tendon reflexes, hypothermia, hyperthermia, choreoathetosis, myoclonus, coma, and death.
   f. Treatment.
      (1) The half-life of CAs in an overdose is greatly prolonged beyond 24 to 36 hours. Serum concentrations correlate with symptoms. Prolongation of the QRS interval beyond 0.12 second is associated with a CA plasma level of 1000 mg/ml, which correlates with severe symptoms.
      (2) Because of delayed GI tract motility resulting from the anticholinergic effect, patients with a major ingestion can initially have relatively minor signs and symptoms of anticholinergic effects.
      (3) Emesis should be induced or gastric lavage instituted after tracheal intubation. Charcoal and a cathartic should be given every 4 hours for 24 hours in mild cases and every 2 hours via nasogastric tube in more severe cases.
      (4) Close surveillance is indicated to look for signs of cardiotoxicity, respiratory depression, and CNS toxicity, with admission to the hospital if necessary.
      (5) Alkalinization of plasma is the principal treatment of CA toxicity and is usually effective in reversing dysrhythmias; use IV sodium bicarbonate, 1 to 2 mEq/kg, to raise the plasma pH to 7.50. Ventilated patients can be alkalinized by hyperventilation.
      (6) Lidocaine is indicated when life-threatening ventricular dysrhythmias fail to respond to alkalinization. Use

1 mg/kg IV as a bolus, and a constant infusion at 3 to 4 mg/min is indicated.

(7) Phenytoin may be effective if lidocaine is ineffective. The adult dose is 1 g IV at 50 mg/min, and for children, 10 mg/kg.

(8) Propranolol is indicated for refractory ventricular dysrhythmias. The adult dose is 1 mg/min to a maximum of 5 mg. The pediatric dose is 0.01 mg/kg IV. Occasionally, this may aggravate conduction disturbances and depress myocardial contractility.

(9) Cardiac pacing may be necessary.

(10) Hypotension requires IV fluids and, if necessary, phenylephrine (Neo-Synephrine), 2 to 4 µg/min.

(11) Diazepam or lorazepam, 0.1 mg/kg, is indicated for seizures (see Chapter 21).

(12) Dialysis or hemoperfusion is not beneficial.

6. PCP.

a. PCP, which is easily made in home laboratories, is one of the most dangerous street drugs available. It is sold under many names and in many forms, and it is often combined with other drugs. PCP is a dissociative anesthetic with sympathomimetic and hallucinogenic properties. Its rapid onset of action, enteric recirculation, and affinity for adipose tissue make treatment difficult. Close observation and the availability of toxicologic studies are important.

b. Clinical presentation.

(1) Low-dose intoxication is often an unpredictable state resembling drunkenness. Disorientation, agitation, and sudden rage are common. Mutism; ataxia; diminished response to painful stimuli; and intermittent horizontal, vertical, or rotatory nystagmus are characteristic. Catatonic rigidity or myoclonus with muscle rigidity on stimulation may occur, as can flushing, diaphoresis, facial grimacing, hypersalivation, and vomiting. Death in this setting is usually due to accidents, especially drowning, fire, automobile accidents, and police encounters with violent subjects who are anesthetized to pain.

(2) High-dose intoxication often induces coma lasting hours to days. The person is unresponsive to pain. Respiratory depression, hypertension, and tachycardia occur, occasionally producing cardiac failure, hypertensive encephalopathy, or intracerebral hemorrhage. Intense muscle rigidity, opisthotonos, and decerebrate rigidity can be found with myoclonus and generalized tonic-clonic seizures. Hyperthermia and rhabdomyolysis are also possible. As the plasma level falls, symptoms of low-dose toxicity appear.

c. Treatment.
   (1) Low-dose intoxication.
       (a) An atmosphere of minimal stimulation is ideal while the patient is observed.
       (b) A patient's stomach should be emptied only when a large overdose or mixed-drug ingestion is suspected.
       (c) Violent patients may require IV diazepam or IM or IV haloperidol, 5 to 10 mg, if an antipsychotic agent is indicated.
   (2) High-dose intoxication.
       (a) If endotracheal intubation is necessary, it should be done very carefully because of the high risk of laryngospasm, pharyngeal hypersecretion, and aspiration.
       (b) Gastric lavage is followed by charcoal, 1 g/kg, and repeated every 2 to 4 hours. Cathartics and continuous nasogastric suction may be useful.
       (c) IV diazepam, 2 to 5 mg, is indicated to control excessive muscle activity and seizures. Neuromuscular blocking agents may be necessary if muscular relaxation cannot be induced.
       (d) Mannitol should be administered if myoglobinuria is detected.
       (e) Brisk diuresis with IV furosemide, 40 mg, and acidification using ascorbic acid, 1 to 2 mg/L of IV fluid, promotes excretion of phencyclidine but may worsen myoglobinuric damage (see Box 28-2).
       (f) Cooling measures are indicated for hyperthermia.
       (g) Hypertensive crises respond to sodium nitroprusside, starting at 3 μg/kg/min.
       (h) In massive overdoses, ammonium chloride (2.75 mEq/kg in a 1% to 2% solution of saline given IV every 6 hours) may be indicated. Blood gases, pH, serum electrolytes, and ammoniac levels must be monitored.
       (i) PCP psychosis may mimic or reactivate classic schizophrenia (see Chapter 29). Hospitalization and treatment with antipsychotic drugs may be required.

D. Opiates.
   1. Clinical presentation.
      a. Miosis is present, and altered level of consciousness may range from drowsiness to coma, with shallow to absent respiration or cyanosis. IV track marks may be visible.
      b. Pulmonary edema with a normal-size heart on chest radiograph can occur.

2. Treatment.
   a. Institute airway management as needed.
   b. Administer 0.8 to 2 mg naloxone IV. This may be repeated if clinically indicated. A continuous IV infusion may be needed (see below).
   c. If IV access is unavailable, naloxone can be given IM or SC.
   d. Application of restraints before the administration of naloxone may prevent an agitated patient emerging from an overdose from injuring himself or herself or medical personnel.
   e. Pulmonary edema is treated with oxygen and positive-pressure ventilation. Digitalis, diuretics, and phlebotomy are not usually indicated.
   f. Careful observation for clinical relapse is necessary, since the duration of action of naloxone is about 45 minutes and opiate toxicity may reappear. A continuous IV infusion of naloxone may be required. Alternatively, administer nalmefene (Revex), a longer-acting narcotic antagonist, 0.5 mg/70 kg IV. If needed, a second dose of 1.0 mg/kg should be administered.

E. Digitalis.

1. Signs and symptoms of digitalis toxicity depend on the chronicity of the intoxication.
   a. *Acute overdose.* Nausea, vomiting, hyperkalemia, and atrioventricular block are common.
   b. *Chronic intoxication.* Weakness, visual disturbances, ventricular dysrhythmias, and hypokalemia are common.
2. Drug levels: Serum levels should be obtained, but these correlate better with severity of chronic intoxication than with acute ingestion.
3. Treatment.
   a. Monitor the cardiac rhythm, and treat dysrhythmias as indicated (see Chapter 15).
   b. Treat hypokalemia, if present.
   c. Digoxin-specific antibody FAB fragments (Digibind) should be administered for life-threatening dysrhythmias or hyperkalemia.

F. Caustic ingestion.

1. Lye and other caustic materials are used in many households for cleaning drains and similar functions. Caustic or corrosive substances, including Clinitest tablets, may be ingested accidentally by children or purposely by suicidal adults.
2. Burns may be noted on the lips and in the mouth and throat. Excessive salivation may be present. The patient should be hospitalized. The development of esophageal stenosis and stricture is a major risk.
3. Arrangement should be made for esophagoscopy to determine the presence and extent of the lye burn in the esophagus.

4. Management of ammonium hydroxide and permanganate ingestion is similar to that of lye. Bleach, however, almost never causes esophageal burns, and esophagoscopy is rarely indicated.

5. Alkaline battery ingestion can cause mechanical GI tract obstruction and chemical burn. Most pass uneventfully, and periodic surveillance radiographs are required. A stuck or split battery requires removal by endoscopy or surgery.

G. Poisoning with kerosene and related hydrocarbons.

1. Kerosene and other compounds that contain hydrocarbons are common causes of poisoning in young children. Products frequently involved are furniture polish, turpentine, lighter fluid, and benzene. A history of ingestion is usually elicited. These children may develop pneumonia, pneumonitis, and pulmonary edema. The hydrocarbon may be the vehicle for other drugs, for example, organophosphates, and thus there may be additional symptoms.

2. Hydrocarbon ingestion signs and symptoms usually include choking and gagging, cough, nausea, characteristic breath odor, fever, weakness, and CNS depression. A chest roentgenogram may reveal pulmonary infiltration.

3. Treatment.
   a. In this type of poisoning, decisions regarding gastric lavage are based on the viscosity, surface tension, and volatility of the substance ingested. When the risks of toxicity outweigh those of aspiration, lavage is indicated (see Box 28-1).
   b. It may be necessary to administer oxygen, high humidity, and IV fluids.

H. Organophosphate poisoning.

1. Organophosphates are commonly used as insecticides, and both are a common and important source of poisoning in children and adults. Among the organophosphates are malathion, parathion, tetraethylpyrophosphate (TEPP), and octamethyl pyrophosphoramide (OMPA). These compounds may be ingested, inhaled, or absorbed through the skin or eye. They inactivate acetylcholinesterase and cause an accumulation of acetylcholine.

2. Symptoms include blurred vision, headache, profuse sweating, abdominal cramping, nausea, and vomiting. Respiratory distress, convulsions, cyanosis, shock, or coma may develop.

3. *Physical examination.* Miosis is usually present, although mydriasis may develop terminally.

4. Mental confusion, muscular incoordination, and areflexia are common.

5. A history of exposure to an organophosphate pesticide 6 hours or less before the onset of symptoms can usually be elicited.

6. Treatment.
   a. Gastric lavage should be used, activated charcoal instilled, and a cathartic administered if the pesticide has been ingested.

  b. Skin and clothing should be decontaminated promptly. Use tincture of green soap if available.
  c. If there is respiratory difficulty, maintenance of an adequate airway is essential, and assisted respiration may become necessary.
  d. Anticonvulsants may be indicated (see Chapter 21).
 7. A specific antidote for organophosphate poisoning is IV atropine. The dose is 0.05 mg/kg slowly every 10 to 30 minutes to ensure atropinization (decreased bronchial secretions). For adults, give 2 to 5 mg slowly, and repeat every 10 to 30 minutes to maintain atropinization (decreased bronchial secretions). Very large total doses may be required.
 8. Pralidoxime (Protopam Chloride) is given after atropine. This drug reactivates cholinesterase. For adults, give 1 g IV (500 mg/min). Repeat every 8 to 12 hours for three doses if muscle weakness persists. For children, give 25 to 50 mg/kg IV, and repeat every 8 to 12 hours for three doses if muscle weakness persists.

I. Heavy metals.

 1. Lead poisoning.
   a. Lead poisoning occurs primarily among children 12 to 36 months old in urban areas, and in adults through industrial exposure. In children, there may be a history of ingestion of paint chips.
   b. Industrial exposure may occur in various occupations, including demolition workers, pigment makers, foundry workers, and welders.
   c. Findings include vomiting, ataxia, change in personality, anorexia, constipation, anemia, incoordination, lethargy, apathy, convulsions, and stupor.
   d. Diagnosis.
     (1) Roentgenograms of the abdomen often show radioopaque material in the stomach. In chronic cases, films of the long bones reveal "lead lines"—areas of increased density at the metaphyses.
     (2) Microcytic or normocytic anemia is usually present in chronic cases, and in some cases basophilic stippling may be seen in erythrocytes.
     (3) Coproporphyrin is found in the urine in most patients.
     (4) The best test for the diagnosis of lead poisoning is the whole blood lead level. A blood lead level higher than 50 μg/100 ml indicates significant exposure. A level above 60 μg/100 ml indicates lead poisoning.
   e. Rapid deterioration may occur, and prompt treatment is therefore essential. Most children with lead poisoning should be hospitalized.
     (1) Urine flow is established by the administration of 10% dextrose in water in a dose of 10 to 20 ml/kg

over a period of 2 hours. Fluids are then continued on a maintenance basis so that the urine output ranges between 350 and 500 ml/day. Overhydration is dangerous in persons with lead poisoning and may induce seizures.

(2) Shortly after the urinary flow is established, dimercaprol (BAL) is given IM in a dose of 4 mg/kg. Four hours later the dose of dimercaprol is repeated, and calcium disodium edathamil (CaEDTA) in a dose of 12.5 mg/kg is also given IM. A small amount of procaine added to the CaEDTA will reduce local pain. Dimercaprol and CaEDTA are then administered every 4 hours for 5 days. If convulsions occur, anticonvulsants may be given (see Chapter 21).

(3) If severe cerebral edema develops, IV mannitol, 20% solution, may be administered at an initial dose of 3 ml/kg, and dexamethasone (Decadron), 20 mg, should be administered IV immediately and followed by 10 mg every 4 hours over a period of 24 hours (in adults).

(4) Respiratory arrest is a constant threat, and preparations should be made for resuscitation and assisted ventilation if they become necessary.

2. Iron poisoning.
   a. Iron poisoning is common in young children. Tablets that contain iron, particularly ferrous sulfate, are often mistaken for candy by children. Occasionally poisoning may occur from liquid preparations that contain iron. A history of ingestion can usually be elicited.
   b. The symptoms and signs include vomiting, abdominal pain, pallor, diarrhea, and dehydration. Acidosis and shock may develop.
   c. The toxicity of iron poisoning is dependent on the amount of elemental iron ingested.
   d. The following measures are indicated:
      (1) Gastric lavage is of doubtful efficacy. Activated charcoal does not adsorb iron and is not recommended.
      (2) Blood should be drawn for serum iron content and iron-binding capacity. Patients ingesting adult iron preparations need levels determined at least 4 to 6 hours after ingestion. For pediatric preparations, levels determined at 2 hours postingestion are adequate.
      (3) A radiograph of the abdomen should be taken. Iron-containing tablets are radioopaque and can often be seen in the roentgenogram.
      (4) Deferoxamine should be administered IV or IM for levels above 500 μg/dl and for levels above 350 μg/dl if there are clinical signs of toxicity. Administer 10 to 15 mg/kg/hr by constant IV infusion. The recom-

mended maximum daily dose is 6 g. The end point in therapy is the resolution of rose-colored urine, resolution of clinical symptoms of intoxication, or serum iron level less than 350 μg/dl. Deferoxamine can cause hypotension, and careful monitoring is essential.

(5) All urine should be collected, and any color change after administration of the drug should be noted. Red indicates a heavy excretion of iron and the need for additional deferoxamine. If the urine does not change color or it returns to a normal color, therapy may be discontinued.

(6) Symptomatic therapy should be carried out as indicated. Occasionally treatment for shock is necessary. The chelation therapy with deferoxamine is effective only if there is good urinary output. If severe oliguria or anuria develops, dialysis should be considered to remove the iron chelate.

(7) In rare cases when iron levels are greater than 1000 μg/dl, the risk of massive liver damage necessitates the consideration of exchange transfusion and endoscopic or surgical removal of aggregated iron pills in the stomach.

3. Mercury poisoning.
   a. Metallic mercury is not absorbed and does not cause mercury poisoning. Mercury salts, however, are extremely toxic.
   b. *Symptoms.* Throat and esophageal lesions develop, and there may be abdominal pain, vomiting, bloody diarrhea, and signs of renal failure.
   c. Therapy includes copious lavage after a protein-containing food such as milk or raw egg has been introduced into the stomach.
      (1) Between 15 and 30 ml of magnesium sulfate may be administered in 6 oz of milk. Activated charcoal (1 g/kg) should follow.
      (2) The major therapy is dimercaprol, which is administered in a dose of 3 mg/kg every 4 hours for six times for a 2-day period, then in a dose of 3 mg/kg every 6 hours for four times, and subsequently in a dose of 3 mg/kg every 12 hours for 2 days. In less severe cases, a smaller dose may be used.
      (3) Urinalysis should be performed daily and the BUN level monitored.

J. Noxious gases.
   1. Several noxious gases are toxic to humans. The major gases are carbon monoxide (CO), carbon disulfate, hydrogen sulfide, cyanide, and the products of fire damage to plastic and other synthetic materials.

2. Hydrogen sulfide and carbon disulfide.
   a. These gases are found in petroleum refineries, tanneries, mines, and rayon factories.
   b. Clinical presentation.
      (1) Slight exposure causes skin and eye irritation, nausea and vomiting, headache, dysphagia, and stupor.
      (2) Extensive exposure causes nausea and vomiting, blurred vision, coma, pulmonary edema, and respiratory paralysis.
   c. Treatment.
      (1) Administer 100% oxygen.
      (2) Follow the principles of management given in Section V.
      (3) Administer amyl nitrite and sodium nitrite as outlined below for cyanide poisoning.
      (4) Reduce the sensory input to the patient to avoid precipitating convulsions.
3. Carbon monoxide: see Chapter 17.
4. Cyanide.
   a. Cyanide is widespread in our environment, for example, in fertilizer, synthetic rubber, metal-cleaning solutions, fruit seeds, and medications. Its toxicity is due to inhibition of the cytochrome oxidase system.
   b. Clinical presentation.
      (1) Ingestion or inhalation of large amounts causes immediate unconsciousness, convulsions, and death within 1 to 15 minutes.
      (2) Ingestion, inhalation, or skin absorption of smaller amounts causes dizziness, tachypnea, drowsiness, hypotension, tachycardia, and unconsciousness.
      (3) Usually convulsions followed by death occur within 4 hours with all cyanide derivatives except sodium nitroprusside, which may cause death as late as 12 hours after ingestion.
   c. Treatment.
      (1) Administer 100% O_2.
      (2) Start amyl nitrate inhalation, 1 ampule every 5 minutes. Stop only if the patient is hypotensive.
      (3) Delay gastric lavage until an antidote is given.
      (4) Immediately give sodium nitrite, 3% solution IV at 2.5 to 5 ml/min, stopping only for severe hypotension. Read the cyanide kit package insert for dosage details.
      (5) After sodium nitrite, give sodium thiosulfate, 25% solution IV at 2.5 to 5 ml/min.
      (6) Nitrite and nitrate administration produces methemoglobin, which combines with cyanide to form cyanmethemoglobin. Thiosulfate converts cyanide to thiocyanate, which is excreted in the urine.

5. Arsenic and arsine gas.
   a. Arsenic is found in ant poisons, insecticides, weed killers, paint, and medicines. Arsine gas is formed when acid acts on metals in the presence of arsenic. Arsenic and arsine appear to cause toxicity by combining with sulfhydryl enzymes and interfering with cellular metabolism.
   b. Clinical presentation.
      (1) Massive ingestion leads to violent gastroenteritis, with burning esophageal pain, vomiting, and watery or bloody diarrhea. Shock follows, with convulsions and coma as terminal signs. Smaller doses cause nausea and vomiting, cramps, and variable paralysis. Ventricular dysrhythmias can occur.
      (2) Inhalation of arsenic dust can induce acute pulmonary edema.
      (3) Inhalation of arsine gas causes hemolysis.
   c. Laboratory findings.
      (1) In arsenic poisoning, proteinuria, hematuria, and cylindruria occur. In arsine gas inhalation, hemoglobinuria may be present.
      (2) Arsenic compounds may appear as bariumlike radioopaque material in the GI tract.
      (3) Massive toxicity correlates with blood levels in a range of 0.1 to 1.5 mg/dl.
   d. Treatment.
      (1) Follow the principles of management given in Section V.
      (2) Give dimercaprol, 3 to 4 mg/kg every 4 hours for the first 2 days, then 3 mg/kg every 12 hours for a total of 10 days. If dimercaprol causes severe nausea and sweating, use ephedrine or diphenhydramine.

K. Methanol and ethylene glycol.

1. Methanol (methyl alcohol, wood alcohol) and ethylene glycol are found in antifreeze, paint remover, shellac, varnish, and denatured alcohol. For unexplained reasons, preparations with denatured methanol often cause toxicity greater than that expected from the methanol concentration.
2. The toxicity of methanol is due to the metabolism of methyl alcohol to formic acid and formaldehyde, which are toxic to most major organs, especially retinal cells. Ethylene glycol toxicity is due to its metabolism to calcium oxalate, formic acid, and other metabolites.
3. Clinical presentations.
   a. Mild and moderate acute poisoning produces headache, nausea, vomiting, and blurred vision; the severity depends on the dose.
   b. Severe acute poisoning causes the progression of these symptoms to cyanosis, tachypnea, hypotension, and

coma. Papilledema and mydriasis are present. Severe metabolic acidosis occurs and is often fatal. Urinalysis shows crystals and ketones.

c. Evaluation of serum osmolality and electrolytes is very helpful when toxicity with these substances is suspected.
    (1) Serum osmolality calculations.
        (a) Calculated serum osmolality =
$$2 \times Na + \frac{BUN}{2.8} + \frac{glucose}{18}.$$
        (b) Osmolal gap = measured osmolality − calculated osmolality.
        (c) Normal = <10 mOsm/kg.
        (d) These solutes increase the osmolal gap, and their molecular weights can be used to estimate blood concentrations.

Alcohol	Molecular weight
Ethanol	46
Isopropanol	60
Ethylene glycol	62
Methanol	32

        (e) Estimated blood concentration in mg/dl =
$$osmol\ gap \times \frac{molecular\ weight}{10}.$$
    (2) Electrolyte calculations.
        (a) Anion gap = Na − (Cl + HCO$_3$).
        (b) Normal = <12 mEq/L.
        (c) An elevated anion gap is usually due to one of the following (A MUDPIE):
            A = Aspirin
            M = Methanol
            U = Uremia
            D = Diabetic ketoacidosis
            P = Paraldehyde or phenformin
            I = Idiopathic lactic acidosis, iron, or isoniazid
            E = Ethanol or ethylene glycol

4. Treatment.
    a. Immediately institute the principles of management given in Section V, and add sodium bicarbonate (20 g/L) to the lavage fluid. Do not give activated charcoal if oral ethyl alcohol is to be used.
    b. Administer ethyl alcohol, 1 to 1.5 ml/kg orally (50%) or IV (10%) initially and 0.5 to 1 ml/kg every 2 hours for as long as 4 days. Ethyl alcohol reduces methanol toxicity by inhibiting the metabolism of methanol to formaldehyde and formic acid. Check the blood level often enough to keep the blood ethanol level between 100 and 200 mg/dl.

    c. Aggressively treat the metabolic acidosis.

    d. Carefully monitor serum glucose levels in children because ethanol-induced hypoglycemia is much more common than in adults.

    e. Hemodialysis should be considered when the blood methanol level is higher than 50 mg/100 ml.

VII. ANIMAL VENOMS.

A. General considerations.

1. Animal venoms are mixtures of many different substances that may produce several different toxic reactions in humans.
2. Few venoms are specific to one organ; some have an effect on almost every organ. Occasionally, the patient may release pharmacologic substances that increase the poison's severity.
3. Venom composition depends on how the animal uses the toxin. Mouth venoms are offensive and are intended to immobilize prey; they often contain lethal factors. Tail venoms are defensive and are intended to drive away predators; the venom is less toxic and destroys less tissue.

B. Snakebite.

1. The majority of poisonous snakes are pit vipers, and in the United States they are rattlesnakes, copperheads, and cottonmouths. Coral snakes, a small but dangerous group, are found mainly in the southern and southwestern states (Fig. 28-3).
2. Identification and clinical presentation.

    a. Pit vipers.

        (1) Identification of the snake is made by noting the facial pit, the vertical elliptic pupils of the eye, a single row of subcaudal scales, and a triangular head.

        (2) Clinical presentation.

            (a) Initial symptoms are one or more fang marks, burning, mild pain, and progressive local swelling. If paresthesia, perioral tingling and numbness, or facial muscle fasciculations occur, significant envenomation has occurred.

            (b) Although swelling will progress very rapidly throughout the limb without treatment, it usually occurs slowly over 8 to 36 hours. Tissue destruction and tissue hemorrhage occur variably, depending on the species.

            (c) Death may be caused by hypovolemic shock and pulmonary edema. Severe coagulopathy may occur within 6 hours. Occasionally neuromuscular toxins cause respiratory failure.

    b. Coral snakes.

        (1) Identification of the snake is by the three-color ring pattern; snakes with red zones bordered by yellow or white are venomous, and those with red zones bordered by black are nonvenomous.

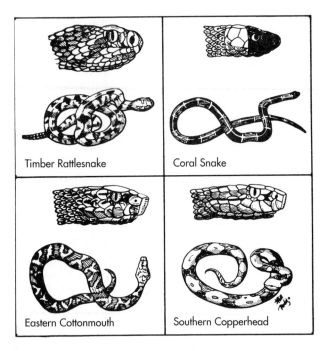

Timber Rattlesnake

Coral Snake

Eastern Cottonmouth

Southern Copperhead

FIG. 28-3 Some venomous snakes found in the United States.
(From *Emergency management of poisonous snakes,* Chicago, 1981, American College of Surgeons.)

    (2) Clinical presentation.
        (a) Early signs within 4 hours include tremors, drowsiness, euphoria, and marked salivation.
        (b) After 5 to 10 hours, cranial nerve involvement leads to slurred speech, ocular muscle palsies, fixed miotic pupils, ptosis, dysphagia, and dyspnea. Survival past 24 hours is a favorable prognostic sign.
  3. Management.
    a. First aid, although important, should not delay transportation to a hospital. If medical care is available within a few hours, the only care in the field is patient immobilization and prompt transportation. If care is more than 3 to 4 hours away and if envenomation is certain, then reassurance, the application of a lymphatic tourniquet immedi-

ately, incision and suction within 30 minutes of the bite (controversial), immobilization, and rapid transportation, preferably on a stretcher, are the most useful measures. If possible, keep the limb level with the heart. Kill the snake, if possible to do so safely, for identification.

b. Perform a complete clinical evaluation and order baseline laboratory studies, CBC, a blood type and crossmatch, PT, PTT, platelet count, urinalysis, and determinations of the levels of blood sugar, BUN, and electrolytes. For severe bites, consider ordering tests for fibrinogen, red cell fragility, clotting time, and clot retraction time. Administer tetanus prophylaxis if more than 5 years has elapsed since last tetanus toxoid.

c. The degree of envenomation must be assessed, and 6 hours of observation is necessary to avoid underassessing severe envenomation.

(1) *Minimal envenomation (Grades O-I).* Local symptoms and signs, few systemic signs and symptoms, and minimally abnormal laboratory test results.

(2) *Moderate envenomation (Grade II).* Swelling progressing beyond the bite area, some systemic symptoms and signs, abnormal laboratory findings, especially abnormal clotting factors, falling hematocrit reading, and falling platelet count.

(3) *Severe envenomation (Grades III-IV).* Marked local and severe systemic symptoms and signs with significant laboratory test abnormalities.

(4) Start IV saline in all patients; give oxygen, and treat shock if present.

(5) Keep the limb level with the heart; remove the tourniquet *only* after shock is treated and antivenin is available.

(6) Some sources recommend early surgical exploration to determine the depth and amount of tissue destruction.

(7) For antivenin, read the package insert carefully, and perform a skin test. Antivenin should not be given to patients who have no signs and symptoms or even to those with local but no systemic symptoms and signs. Administer antivenin IV on the basis of a clinical grading of envenomation.

(a) Grade II—up to 4 vials.

(b) Grade III—5 to 15 vials, especially in children and the elderly.

(c) Grade IV—more than 15 vials.

(d) The amount of antivenin is based on improvement of the clinical picture, not the patient's weight. Children may need more antivenin than adults. Severe envenomation may require a rapid

IV infusion of antivenin in large doses. Use poly-valent antivenin for all bites with the exception of eastern coral snake bites, for which North American coral snake antivenin is issued.

(8) Hospitalize any patient who is receiving antivenin, and observe carefully for vascular insufficiency or compartment syndrome.

C. Arthropod bites. Arthropod venom is variable and complex. Some venoms, like that of the black widow, affect neuromuscular transmission, whereas others produce tissue necrosis only.

1. Black widow.

   a. The venom increases the amount of acetylcholine released from myoneural junctions, which exhausts end-plate activity and blocks synaptic transmission by depolarizing the postsynaptic membrane.

   b. *Identification.* A shiny, coal-black spider with a red hour-glass on the abdomen; the body is 1 to 5 cm long with up to a 5-cm leg span.

   c. Clinical presentation.

      (1) There is usually a history of a sharp pinprick bite followed by a dull, numbing pain in the affected extremity or body area.

      (2) Severe pain is followed by muscle rigidity of the limb or body area.

      (3) Other symptoms include headache, dizziness, ptosis, eyelid edema, conjunctivitis, skin rash and pruritus, nausea, vomiting, sweating, salivation, weakness, and oliguria. In severe cases, hypotension and ECG abnormalities similar to those of a digitalis overdose are present.

      (4) The only local sign may be two fang marks with little local swelling. Multiple bites are rare.

   d. Treatment.

      (1) Clean the wound and apply cool compresses (not ice).

      (2) For severe muscular spasms, give 2 to 10 ml of 10% calcium gluconate IV for immediate muscle relaxation. Methocarbamol (Robaxin), 1 g, is given at 100 mg/min IV as an alternative. For milder symptoms in adults and children over the age of 6, diazepam may be sufficient.

      (3) In severe cases, in the elderly, and in children under the age of 6, give antivenin (Lyovac *Latrodectus*), 1 ampule (2.5 ml) IV in 50 ml of saline. Perform a skin test first.

2. *Loxosceles* (brown recluse).

   a. Venom is a complex mixture of multiple enzymes that damage the endothelium of the arterioles and venules, causing thrombosis. Lysis of polymorphonuclear and mast cells leads to release of substances that damage tissue.

b. *Identification.* The spider is fawn to dark brown. The body is 9 to 12 mm long. There are six white eyes in a semicircular head and a dark violin-shaped marking on the cephalothorax.
c. Clinical presentation.
  (1) There is no significant pain initially, but later, localized pain and erythema occur.
  (2) In a few hours, a blister develops that is surrounded by an ischemic ring and further outlined by an erythematous ring—a "bulls-eye" lesion.
  (3) After several days, the area enlarges, necrosis occurs, and the center ruptures into an ulcer that may extend deep into the muscle layer.
  (4) At 7 to 8 days, an eschar develops, sloughs, and leaves a tissue defect.
d. Treatment.
  (1) Clean the wound and administer tetanus prophylaxis if indicated.
  (2) Some authorities recommend the use of dapsone (50 to 200 mg/day). This is a leukocyte inhibitor and reduces erythema and induration. Dapsone is contraindicated in children.
  (3) Some sources recommend excision of the bite. Obtain surgical consultation for wound care.

D. Mushroom poisoning.
1. Identifying mushroom species is very difficult and should be left to expert mycologists. Gastric contents should be examined microscopically to differentiate deadly toxic mushrooms from mildly toxic ones. High-power examination will show hyphae, and oil immersion examination will show spores the size of RBCs. Staining the aspirate with Melzer's reagent will demonstrate the *Amanita* organisms as blue.
2. Clinical presentation (Table 28-3).
  a. Whereas many types of mushrooms may cause nausea, vomiting, abdominal cramping, and diarrhea, persons who ingest the lethal *Amanita* species may have a latent period of 6 hours before symptoms occur.
  b. Severe vomiting, watery diarrhea, elevated liver enzyme and bilirubin levels, and hypoglycemia suggest *Amanita* poisoning. Death results from liver failure.
  c. Symptoms that occur immediately or within 2 hours of ingestion make diagnosis more difficult. Treatment should start and be accompanied by close surveillance.
3. Treatment.
  a. Specific treatment is based on the identification of the mushroom group and signs and symptoms.
  b. Induce emesis or perform gastric lavage, with endotracheal intubation if necessary.

TABLE 28-3
Mushroom Groups

Chemical groups	Onset of symptoms	Treatment
I. Cyclopeptides	6-24 hr, typically 10-14 hr	Thioctic acid, 50-150 mg/kg q6h IV with glucose (questionable benefit) and penicillin G, 250 mg/kg/day in continuous IV infusion (controversial value as a displacer). Vitamin K, 40 mg IV daily. Massive doses of corticosteroids, e.g., dexamethasone 20-40 mg IV daily. Maintain fluid and electrolyte balance. Follow liver and renal parameters and blood sugar levels. Death may occur on the 4th-7th day, or recovery may take as long as 2 weeks.
II. Ibotenic acid, muscimol (isoxazoles)	½-2 hr	Physostigmine, 0.5-2 mg slowly IV, repeated hourly as needed for anticholinergic symptoms. Do *not* give atropine unless definite cholinergic symptoms are present. Recovery in 4 to 24 hr.
III. Gyromitrin, monomethyl-hydrazine (MMH)	6-12 hr	Pyridoxine HCl, 2.5 mg/kg IV titrated with the patient's symptoms. Follow methemoglobin and free hemoglobin levels and hepatic parameters. Death may occur on the 5th-7th day. In mild poisonings, recovery may occur in 1 day.
IV. Muscarine and other muscarinic compounds	½-2 hr	Atropine, 1-2 mg IV, repeated as needed. Symptoms subside within 6 to 24 hr.
V. Corpine (Antabuse-like)	About 30 min after drinking alcohol, as long as 5 days after eating mushrooms	Avoid elixirs and tinctures. Propranolol (Inderal) may be necessary to control arrhythmias. Recovery is usually spontaneous within 2-4 hr.
VI. Psilocybin and psilocin (indoles)	30-60 (180) min*	Diazepam (Valium), 5-10 mg for seizures. Chlorpromazine (Thorazine), 50-100 mg IM for psychosis. Reassurance for apprehension. Recovery is usual within 6 hr.
VII. Gastrointestinal irritants	½-2 hr	Death is rare; recovery varies according to species from 1 hr to several days or 1 wk.

From Rumack B, Peterson G: Diagnosis and treatment of mushroom poisoning. *Topics in Emergency Medicine* 1(3):85-95, 1979, Aspen Systems Corp.
*Three hours is usually the latest onset.

   c. Monitor blood sugar and liver enzyme levels and renal functions.
   d. Administer analgesics and occasionally opiates for pain.
   e. Severe seizures may occur (see Chapter 21).

E. Plant toxins.

1. Although approximately 700 species of North American plants are considered poisonous, the number of related deaths is low given that plants are among the three most common substances ingested by children (Table 28-4).
2. Toxicity varies with region, plant maturity, quantity ingested, weight of the patient, degree of systemic absorption, and whether ingested seeds are cracked.
3. Specific antidotes for plant poisons are rare; care is usually supportive (see Section V). The symptoms usually appear in 4 hours, and no treatment is necessary if they do not appear within 12 hours. Symptoms are related to the GI tract in 75% of cases, but alkaloids produce systemic reactions as well. The toxic contents of commonly ingested plants are listed in Box 28-5. Actual plant identification is often difficult. Reference should be made to recent toxicology textbooks or *Poisindex* for assistance.
4. Major toxic categories.
   a. Alkaloids.
      (1) The principal effect is on the nervous system, and the rate of onset varies with the mode of ingestion. Systemic effects vary with the chemical structure.
         (a) Atropine-containing plants produce an anticholinergic picture. Treatment is supportive, and in severe cases, physostigmine, 1 to 2 mg IV, repeated as needed, is useful.
         (b) Colchicine produces severe dysphagia, nausea and vomiting, and profound fluid loss. Treatment is supportive, including fluid and electrolyte replacement.
         (c) Aconitine is rapidly absorbed and produces oral paresthesia, visual disturbances, respiratory difficulties, convulsions, and ventricular fibrillation. Treatment is rapid gastric lavage; for sensory or muscular disturbances, calcium chloride, 250 to 500 mg IV slowly, may be useful. Cardiac dysrhythmias should be treated as described in Chapter 15.
         (d) Solanine is poorly absorbed and in mild intoxication produces primarily gastrointestinal symptoms: vomiting, diarrhea, abdominal pain. In more severe intoxication, fever, depression, and headache may be seen.
      (2) Polypeptides and amines.
         (a) The major sources are the akee plant, which is not found in the United States, and mistletoe.

TABLE 28-4
The 11 Most Ingested Toxic Plants

Plant	Toxic part	Toxin	Symptoms	Treatment
Philodendron	All parts	Oxalates	See oxalates in text	See oxalates in text
Yew	All parts, especially seeds	Alkaloid taxine	See alkaloids in text	See alkaloids in text
Nightshade (includes bittersweet, eggplant, Jerusalem cherry, potato)	Green fruit and spoiled sprouts; ripe fruit is harmless	Alkaloid alkaloids	See alkaloids in text	See alkaloids in text
Holly	Berries	Ilicin, ilexanthin, and ilex acid; not identified as to structure and exact action	Nausea, vomiting, diarrhea, and stupor	Gastric lavage and symptomatic care
Poinsettia	White latex exuding from all parts of plant when broken	Not identified	Very similar to oxalates	See oxalates in text
Dieffenbachia	All parts	Oxalates	See oxalates in text	See oxalates in text

Black elder	All parts except berries	Cyanogenic glycoside sambunigrin	See cyanogenic glycoside in text	See cyanogenic glycoside in text
Oleander	All parts	Cardiac glycosides (nerioside and oleandroside)	See glycosides in text	See glycosides in text
Jerusalem cherry	Berries	Alkaloid solanine	See solanine in text	See solanine in text
Jimsonweed	Seed	Atropine alkaloids	See atropine alkaloid in text	See atropine alkaloid in text
Mistletoe	All parts, especially berries	Tyramine and β-phenylethylamine	Increased blood pressure, bradycardia, increased contractions of uterus and intestine	Gastric lavage, supportive care potassium, procainamide, or quinidine

From Burton D, Hanenson IB: Plant toxins. In Hanenson IB, editor: *Quick reference to clinical toxicology*, Philadelphia, 1980, JB Lippincott.

BOX 28-5
Commonly Ingested Plants

PLANT	TOXIN
Aconitum (monkshood)	Aconitine alkaloid
Amaryllis	Lycorine alkaloid
Angel's trumpet	Atropine alkaloid
Apple (seed)	Cyanogenic glycoside
Apricot (seed)	Cyanogenic glycoside
Autumn crocus	Colchicine alkaloid
Azalea	Andromedotoxin alkaloid
Beet	Oxalates
Belladonna (deadly nightshade)	Atropine alkaloids
Bitter almond	Cyanogenic glycoside
Black locust	Phytotoxins
Buckeye	Saponins
Buttercup	Irritant oils
Caladium (elephant's ear)	Oxalates
Calla lilly	Oxalates
Castor bean	Phytotoxins
Cherry (seed)	Cyanogenic glycoside
Daffodil	Lycorine alkaloid
Delphinium	Aconitine alkaloid
Devil's ivy (pothos)	Oxalates
English ivy	Saponins
Foxglove	Cardiac glycosides
Glory lilly	Colchicine alkaloid
Hemlock, poison	Coniine alkaloid
Hyacinth	Lycorine alkaloid

From Burton D, Hanenson IB, editors: Plant toxins. In Hanenson IB, editor: *Quick reference to clinical toxicology,* Philadelphia, 1980, JB Lippincott.

    (b) Mistletoe is toxic in all forms, especially the berries, and causes hypertension, bradycardia, and smooth muscle contractions because of the toxins tyramine and β-phenylethylamine. Treatment is supportive and similar to that for digitalis intoxication.

  (3) Glycosides.

    (a) Cyanogenetic glycosides yield hydrocyanic acid (see Section VI, J, 4, C, for the treatment of cyanide poisoning).

    (b) Cardiac glycosides produce GI tract irritation and digitalis intoxication. Treatment is supportive, with dysrhythmia treatment based on the ECG and clinical presentation.

  (4) Oxalates.

    (a) Soluble oxalates occur in high concentration in plants in the summer and fall. Rapid absorption

---

BOX 28-5
Commonly Ingested Plants—cont'd

PLANT—cont'd	TOXIN—cont'd
Hydrangea	Cyanogenic glycoside
Hyoscyamus (henbane)	Atropine alkaloids
Iris	Resins
Jack-in-the-pulpit	Oxalates
Jonquil	Lycorine alkaloid
Larkspur	Aconitine alkaloid
Lilly-of-the-valley	Cardiac glycosides
Lima bean	Cyanogenic glycoside
Matrimony vine	Atropine alkaloids
Mayapple	Resins
Milkweed	Resins
Monkshood *(Aconitum)*	Aconitine alkaloid
Monstera species	Oxalates
Narcissus	Lycorine alkaloid
Peach (seed)	Cyanogenic glycoside
Plum (seed)	Cyanogenic glycoside
Pokeweed	Saponins and resins
Pothos (devil's ivy)	Oxalates
Privet	Andromedotoxin alkaloid
Rhododendron	Andromedotoxin alkaloid and resins
Rhubarb	Oxalates
Spider lily	Lycorine alkaloid
Syngonium (tri-leaf wonder)	Oxalates
Tuberose	Lycorine alkaloid
Wisteria	Resins

---

leads to a decrease in the amount of blood-ionized calcium. Although the kidneys can handle moderate amounts of soluble oxalates, large amounts precipitate oxalate crystals in tubules and cause proteinuria, hematuria, and crystalluria.

(b) Symptoms include dysphagia, colic, dyspnea, and oropharyngeal edema, which can be severe.

(c) Treatment is with 30 ml of aluminum magnesium hydroxide every 2 hours, gargled and swallowed.

(5) Resins.

(a) These act on nervous and muscle tissue and cause GI tract distress.

(b) Treatment is supportive and based on the symptoms.

(6) Phytotoxins or toxalbumins.

(a) These are similar to bacterial toxins and elicit an antibody response and GI tract distress, with hemorrhagic lesions of the GI tract mucosa.

(b) Treatment is supportive and based on the symptoms.

F. Rodenticides. The most common rodenticide ingested is warfarin. This compound is not very toxic to humans and produces only hypoprothrombinemia after repeated administration. In most cases, because the ingested dose is usually fairly low, therapy after ingestion is not necessary, although vitamin K can be administered.

29

Psychiatric Emergencies*

I. INTRODUCTION.

A. Emergency management of psychiatric patients includes the following:

1. Ensuring protection of the patient and the medical staff.
2. Ruling out serious medical illness that is manifested psychiatrically (characterized by abnormal cognitive function on mental status examination [MSE] and frequently referred to as *organic mental disorders*). Such organic disorders may be classified as follows:
   a. Acute cognitive dysfunction (*delirium,* sometimes referred to as *acute encephalopathy*).
   b. Chronic or gradual intellectual deterioration (*dementia*).
3. Ruling out life-threatening psychiatric conditions.
   a. Suicidal risk.
   b. Homicidal or assaultive risk.
   c. Grave mental disability.
4. Formulating a working psychiatric diagnosis.
5. Selecting the appropriate treatment and disposition.

B. Decisions are made primarily on the basis of the history, physical and neurologic examination, and MSE. The latter is crucial; it will enable the examiner to distinguish between psychiatric presentations that require medical, neurologic, or surgical treatment, and those that require primarily psychiatric treatment.

C. This chapter discusses the following areas:

1. Physical protection.
2. MSE.
3. Specific psychiatric syndromes—diagnosis and treatment.
4. Differential diagnosis and disposition.

II. PHYSICAL PROTECTION.

A. Violent patients are seen frequently in the ED. Ensuring physical protection of the medical staff and the patient is a high priority.

---

*Robert S. Hoffman, M.D., Neurologist, Seton Medical Center, Daly City, Calif., contributed to this chapter.

B. Early recognition of the violence-prone patient is essential.
   1. Beware of the patient who is agitated, angry, suspicious, hostile, or delusional.
   2. Have a high index of suspicion for the violence potential of patients taking alcohol, amphetamines, cocaine, or hallucinogens (especially phencyclidine [PCP]).
   3. In this setting, have extra staff present during your examination or ensure immediate access to them by leaving the door ajar.
C. Two principles of management are crucial.
   1. Adopt a calm, reassuring, businesslike manner that communicates recognition of the patient's needs and a clear intent to help.
   2. Ensure adequate physical controls.
      a. If the patient arrives accompanied by the police, ask them to remain until controls are instituted or the patient is examined and found to be calm.
      b. If the patient arrives in restraints, *do not* remove them until a preliminary assessment is made. Ignoring this rule is the most frequent cause of injury.
D. If a patient unexpectedly becomes threatening or violent, *maximal force* should be deployed.
   1. Frequently a simple show of force (appearance of several burly staff members) will suffice by convincing the patient that any struggle is pointless.
   2. If a threat of force is unsuccessful, the maximum force is *applied* with the humane use of restraints. Ideally, four staff members should be used, one for each extremity.
E. Pharmacologic intervention.
   1. If possible, avoid administering psychoactive drugs to a violent patient before evaluation is performed and a diagnosis achieved. These agents may confuse an evolving neurologic picture and may increase organic confusion or obtundation.
   2. If necessary, agitated patients may be sedated.
      a. If the patient is nonpsychotic or intoxicated with CNS stimulants, a benzodiazepine may be effective (e.g., diazepam, 10 mg IM or 5 to 10 mg IV, or lorazepam, 4 mg IM or 2 mg IV in the average-size adult). Beware of excess sedation, especially if other drugs have been taken.
      b. If the patient is psychotic and agitated, haloperidol, 5 mg, or chlorpromazine, 50 mg, may be administered IM and repeated every hour until the patient is calm. Haloperidol may be given IV, 3 to 5 mg over a period of 1 minute and repeated several times as needed at intervals of at least 20 minutes. Monitor the patient for hypotensive response, particularly with chlorpromazine, which should not be given IV.

III. MSE.

A. Before performing the MSE, it is essential to obtain an adequate history from family and friends, as well as the patient. This should include the following:
   1. Presenting symptoms, precipitating factors, and chronology of events.
   2. Associated symptoms (e.g., Is the patient depressed? Is there also anorexia, weight loss, insomnia, or suicidal ideation?).
   3. Prior psychiatric history, medical history, and medications (legal and otherwise).
   4. Situational resources such as family, friends, physicians, counselors, and living arrangements. Knowledge of these greatly simplifies disposition.

B. A physical and neurologic examination should be done to rule out possible neuromedical disorders.

C. The MSE assesses the following (the first four of which are usually evaluated automatically during the initial conversation and history taking, whereas cognitive function must be tested separately and specifically):
   1. General description and behavior.
   2. Mood and affect.
   3. Insight and judgment.
   4. Thought and language.
   5. Cognition.

D. **General description and behavior.** Note general appearance, psychomotor agitation or retardation, restlessness, dishevelment, inattentiveness, or unusual posturing.

E. **Mood and affect.** The patient's mood may be anxious, depressed, euphoric, hostile, withdrawn, suspicious, inappropriate, "speeding," or labile.

F. **Insight and judgment.** Understanding of current situation, personal options and responsibilities, appropriate perspective, etc.

G. **Thought and language.** Comprehension and output.
   1. Abnormal thought process.
      a. Looseness of associations, that is, varying degrees of slippage in logical connections. This may range from mild rambling (tangential or circumstantial speech) to incoherence ("word salad"), as opposed to normal goal-directed conversation. Note that apparent looseness may result from memory dysfunction in cases of organic mental disorder.
      b. Looseness should be distinguished from the flight of ideas or pressured speech of mania (fast but understandable if one slows the patient down).
      c. Various types of faulty logic may also be seen.
   2. Abnormal thought content.
      a. *Delusions.* Fixed false beliefs that are not amenable to change via persuasion or evidence. Types are persecutory, grandiose, somatic, and depressive.

      b. *Ideas of references.* Interpreting events falsely as related to oneself. ("The TV anchorman is sending me personal messages.")

      c. *Feelings of influence.* Belief that one's thoughts or actions are controlled by other persons or uncanny forces.

      d. *Thought broadcasting.* Belief that one's thoughts are audible to others or that one's mind can be read.

      e. *Somatic preoccupations.* Unrealistic concern with one's body or fear of disease that is not responsive to facts or reassurance.

      f. *Derealization.* Feeling that the world is unreal, as if in a dream.

      g. *Depersonalization.* Feeling that oneself is unreal, for example an inanimate object.

      h. *Suicidal thoughts.* Inquire about these in *every* depressed patient.

      i. Homicidal thoughts.

   3. Abnormal perception.

      a. *Illusions.* False interpretations of actual perceptions, for example, belief that a passing cloud represents a radioactive vapor (compare with delusions).

      b. *Hallucinations.* False perceptions in the absence of external stimuli.

         (1) *Auditory.* Most common in schizophrenia.

         (2) *Visual, gustatory, olfactory, or tactile.* Most common in organic mental disorders including drug intoxications. *If present, assume an organic cause until proven otherwise.*

H. Cognition.

   1. Testing cognitive (intellectual) function is perhaps the most crucial factor in evaluating psychiatric patients. *Impairment of cognition is pathognomonic of medical, neurologic, pharmacologic, or surgical pathology* (often referred to as *organic mental disorders*). It is thus extremely important to evaluate cognitive function to accurately diagnose and treat the illness. Many people have died because treatable medical or surgical illnesses were not considered in patients with psychiatric symptoms.

   2. Cognitive function testing includes evaluation of the following:

      a. Level of consciousness.

      b. Orientation.

      c. Attention.

      d. Memory.

      e. Fund of information.

   3. The level of consciousness may vary from full alertness, through various levels of obtundation, to frank coma.

   4. Orientation.

      a. The patient should be "oriented $\times$ 4," that is, to situation, time, place, and person.

b. Impaired orientation indicates severe cognitive dysfunction. However, the presence of orientation × 4 does *not* rule out organic mental disorder.

5. Attention.

a. When attention is grossly impaired, wandering attention and distractibility are obvious.

b. Subtle degrees of impairment are tested by asking the patient to repeat a series of numbers. (A normal person can repeat six digits in the same order as spoken by the examiner and four in reverse order.) Simple two-digit arithmetic calculations can also be tested.

6. Memory.

a. Immediate memory is evaluated by the examiner mentioning three words or objects; the patient should be able to remember these at 1- and 5-minute intervals.

b. Recent memory is tested by asking the patient about events of the last few hours or days. Confabulation is ruled out by asking the same question more than once.

c. Remote memory is reflected in the capacity to give a past medical history. The examiner should be sure that failure is due to the inability to remember as opposed to a lack of interest or cooperation.

7. Fund of information.

a. The patient should have a knowledge appropriate to his or her age and social situation.

b. Information can include current events, political figures or others in the news, or local geography.

IV. DIAGNOSTIC CATEGORIES OF PSYCHIATRIC SYNDROMES.

A. DSM-IV.

1. *The Diagnostic and Statistical Manual of Mental Disorders,* fourth edition, revised (Washington, DC, 1994, American Psychiatric Association) is the official psychiatric classification system of the American Psychiatric Association. It is frequently revised in accordance with the continuing evolution of our understanding of mental disorders. The actual definitions of the various psychiatric terms thus have changed over the years and continue to do so with each new edition of the DSM. For example, the categories *organic mental disorders* (medical pathology) and *functional disorders* (the schizophrenias and affective/mood disorders) have been eliminated in the fourth edition because it is now felt that all psychotic disorders may involve underlying brain dysfunction.

2. Because the diagnostic and therapeutic goals in emergency medicine are somewhat different from those in general psychiatry, we have elected in this book to emphasize the difference between those disorders previously called *organic*

and all other psychiatric abnormalities. We also stress the difference between acute vs. chronic organic mental disorders (i.e., delirium vs. dementia) because immediate treatment and disposition in the ED are largely functions of the degree of acuity.

3. The terminology in the chapter generally follows that of the DSM-IV but is not identical. It is convenient for us to continue to use the term *organic* when referring to disorders with medical, surgical, neurologic, or pharmacologic etiology. Such disorders are differentiated from all others by abnormal cognitive function on MSE.

B. Psychiatric presentations are broadly divided between nonpsychotic and psychotic disorders (Fig 29-1).

C. Nonpsychotic disorders.
   1. The MSE findings are normal. The patient is neither confused nor psychotic.
   2. ED visits are often due to acute anxiety reactions.

D. Psychotic disorders are further divided into two general categories depending on whether cognitive function is abnormal (organic disorders) or normal (all others).
   1. Disorders with abnormal cognitive function (organic).
      a. Organicity may be acute (delirium) or chronic (dementia).
      b. Medical, surgical, neurologic, or pharmacologic causes underlie many organic disorders. A correct diagnosis is therefore crucial.
   2. Disorders with normal cognitive function.
      a. Other parts of the MSE may show substantial impairment. The nonorganic psychoses include the following:
         (1) The schizophrenias.
         (2) Mood (previously called *affective*) disorders (major depression and bipolar disorders).

V. COGNITIVE (ORGANIC) DISORDERS.
A. General considerations.
   1. Etiology. Medical illness presenting psychiatrically (Box 29-1).
      a. Medications or abused drugs.
      b. Endocrine or metabolic disorders.
      c. Infections: systemic or CNS.
      d. Neurologic degenerative diseases.
      e. Seizure disorders.
      f. Chronic subdural hematoma.
      g. Oncologic diseases including cerebral metastases or hormone-producing tumors.
      h. Autoimmune disorders.
      i. Vascular occlusion.
   2. A frequent error is neglecting to perform an adequate medical workup in patients who already carry a psychiatric diagnosis and now have new symptoms, particularly impaired cognitive function.

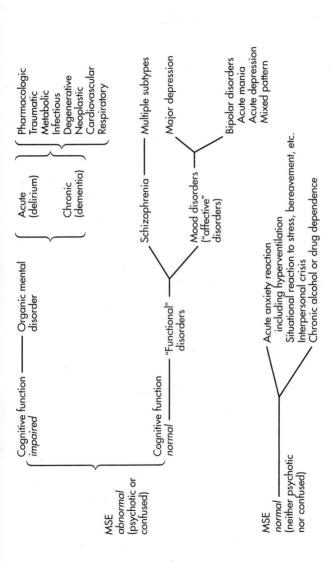

FIG. 29-1 Diagnostic flowchart.
Note that testing of cognitive function part of the mental status examination (MSE) is crucial to the differential diagnosis.

BOX 29-1
Common Medical Illnesses Presenting as "Psychiatric" Disorders

---

METABOLIC DISORDERS

Glucose, sodium, calcium, or magnesium imbalance, acid/base imbalance, acute hypoxia or posthypoxic encephalopathy, renal failure, hepatic failure, anemia, copper disorders (Wilson's disease)

ENDOCRINE DISORDERS

Thyroid disease, parathyroid disease, adrenal hormone imbalance (corticosteroids, mineralocorticoids, catecholamines [pheochromocytoma]), other catecholamine disorder (carcinoid), insulinoma

INFECTIOUS DISEASES

Encephalitis, meningitis, brain abscess, tertiary syphilis, generalized sepsis, or any severe systemic infection

TRAUMA

Concussion or postconcussive syndrome, intracranial hematoma (especially occult subdural hematoma)

CARDIOVASCULAR DISORDERS

Cardiac dysrhythmia, hypotension, TIA, CVA, migraine, vasculitis (temporal arteritis, lupus, periarteritis nodosa), hypertensive encephalopathy, multiinfarct dementia

NEOPLASTIC DISEASES

CNS tumors or metastases, remote tumors with hormonal secretion (insulin, ADH, ACTH)

DEGENERATIVE DISEASES

Senile or presenile dementia of the Alzheimer type

DRUG ABUSE

Alcohol, barbiturates, sedative hypnotics, amphetamines and other stimulants, hallucinogens

DRUG REACTIONS

L-Dopa, steroids, β-adrenergic blockers, antihypertensives (reserpine, α-methyldopa, hydralazine), cardiac drugs (digoxin, quinidine, procainamide, lidocaine), bronchodilators (methylxanthines [aminophylline], β-adrenergic agonists [ephedrine, terbutaline]), anticonvulsants, thyroid preparations, cimetidine, isoniazid, rifampin

---

From Bresler MJ, Hoffman RS: Behavioral emergencies. In Callaham M, editor: *Current therapy in emergency medicine,* Philadelphia, 1987, BC Decker.
TIA, transient ischemic attack; CVA, cerebrovascular accident; ADH, antidiuretic hormone; ACTH, adrenocorticotropic hormone.

3. Early recognition of the underlying medical or surgical cause is essential. Clues to an underlying medical or surgical cause include the following:
   a. Personality change after the age of 40.
   b. Onset of psychiatric symptoms related in time to the onset or exacerbation of medical illness or trauma, or to a change in medications.
   c. Prominent cognitive dysfunction (disorientation, inattention, memory loss).
   d. Hallucinations other than auditory.
   e. Brief or transient behavioral aberrations lasting minutes or hours (rule out especially psychomotor seizures or postictal states after major motor seizures).

B. Delirium.

   1. Definition. An *acute* global impairment of brain function, usually transient and treatable. Although delirium can mimic any major psychiatric disorder, the hallmark is that cognitive function is acutely impaired over a period of several hours to days. The level of consciousness is often diminished.

   2. Characteristics.
      a. Impaired cognition is demonstrated on MSE (disorientation, memory dysfunction, decreased level of consciousness, or reduced fund of information).
      b. Sudden or recent onset in the context of medical illness, trauma, or drugs. However, these factors may not be apparent initially.
      c. Fluctuation of signs, even minute to minute, which tends to increase at night.
      d. Disorders of any of the following: behavior (psychomotor agitation, apathy), mood (excited, apathetic, labile), thought process (disordered speech), thought content (delusions), or perception (hallucinations).

   3. Etiology. Often lies outside the CNS. Causes include systemic infections, metabolic disorders, hepatic or renal disease, thiamine deficiency, drug intoxication or withdrawal, hypertensive encephalopathy, hypotension, hypoxia, encephalitis, postictal state, and subdural hematoma.

   4. Differential diagnosis. Nonorganic disorders such as schizophrenia, mania, or major depression.

   5. Management.
      a. An expeditious medical workup is indicated, including metabolic and toxicologic studies as indicated.
      b. The major danger is to misdiagnose acute organic disorders as nonorganic psychosis. *Testing of cognition on MSE will avoid this pitfall.*
      c. Another error is to misdiagnose an acute, potentially treatable delirium as chronic dementia. Taking an accurate history is crucial. Remember that dementia proceeds very slowly; if a known demented patient *acutely* becomes

worse, a superimposed delirium is usually present, and
the cause must be found.

C. Dementia.

  1. Definition. A progressive impairment of cognitive function,
  usually of insidious onset and gradual course. The level of consciousness is stable.

  2. Characteristics.

  a. Impaired cognition (especially memory).

  b. Subtle or major personality change, impaired judgment,
  and occasionally frankly psychotic symptoms (*nonaudi-
  tory* hallucinations, delusions).

  3. Etiology.

  a. Most common are dementia of the Alzheimer's type and
  vascular (multiinfarct) dementia.

  b. Other causes—many of which are treatable—may be CNS-
  or non–CNS-related.

   (1) *CNS.* Hemorrhage (especially chronic subdural
   hematoma), cerebral infarct, low-pressure hydrocephalus, brain tumors.

   (2) *Non-CNS.* Neoplasm, nutrition (vitamin B_{12}, or fo-
   late deficiency), endocrine, toxic, metabolic.

  4. Differential diagnosis.

  a. *Major depression.* Depressed patients may perform poorly
  on cognitive testing resulting from a lack of motivation
  (pseudodementia).

  b. *Delirium.* Elderly patients, even with a clear history of
  progressive dementia, may have a rapid onset of confusion, clouded consciousness, delusions, hallucinations,
  or agitation. This most often represents a superimposed
  delirium related to underlying medical illness.

  c. *Chronic schizophrenia.* In late stages of schizophrenia, apathy may lead to poor performance on cognitive testing.

  5. Management. Admission as indicated to a psychiatry or neu-
  rology service for a definitive workup.

VI. PSYCHOSES WITH NORMAL COGNITION.

Previously called *functional psychoses,* schizophrenia and the
mood (affective) disorders are distinguished by abnormal findings
on the MSE but *normal cognitive function.*

A. Schizophrenia.

  1. Definition. A psychotic disorder that may be acute or chronic,
  often relapsing or remitting, with impaired behavior, mood,
  thought process, thought content, perception, or judgment, but
  without clouding of consciousness or cognitive dysfunction. If
  the latter is present, the diagnosis is much more likely to be dementia or delirium.

  2. Characteristics.

  a. Onset in adolescence or early adulthood. The new onset
  of psychosis after age 45 is not due to schizophrenia.

    b. Poor premorbid history, for example, a long history of social withdrawal, eccentricity, and impaired educational or vocational function.

    c. Family history of schizophrenia often positive.

    d. *Psychotic symptoms.* Bizarre delusions (usually persecutory); *auditory* hallucinations; loose associations or incoherence; blunted, flat, or inappropriate affect; bizarre motor mannerisms, for example, catatonic posturing or unresponsiveness.

    e. *No* clouding of consciousness, disorientation, confusion, or cognitive impairment as in delirium or dementia.

3. *Management.*

    a. Decide whether psychiatric hospitalization, urgent or elective, is indicated. If not, provide for psychiatric follow-up.

    b. Psychotic agitation may be treated with haloperidol (Haldol), 5 mg IM or IV. Chlorpromazine (Thorazine), 50 mg, PO or IM may be used instead. These agents may be repeated every hour until the patient is calm.

        (1) Postural hypotension may occur, especially with chlorpromazine. Monitoring of the BP is therefore important.

        (2) Dystonic (extrapyramidal) side effects may also occur, especially with haloperidol. These may be controlled with benztropine mesylate (Cogentin), 1 to 2 mg, or diphenhydramine (Benadryl), 25 to 50 mg, either PO, IM, or IV.

    c. Treatment will eventually include an antipsychotic agent; haloperidol or chlorpromazine may be started on a two- or three-times-a-day schedule pending referral.

B. Mood disorders (previously called *affective disorders*).

  1. There are two types: bipolar disorder, consisting of recurrent episodes of mania and depression, and unipolar depressive disorder, consisting of depression alone. At a given time, a patient is said to be suffering a manic episode or a depressive episode, depending on the direction of the mood swing.

  2. Characteristics of **manic episodes.**

    a. Euphoric or irritable mood.

    b. Pressure of speech, flight of ideas, racing thoughts.

    c. Inflated self-esteem, often to point of grandiose delusions.

    d. Restlessness, increased activity, decreased need for sleep.

    e. Self-destructive activities, for example, spending sprees, hypersexuality, foolish investments or projects, reckless driving, all inconsistent with previous behavior.

    f. With severe impairment, bizarre delusions, hallucinations, and incoherence.

    g. A useful point to remember is that manic patients can be humorous, whereas schizophrenic patients generally cannot.

3. Characteristics of **major depressive episodes.**
    a. A depressed mood with a loss of interest in usual activities; must be prominent, persistent (not momentary mood shifts from day to day), and severe enough to impair daily functioning.
    b. Poor appetite and weight loss or increased appetite and weight gain.
    c. Insomnia or hypersomnia.
    d. Psychomotor retardation or agitation.
    e. Fatigue, loss of energy, and multiple somatic complaints.
    f. Feelings of worthlessness, self-reproach, or guilt. These may be of delusional proportions but are consistent with depression and not bizarre as in schizophrenia.
    g. Suicidal ideation.
    h. *No* cognitive dysfunction suggesting delirium or dementia (distinguish depressive refusal to answer test questions from actual cognitive impairment).
4. Management.
    a. Psychiatric hospitalization is usually indicated.
    b. Always assess for suicidal intent in patients with any level of depression.
    c. Definitive treatment may include a number of modalities. However, the initial use of antipsychotic agents may be helpful, especially in emergency situations involving agitation, for example, haloperidol or chlorpromazine in the same doses as for schizophrenia (see Section VI, A, 3).
5. *Note:* Patients with major mood (affective) disorders usually function normally between acute episodes of mania or depression. By contrast, schizophrenic patients often appear abnormal or eccentric and function poorly between acute exacerbations of their illness. Such history greatly assists in the diagnosis.

VII. NONPSYCHOTIC DISORDERS.
A. The hallmark of nonpsychotic disorders is an essentially normal MSE (neither confused nor psychotic). Nonpsychotic behavioral problems are common in the ED.
B. Acute anxiety reactions.
    1. Acute situational anxiety is a common problem in the ED. The MSE reveals signs of anxiety but not those of psychosis or cognitive dysfunction.
    2. Acute anxiety frequently is accompanied by certain physical symptoms, which may in fact constitute the chief complaint. In addition to feelings of tension, restlessness, or dread, prominent symptoms may include tremulousness, abdominal cramps, diarrhea, headache, and the hyperventilation syndrome (panic, dyspnea, paresthesias, dizziness, carpopedal spasm, and sometimes chest discomfort or syncope).
    3. After appropriate medical workup as indicated (e.g., ECG and a blood gas determination), the principal treatment is

reassurance, with an explanation of how stress or anxiety can produce real physical symptoms. Bag rebreathing has traditionally been used to treat hyperventilation but may actually cause hypoxia. During acute panic states a one-time dose or a short course of benzodiazepines may be useful. Arrangement for follow-up counselling is important in preventing a recurrence.

VIII. SUBSTANCE-RELATED DISORDERS.
A. General considerations.
1. Many drugs can affect mentation. Older patients are particularly susceptible to the side effects of prescription medications. Younger patients are more likely to have used illegal drugs. Alcohol abuse is common in any age-group.
2. Although patients with chronic substances abuse present frequently to the ED with a variety of related medical and emotional problems, the emergencies directly caused by drugs are generally due to either acute intoxication or acute withdrawal.
3. Medical management of intoxication and withdrawal is discussed more fully in Chapter 28. The following section deals primarily with the behavioral manifestations, many of which cause acute encephalopathy (delirium).

B. Specific drug syndromes.
1. Alcohol.
a. *Simple intoxication.* No specific treatment is necessary unless the following occur:
   (1) Deep coma with aspiration or impairment of ventilation.
   (2) Descending level of consciousness. Suspect a mixture with other drugs or associated medical condition, for example, trauma.
   (3) Suicidal or assaultive risk. This generally clears as the alcohol is metabolized.
   (4) Gross disorientation, confusion, agitation, or bizarre psychotic thinking. This may require hospitalization on a psychiatric or medical unit for protection and diagnosis.
b. Intoxication with medical complications of alcohol abuse (e.g., head trauma, GI tract bleeding, pancreatitis).
c. *Wernicke-Korsakoff syndrome.* In a chronic drinker after a binge: confusion, memory deficit, ataxia, nystagmus, ocular palsies. Treat with IV thiamine after drawing blood for a serum level to confirm the diagnosis.
d. *Alcohol withdrawal* (see Chapter 21 for full discussion). Escalating tremulousness, weakness, ataxia, confusion, agitation, delusions, visual or tactile hallucinations, seizures.
   (1) In early stages of tremulousness, give diazepam IV in 5-mg increments until a response occurs.

(2) Full-blown delirium tremens has more than a 15% mortality. Admit the patient to an inpatient service that can provide medical treatment including benzodiazepines and electrolyte and fluid management.

2. Opiates.

a. *Intoxication.* Naloxone and supportive care as indicated (see Chapter 28).

b. *Withdrawal.* Uncomfortable but not dangerous; rarely requires admission; refer to treatment program for detoxification and counselling.

3. Barbiturates and other sedative hypnotics *(see Chapter 28).*

a. *Intoxication.* Supportive care.

b. *Withdrawal.* Resembles alcohol withdrawal with restlessness, diaphoresis, vomiting, tremors, hypotension, fever, potentially fatal seizures, and/or toxic psychosis.

c. Hospitalize for treatment.

4. CNS stimulants (amphetamines, cocaine).

a. *Intoxication.* Insomnia, euphoria or irritability, belligerence, panic reactions, paranoid ideation, hallucinations (especially visual and tactile), tachycardia, hypertension; eventually arrhythmias, fever, seizures, coma. Cardiac dysrhythmias and coronary artery spasm with or without MI may also occur (see Chapter 15).

(1) The toxic psychosis may be indistinguishable from paranoid schizophrenia.

(2) Immediate treatment is often required: diazepam IV in 5-mg increments may be effective. Haloperidol IV in 5-mg increments may be useful for frankly psychotic behavior, although this may theoretically lower the seizure threshold. Fever is an ominous sign.

(3) Respiratory support if indicated.

b. *Withdrawal.* Fatigue, weakness, hypersomnia. Severe depression can be a complication, but it is treatable. Hospital admission is often necessary.

5. Hallucinogens (LSD, PCP, marijuana) *(see Chapter 28).*

a. Medical complications are relatively benign, but psychiatric ones can be severe and lethal, for example, falls or accidents.

b. *Mild "bad trip."* Extended period of intoxication, panic reactions.

c. *Severe intoxication.* Toxic delirium with agitation, thought disorder, delusions, and hallucinations. PCP produces a virulent picture of extreme agitation and violence plus neurologic findings. Death can result from violence or suicide (acute renal failure from rhabdomyolysis has been reported).

    d. *Management.* For mild bad trips, "talking down" often suffices. For severe reactions, admit to psychiatry service. Sedation is acceptable with agents such as diazepam or diphenhydramine.

IX. LIFE-THREATENING PSYCHIATRIC CONDITIONS.
Patients may require hospitalization involuntarily if their condition appears to be life-threatening. Such risk generally falls within three categories.

A. Suicide risk. The following factors are associated with higher risk:
1. Detailed plan or recent attempt.
2. Previous serious attempt.
3. Advanced age, living alone, unemployed, with no money or other resources.
4. Major depressive illness, schizophrenia, chronic alcoholism, or delirium.
5. Immobilization and feeling of life impasse without solutions persisting after interview; no response to helpful advice, interventions, and referrals.

B. Homicidal risk. Factors associated with high risk are as follows:
1. Concrete plans and preparations.
2. Past history of violence—the best predictor.
3. Persecutory delusions, with the potential victim seen as the main persecutor.
4. Intoxication or chronic use of drugs thought to stimulate or release violent behavior: alcohol, amphetamines, cocaine, or hallucinogens (especially PCP).
5. A provocative victim (e.g., spouse who goads patient with statements such as "You'd never have the guts" or who repeatedly starts violent arguments).
6. Postpartum depression, which is associated with the risk of injury to the newborn.
7. Factors associated with a loss of control: constant preoccupation with the homicidal ideas, no concern about expected legal consequences, state of agitation or rage objectively evident, no response to the interview in terms of relaxation and increased control.

C. Grave mental disability. Defined as a state of impaired judgment such that the patient is unable to provide for basic needs such as food, clothing, and shelter.
1. Many patients with a functional psychosis or organic mental disorder are gravely disabled, but many are not and function quite well.
2. In contrast, persons without psychiatric illness who are under severe stress may occasionally develop acute panic reactions that disable them as much as would a psychosis.

3. Assessment is carried out by attention to three sources of information.
   a. MSE evidence of gross impairment in thought processes (looseness, incoherence), thought content (extensive delusions), perception (hallucinations), and especially cognitive function (disorientation, confusion, memory loss).
   b. Questions posed to the patient to test judgment. Inquire in detail about the patient's immediate plans: destination after leaving the ED; method of transportation; arrangements for meals, sleeping, income, etc. If the answers are unintelligible or unconvincing, a grave disability is presumed.
   c. Information from family, friends, and other professionals who know the patient. Some seriously impaired patients may converse normally, whereas such collateral information may reveal severe deterioration in life functioning.

X. DIFFERENTIAL DIAGNOSIS AND DISPOSITION.
A. Differential diagnosis (see Fig. 29-1).
1. The essential distinctions are between the following:
   a. Psychotic and nonpsychotic.
   b. If psychotic or confused, the differential diagnosis is between a cognitive (organic) mental disorder and a noncognitive (functional) disorder (schizophrenia or mood disorder).
   c. If organic, the differential diagnosis is between delirium and dementia.
2. The distinction between psychotic and nonpsychotic is frequently made immediately and intuitively when the patient is severely disturbed. The psychotic patient is recognized by thought disorder, gross confusion, or inappropriate, bizarre, or unexpected behavior. In questionable cases, the best way to elicit psychotic material is to permit the patient to speak freely and encourage him with broad-focus questions.
3. Once a patient is determined to be psychotic, the distinction must be made between organic (delirium or dementia) and functional (schizophrenia or affective) disorders. This distinction rests primarily on the findings of cognitive dysfunction (consciousness, orientation, attention, memory, fund of information, and abstraction). Accordingly, the MSE with these test questions should never be omitted with any seriously disturbed patient. Misdiagnosis in either direction may result in inappropriate treatment.
4. If cognitive testing reveals the patient to have an organic mental disorder (impaired cognitive function), the distinction between acute (delirium) and chronic (dementia) is made by history. This may require collateral information from others.

5. If the patient is found to have normal cognition, further distinction is made among schizophrenia, mania, and major depression with the help of the history and the MSE.
   a. If the disturbance recurs as discrete episodes lasting weeks to months with excellent function between, it is probably an affective mood disorder (mania or depression).
   b. If the patient has residual symptoms or signs and poor functioning between acute episodes, the disturbance is probably schizophrenia.
   c. A number of medical illnesses and drugs produce secondary depression, mania, or psychosis; these should always be considered.
6. In a nonpsychotic patient, further diagnostic distinctions are made by history; the categories in Figure 29-1 are self-explanatory. The major goal with such patients is correct evaluation and referral for psychotherapy, special treatment programs, social services, or psychiatric hospitalization in the case of grave mental disability or suicidal or homicidal ideation.
7. When evaluating the elderly, one should always maintain a high index of suspicion for treatable disorders. The major pitfall with the elderly is failing to distinguish between chronic dementia and more treatable problems such as acute delirium or major depression, either of which may be superimposed on chronic dementia. Although affective symptoms such as depression or anxiety may occur in patients with dementia, elderly patients with major depression may be too inert and unmotivated to make any effort to answer cognitive test questions and thus may be mistakenly diagnosed as demented. Such patients with "pseudodementia" may then be denied effective antidepressant treatment—and worse, be consigned to a nursing home or a state hospital, when they might have been able to lead normal lives with proper treatment. These facts again emphasize the importance of adequate cognitive testing in the elderly.

B. Disposition.

1. Indications for *medical* hospitalization.
   a. Delirium resulting from medical illness, trauma, or unknown cause.
   b. Serious drug intoxication.
   c. Withdrawal syndrome from alcohol (delirium tremens), barbiturates, or other sedative hypnotics.
   d. Certain medical illnesses manifesting themselves psychiatrically, for example, endocrine or metabolic encephalopathies or temporal lobe epilepsy.
2. Indications for urgent (involuntary if necessary) *psychiatric* hospitalization.
   a. Suicidal risk.
   b. Homicidal or assaultive risk.

      c. Grave mental disability.

      d. Initial presentation of acute behavioral changes in an elderly patient.

3. Indications for elective psychiatric hospitalization depend on the individual's medical, emotional, and social situation.

4. If hospitalization is not indicated, decide on immediate treatment (reassurance or medication) and arrange for appropriate follow-up (psychiatric referral, medical referral, drug or alcohol treatment program, or social service involvement).

30

Pediatric Emergencies

I. EVALUATION OF THE FEBRILE CHILD.

Serious illnesses in the child, especially in the young infant, are often characterized by an abrupt onset that may have fever as the only sign. Important accompanying symptoms may be a refusal to eat, vomiting, unusual fussiness, or lethargy. If physical examination fails to reveal a focus of infection, the following approach is suggested.

A. Newborn infants.

1. Specific clinical signs and symptoms are often absent in the infant under 3 months old.
2. Sepsis, meningitis, pneumonia, or UTI should be strongly suspected.
3. Appropriate diagnostic studies may include a CBC; urinalysis; blood and urine cultures; chest radiograph; and lumbar puncture for cell count, Gram's stain, protein, glucose, and culture.
4. The WBC and the differential can be misleading in determining whether a fever is of bacterial or viral origin.
5. Young infants with fever should be strongly considered for hospitalization and antibiotic therapy pending culture results.

B. Older infants and children under the age of 3 years.

1. The inability to communicate symptoms, for example, headache, earache, sore throat, or abdominal pain, is characteristic of many children in this age-group.
2. If the physical examination is normal but it is nevertheless thought that the child is severely ill, investigation should include the studies discussed in Section I, A, 2.
3. Significant fever should be treated with acetaminophen, 15 mg/kg PO q4h (or 45 mg PR for the initial dose), and/or ibuprofen, 5 to 10 mg PO q6h. Tepid water sponging has traditionally been used for significant fever in children but is often not well tolerated and frequently unnecessary.

C. Older children.
The older child with fever is often able to relate a specific complaint. Laboratory studies are less important in the older child. They should, however, be obtained as indicated.

II. ACCESS FOR DRUG DELIVERY.

IV cannulation may be quite difficult in children. In neonates, the umbilical veins can be used. For infants and older children, the rectal and intraosseous drug routes offer alternatives to IV or oral administration. Endotracheal delivery may be used for some medications.

A. Endotracheal medication.

1. The following drugs can be delivered via an endotracheal tube:
   a. Epinephrine.
   b. Atropine.
   c. Lidocaine.
   d. Naloxone.
   e. Diazepam.
2. In general, the standard IV dose of medication is added to several ml of saline (5 to 10 ml for an adult, less for children) and injected through a catheter threaded just beyond the distal tip of the endotracheal tube. This is followed by several large-volume breaths via bag-valve-tube.

B. Rectal medication.
The rectal route is readily accessible. A lubricated small syringe or feeding tube can gently be inserted several centimeters beyond the anus and the drug injected. In general, the recommended rectal dose is often triple the oral or IV dose. Absorption may be erratic, however, and individual recommendations should be followed for the given drug.

C. Intraosseous medication.

1. Fluid and medication may be absorbed from the bone marrow nearly as fast as through the veins. This route can be lifesaving if venous access cannot rapidly be achieved in the critically ill child.
2. The tibea offers a flat, easily palpable, superficial, and readily accessible location for intraosseous infusion. Either of two sites may be used:
   a. Proximal tibea below the knee but distal to the growth plate.
   b. Distal tibea above the medial malleolus.
3. An intraosseous needle with a stylet is optimal, but an IV needle can be utilized. A twisting motion is used, with care taken not to penetrate the posterior aspect of the tibea. Aspiration of bone marrow confirms the location.

III. MANAGEMENT OF SPECIFIC DISORDERS IN CHILDREN.

A. Cardiopulmonary arrest (see also Chapter 15).

1. Unlike adults, for whom cardiac arrest is usually a sequela of arteriosclerotic ischemic disease, children develop cardiac arrest primarily as a result of respiratory arrest, often caused by upper airway obstruction. Immediate restoration of airway and ventilation is crucial. Other causes include trauma, sudden infant death syndrome, drowning, fluid and electrolyte

disorders, congenital heart disease, sepsis, and meningitis or encephalitis.
2. External cardiac compression.
   a. *Infant.* With two to three fingers positioned over the midsternum, compress the sternum ½ to 1 inches, 100 times per minute.
   b. *Child.* With the heel of one hand, compress the sternum 1 to 1½ inches, 80 times per minute.
3. Ventilation.
   a. *Infant.* 20 times per minute.
   b. *Child.* 15 times per minute.
4. Drug dosages.
   a. *Epinephrine.* 0.01 ml/kg (1:10,000, 1 mg in 10 ml).
   b. *Atropine.* 0.02 mg/kg, repeated as needed to a maximum of 0.5 mg in children or 1 mg in young adolescents. A minimum of 0.1 mg should be given regardless of size or age.
   c. *Lidocaine bolus.* 1 mg/kg per dose; maintenance, 30 μg/kg/min.
   d. *Dopamine.* 1 to 5 μg/kg/min, β-effect; 5 to 12 μg/kg/min, mixed effect; more than 15 μg/kg/min, α-effect.
   e. *Norepinephrine.* Begin the infusion at 0.1 μg/kg/min and titrate to effect.
   f. *Isoproterenol.* Begin at 0.1 μg/kg/min and titrate to effect.
   g. *Sodium bicarbonate.* Administration is controversial and, if given at all, should be administered 1 mEq/kg only if significant metabolic acidosis persists (pH < 7.1) despite resolution of respiratory alkalosis with adequate ventilation.
   h. *Calcium chloride.* 25 mg/kg per dose. (Calcium gluconate, 60 mg/kg per dose.) Calcium is no longer used in cardiac arrest but may be helpful with documented hypermagnesemia, hypocalcemia, or calcium channel blocker overdose.
B. Dehydration. (See Chapter 2 for discussion of electrolyte and acid-base disorders.)
1. Dehydration in children, often with an accompanying electrolyte imbalance, may result from a variety of causes, especially GI tract loss from vomiting or diarrhea, or decreased fluid intake caused by acute illness.
2. Dehydration is defined as isotonic (serum sodium concentration 130 to 150 mEq/L, hypotonic (serum sodium concentration < 130 mEq/L), or hypertonic (serum sodium content > 150 mEq/L). The type of dehydration is dependent on the source of the fluid and salt loss and dictates the type of fluid used to replace the deficit.
3. Unless there is good evidence of excessive fluid intake or a high solute load that leads one to suspect either hypotonic or hypertonic dehydration, it is reasonable to assume initially that dehydration is isotonic.

4. The amount of fluid deficit in mild dehydration is approximately 30 to 50 ml/kg; for moderate dehydration, 50 to 100 ml/kg; and for severe dehydration, 100 to 150 ml/kg.

5. Obtain a blood sample to measure electrolyte levels and other laboratory tests, and start IV fluids in the most accessible vein.

6. Administer normal saline or lactated Ringer's solution, 20 ml/kg over 30 to 60 minutes.

7. Replacement of fluid loss should then be continued, with half the calculated deficit infused in the first 8 hours. One-third or one-quarter normal saline should be used, with 15 to 20 mEq of potassium added to each liter if needed.

8. The sodium deficit in hyponatremic dehydration should be calculated by the following formula:

mEq sodium deficit
$$= (135 \text{ mEq/L} - \text{measured serum sodium}) \times 0.6 \times \text{kg weight}$$

The number 0.6 is the distribution coefficient for sodium. Normal or two-thirds–normal saline should be used.

9. In hypernatremic dehydration, the amount of fluid administered should be calculated to reduce the serum sodium level to 145 mEq/L. The amount of free water necessary to do this may be calculated by the following formula:

Free water
$$= (\text{measured serum sodium} - 145 \text{ mEq/L}) \times 4 \text{ ml} \times \text{kg weight}$$

The amount of free water necessary to lower the serum sodium concentration by 1 mEq is 4 ml/kg. It is essential that the sodium concentration not be reduced too precipitously because cerebral edema may result. Therefore quarter-normal saline in 5% dextrose should be infused slowly, with an aim of returning the serum sodium level to 145 mEq/L over a period of approximately 48 hours.

10. Vital signs, urinary output, and serum electrolytes should be monitored to determine the effectiveness of fluid replacement.

C. Seizures. (See Chapter 21 for further discussion of seizures.)

1. Convulsions associated with febrile illness occur frequently in young children. They may indicate a CNS infection or merely a benign febrile seizure. If the temperature is higher than 38.5° C, it should be lowered as described in Section I, B, 3.

2. Convulsions in afebrile children can be due to a variety of causes, including the following:
   a. Infection, including meningitis.
   b. Metabolic disorders.
      (1) Electrolyte imbalance.
      (2) Hypoglycemia.
      (3) Hypocalcemia.

    c. Intoxication.
      (1) Lead.
      (2) Phenothiazine.
      (3) Theophylline.
    d. Intracranial hemorrhage.
      (1) Vascular disorders.
      (2) Coagulation disturbances.
    e. Brain tumor.
    f. Degenerative diseases.
    g. Trauma.
    h. Idiopathic epilepsy.
3. Immediate management of the child during the convulsion consists of the following:
    a. Protecting the airway, suctioning secretions, and padding and restraining when necessary.
    b. Most seizures are brief and self-limiting. If major motor seizure activity persists, treatment with one of the following agents is warranted:
      (1) Diazepam, 0.2 to 0.3 mg/kg IV at a rate of 1 mg/min. The maximum IV dose for children under 2 is 4 mg; for older children, it is 10 mg. Diazepam can also be administered rectally if venous access is delayed.
      (2) Lorazepam, 0.05 to 1.5 mg/kg/dose slowly IV, with maximum 5 mg/dose.
      (3) Phenobarbital, 15 to 20 mg/kg loading dose IV, IM, or PO at a rate of less than 1 mg/kg/min IV.
4. A thorough history and physical examination are performed to determine the cause of the convulsion.
5. If the febrile child's mental status is normal after resolution of the postictal state, and if there is no sign whatsoever of serious illness, the cause may be ascribed to a benign febrile seizure and lumbar puncture may not be required. (This does not apply to young infants.) Otitis media or other obvious bacterial infections should of course be treated.
6. If there is any question of serious illness or meningitis, however, lumbar puncture and septic workup are indicated.
7. Unless it is determined that the convulsion was a benign febrile seizure from which the child has fully recovered, consideration should be given to admitting the child to the hospital. The clinical appearance of the child, the results of examination and diagnostic tests, and the response to temperature-lowering measures should be used as guides to the necessity for hospitalization.
8. If the child has a known seizure disorder and is taking anticonvulsant medication, a serum drug level should be obtained to confirm a therapeutic level, with dosage adjusted if indicated.

D. Meningitis.

1. The classic signs and symptoms of meningitis are fever, headache, nuchal rigidity (meningismus), Kernig's and Brudzinski's signs, and a bulging fontanelle. Any combination—or none of these—may be present, especially in the child younger than 6 months, in whom lethargy, irritability, and poor feeding may be the only clues to the diagnosis. *Meningismus is absent in most meningitis patients younger than 18 months.* Meningococcemia may be present without meningitis. A petechial rash is a strong indicator of meningococcemia.

2. Bacteriology.
   a. During the first 2 months of life, the most common organisms include Group B streptococcus and meningococcus *(Neisseria meningitidis),* along with *Escherichia coli* and *Listeria monocytogenes* during the first month, and *Haemophilus influenzae* during the second.
   b. In older children, *H. influenzae,* meningococcus *(N. meningitidis),* and pneumococcus *(Streptococcus pneumoniae)* are the primary causes, with *H. influenzae* less frequently encountered after the age of 6 and in younger children who have been immunized against it.

3. Lumbar puncture is the key to diagnosis and should be performed early in the workup of any patient in whom the diagnosis of meningitis is considered. Cerebrospinal fluid should be evaluated for the following:
   a. WBC and differential.
   b. Gram's stain and bacterial culture.
   c. *Protein.* Normal is 12 to 25 mg/dl.
   d. *Glucose.* Normal is two thirds of the simultaneous serum glucose level.

4. Typical antibiotic regimens for the initial dose of empiric treatment before bacterial identification are as follows:
   a. Neonatal: IV ampicillin, 100 mg/kg to cover *Listeria, plus* either ceftriaxone (Rocephin), 100 mg/kg, cefotaxime (Claforan), 50 to 75 mg/kg, or gentamycin, 2.5 mg/kg.
   b. Children older than 3 months: IV ceftriaxone, 100 mg/kg, or cefotaxime, 50 to 75 mg/kg. An alternative regimen is ampicillin, 100 mg/kg *plus* chloramphenicol, 25 mg/kg.

5. Corticosteroids may blunt the inflammatory response to bacterial cell death, which can lead to deafness after meningitis, especially that due to *H. influenzae.* Dexamethasone, 1.5 mg/kg IV, should be given before antibiotic administration.

E. Pneumonia.

1. Pneumonia may be particularly difficult to diagnose, especially in an infant in whom fever, respiratory distress, irritability, and poor feeding may be the primary findings.

2. Subtle physical signs of flaring nasal alae, costal retractions, and tachypnea are often present but may be obscured by crying. Slightly diminished breath sounds may be the only finding.

3. The older child is more likely to have physical findings such as rales.

4. Viral etiology is common, and it is now recognized that chlamydial pneumonia is frequent as well.

5. Bacterial pneumonia is often due to pneumococcus, but other organisms such as group B streptococcus and *L. monocytogenes* must also be considered in newborns. *H. influenzae* is a common organism in children younger than 6 years old who have not been previously vaccinated against it.

6. Nasopharyngeal, sputum, and blood cultures may reveal the causative organism, but often the exact cause is not found.

7. Hospitalization is generally indicated for infants less than 1 year of age; children with severe respiratory distress; or any child with a predisposing illness such as sickle cell anemia, fibrocystic disease, diabetes mellitus, or immune system deficiency.

8. A typical parenteral regimen for empiric treatment of pneumonia before bacterial identification is as follows:
   a. Ceftriaxone, 50 to 100 mg/kg/day in 1 or 2 divided doses, or cefotaxime, 150 mg/kg/day in 3 doses.
   b. Ampicillin, 100 mg/kg/day in 4 doses, should be added to the cephalosporin in children younger than 3 months to cover *Listeria*.

9. Outpatient oral therapy for children age 3 months to 6 years may include the following:
   a. Amoxicillin, 40 mg/kg/day divided tid, or erythromycin (50 mg/kg/day)/sulfisoxazole (Pediazole) combination, divided tid-qid.
   b. Beyond age 6, and in younger children previously vaccinated against *Haemophilus*, erythromycin (40 mg/kg/day divided qid) or a newer-generation macrolide can be used, such as clarithromycin (Biaxin), 7.5 mg/kg q12h.

F. Diabetes.

1. Hypoglycemic coma.
   a. Hypoglycemia in childhood can be caused by a variety of disorders in addition to excessive hypoglycemic medication. These include sepsis, enzymatic deficiencies, endocrine disorders, malnutrition, malabsorption, poisoning with ethanol or salicylates, and Reye's syndrome. Neonates are particularly susceptible to hypoglycemia.
   b. Symptoms may include restlessness, apathy, seizures, and coma.
   c. After a blood sample is drawn to determine the glucose level, IV glucose should be administered. In neonates, 1 to 2 ml/kg of a 10% dextrose solution should be given.

For older children, 1 ml/kg of 50% dextrose is appropriate. The initial dose should be followed by an IV infusion of 5% or 10% dextrose at 5 mg/kg/min if there is any risk of continuing hypoglycemia.

2. Diabetic ketoacidosis.

   a. Ketoacidosis may occur in a known diabetic or may be the presenting syndrome of new-onset diabetes. Findings include dehydration, hyperventilation, mental status alteration, vomiting, and often abdominal pain. The serum glucose level is elevated, ketones are present in the blood and breath, and both glucose and ketones are found in large concentrations in the urine.

   b. Baseline laboratory studies should include urinalysis and a determination of the levels of serum glucose, ketones, osmolality, electrolytes, and ABGs.

   c. Treatment.

      (1) *Fluid replacement.* In moderate-to-severe cases of ketoacidosis, initial fluid replacement should consist of 20 ml/kg of normal saline for the first hour. This should be followed by the administration of half-normal saline for the next several hours at a rate consistent with the degree of dehydration. The potassium deficit is usually about 6 to 10 mEq/kg. Half this deficit should be replaced during the first day, but potassium replacement should be delayed until renal function is established and the serum potassium level has fallen back into the normal range.

      (2) *Insulin.* The standard regimen has included an initial bolus of regular insulin, 0.1 U/kg, followed by a constant IV infusion of 0.1 U/kg/hr. There has been a trend recently, however, to omit the initial bolus and begin treatment with the constant infusion. As the serum glucose level falls below 300 mg/dl, a solution containing 5% dextrose should be administered and the insulin tapered off to prevent the development of iatrogenic hypoglycemia. The goal is to reduce serum glucose by 75 to 100 mg/dl/hr because more rapid reduction can result in cerebral edema.

      (3) *Sodium bicarbonate.* Administration of sodium bicarbonate is controversial. Its use has been associated with hypokalemia, hypomagnesemia, CSF acidosis, and cerebral edema. If used, it should be reserved for patients with profound acidosis (pH 7.1 or less). Sodium bicarbonate, 2 mEq/kg, can be administered slowly over a period of 1 to 2 hours. No bicarbonate should be given for more moderate acidosis because treatment with fluids and insulin will result in a return to normal pH.

G. Croup.

1. Croup in infants and children is usually due to a viral upper respiratory tract infection. Parainfluenza virus is a common cause. Children affected are generally younger than 2 years old. The onset of the disease is gradual, occurring over 1 or more days, with symptoms particularly severe during the night. Symptoms include a barking cough, hoarseness, and difficulty breathing. Children display a varying amount of respiratory distress. Muscular retraction and stridor are frequently present, but there is no preferred body position. Fever is common, but the temperature is rarely higher than 39° C. Inhalation of cool air is beneficial, and the child has often improved after a ride to the hospital.

2. Treatment of croup.
   a. *Humidity.* Humidification of inspired air is the mainstay of therapy. This may be achieved by face mask, croup tent, vaporizer, or simply steaming up a bathroom with hot shower water. Mild cases may respond to humidified air alone.
   b. *Inhalation of a β-adrenergic agent.* Significant croup generally responds well to inhaled sympathomimetic agents. The traditional treatment is with racemic epinephrine (0.5 ml of a 2.25% solution in 4.5 ml of saline) delivered by nebulization. However, racemic epinephrine has no advantage over 1-epinephrine, which is administered by nebulization as a 5-ml solution of 1:1000 dilution. Recent studies have shown that inhaled albuterol (0.15 to 0.3 mg/kg in several ml of saline) is just as effective as epinephrine. The treatment should last about 15 minutes and the heart rate, rhythm, and BP monitored during this time.
   c. *Corticosteroids.* Steroids have been shown to be beneficial. Dexamethasone, 0.6 mg/kg IM, may be sufficient, but several days of prednisone or prednisolone, 1 to 2 mg/kg/day in divided doses, may also be used.
   d. Croup can usually be managed on an outpatient basis, but children in severe respiratory distress should be admitted to the hospital. If inhaled adrenergic agents are administered, the child should be observed for 2 hours afterward to ensure that repeat treatment is not necessary.

H. Epiglottitis.

1. Epiglottitis is a less common cause of stridor than croup. The causative organism of this supraglottic infection is usually *H. influenzae,* but streptococci or staphylococci may be involved. Children 2 to 6 years old are most commonly affected, but epiglottitis may involve any age-group, including adults. The onset of illness is rapid, usually progressing over several hours. The child is acutely ill, with stridor, severe res-

piratory distress, high fever, and drooling. The upright position is preferred by the patient. A cough is not usually present. The child may be cyanotic.

2. Diagnosis of epiglottitis.
   a. The diagnosis should be made on the basis of the clinical picture. It is generally thought that the oropharynx should not be examined because this may precipitate acute laryngospasm and airway obstruction.
   b. A lateral radiograph of the neck may reveal enlargement of the epiglottis or narrowing of the airway.
   c. Blood cultures are frequently positive for the causative organism.

3. Treatment of epiglottitis.
   a. No effort should be made to place the child supine or to otherwise interfere with ventilation.
   b. Humidified oxygen should be applied if tolerated.
   c. The significantly ill child should be taken to the operating room where direct laryngoscopy and, if necessary, endotracheal intubation or tracheostomy can be carried out.
   d. Antibiotics may be administered parenterally, but they are not the mainstay of therapy. Regimens include ampicillin, 50 mg/kg/day divided into 4 doses, cefotaxime (Claforan), 100 mg/kg/day divided into 3 doses, or ceftriaxone (Rocephin), 50 mg/kg/day in a single dose.

I. Asthma. (See Chapter 17 for complete discussion of asthma.)

Acute asthmatic bronchospasm frequently can be controlled with the following:

1. Albuterol, 1 to 2 puffs by metered-dose inhaler, or 0.15 to 0.3 mg/kg in several ml of saline by nebulization, or in severe cases by positive pressure. The treatment may be repeated as required with monitoring of heart rate. Exact dose is not required, since much of the albuterol from a nebulizer is not inhaled. Younger children can receive 0.25 ml of a 0.5% solution (1.25 mg) in 2.5 ml NS, and older children and adolescents 0.5 ml (2.5 mg) in 2.5 mg NS. Continuous albuterol can also be given at a rate of 0.5 mg/kg/hr (maximum 7.5 mg/hr).

2. Although not usually necessary, in severe cases, aqueous epinephrine (1:1000) can be administered, 0.01 ml/kg per dose subcutaneously (maximum single dose not to exceed 0.5 ml). The onset of action is rapid, and the duration of action is approximately 20 minutes. Injection may be repeated every 15 to 20 minutes to a total of three doses.

3. The concomitant administration of oral or IV fluids to liquify mucus is beneficial and is especially important if the child is dehydrated.

4. In significant cases, steroids may be administered in the ED, prednisolone 1 to 2 mg/kg PO (Prelone) or IV (Solu-Medrol).

5. If the aforementioned measures do not abate the attack, the patient should be admitted to the hospital.

6. If the asthmatic attack responds to treatment, the child may be discharged. Inhaled bronchodilators should be continued, and any significant episode should be treated with a brief course of steroids. Various regimens are used, for example, prednisone or prednisolone, 1 to 2 mg/kg/day in divided doses for 3 days or tapered over 10 days.

7. Sustained-release epinephrine (Sus-Phrine), 0.005 ml/kg, is sometimes administered subcutaneously before discharge, although its use has declined in recent years.

J. Bronchiolitis. This frequent manifestation of viral respiratory tract infection in infants under 2 is characterized by the following:

1. The rapid development of dyspnea, respiratory distress, prolongation of expiration, wheezing, and occasionally rales.

2. Small infants can rapidly develop severe respiratory distress with poor ventilatory exchange. Signs of hypoxia may be subtle and nonspecific, signified only by restlessness and apprehension.

3. The chest radiograph may reveal hyperinflation.

4. Bronchiolitis is usually benign. Treatment consists of the administration of humidified oxygen and fluids and specific supportive measures to ensure high humidity and adequate hydration.

5. Differentiation of bronchiolitis from acute asthma may be difficult, but bronchospasm with either can be treated as described in Section II, E with inhaled albuterol or SC epinephrine.

6. Indications for admission to the hospital include dehydration, severe respiratory distress with a sustained respiratory rate faster than 60 per minute, and age under 6 months.

K. Tonsillitis and pharyngitis.

1. Sore throat is one of the most frequently encountered pediatric illnesses. An accurate diagnosis (viral vs. streptococcal) cannot definitively be made on the basis of the clinical impression alone.

2. While tonsillar exudate and cervical adenopathy are frequent with streptococcal infection, their absence does not exclude streptococcus, and the most impressive physical findings may nevertheless be viral, especially with mononucleosis.

3. Rapid streptococcal screens of pharyngeal swabbings are quite reliable if positive, but they do miss some cases. Negative screens should be followed by definitive streptococcal culture.

4. If β-hemolytic *Streptococcus* (group A) is found or strongly suspected, any of the following regimens may be used:

   a. Phenoxymethyl penicillin (penicillin VK), 25 to 50 mg/kg/day PO divided qid for 10 days.

b. Benzathine penicillin/procaine penicillin (Bicillin C-R) IM, available as 1:1 or 3:1 combinations. Dosage is based on the bezathine component: 300,000 U for children under 30 lb, 600,000 U between 31 and 60 lb, 900,000 U between 61 and 90 lb, and plain benzathine 1.2 million U without procaine (Bicillin L-A) for children over 90 lb.

c. In patients who are allergic to penicillin, erythromycin, 30 to 50 mg/kg/day divided qid for 10 days, is the drug of choice.

L. Otitis media.

1. Otitis media is a common childhood infection. The distinction between purulent otitis and serous otitis may be difficult, however.

2. On examination, the tympanic membrane may be dull, thickened, or erythematous. The fluid-filled ear will not allow the tympanic membrane to move on pneumatic otoscopy.

3. The causative organism is usually pneumococcus *(S. pneumoniae)* or *H. influenzae,* the latter being more frequent in children younger than 6 years who have not been vaccinated against it. *Branhamella catarrhalis* is not uncommon.

4. Treatment should be a 10-day course of any of the following oral agents:

   a. Amoxicillin, 40 mg/kg/day divided tid.

   b. Trimethoprim (8 mg/kg/day)–sulfamethoxazole (40 mg/kg/day) combination (Bactrim, Septra), divided bid.

   c. Erythromycin (50 mg/kg/day)–sulfisoxazole combination (Pediazole), divided qid.

   d. Refractory cases are sometimes responsive to cefaclor (Ceclor), 20 mg/kg/day divided tid.

   e. A single IM dose of ceftriaxone (Rocephin), 50 mg/kg, is also effective for treating otitis, particularly in those for whom compliance might be difficult.

M. The battered child.

1. There has been increasing awareness among health care workers of how common child abuse is. Such children may be identified by a history of frequent "accidents" or a description of an accident that is suspicious. Multiple ecchymoses in the absence of blood dyscrasia is another clue. There often is evidence of neglect.

2. When child abuse is suspected, a detailed physical examination should be undertaken to ascertain the presence of additional injury. Radiographs may reveal skull or long-bone fractures.

3. The parents of such children have severe emotional problems that require professional help, and the children require protection while the family situation is assessed. The mortality and incidence of permanent physical and mental damage are high in abused children.

4. Children who are suspected of being physically abused should be hospitalized immediately and the case referred to the appropriate social service and legal agencies. In many states, such reporting is required by law.

N. Appendicitis.

1. Appendicitis in young children is a rapidly progressive disease that can go on to rupture within a few hours. It is not at all unusual for children with even equivocal preoperative findings to be discovered at surgery to have already ruptured their appendix.

2. Appendicitis should always be considered in the child with abdominal pain. The diagnosis is particularly suggested if the pain is at first vague and diffuse and then localizes in the right lower quadrant. Anorexia, nausea, and vomiting are usually, but not always, present.

3. The right lower quadrant is usually tender on palpation, but the abdominal findings may be surprisingly benign. A retrocecal appendix may simulate pyelonephritis. If the appendix is deep in the pelvis, the child may have only rectal tenderness. Psoas and obturator signs may be positive, reflecting posterior peritoneal inflammation.

4. Many diseases cause abdominal pain in children and may mimic appendicitis. Common offenders are acute pharyngitis with viral enteritis, mesenteric adenitis, and acute pyelonephritis.

5. Diagnostic studies are often of little assistance. If appendicitis is strongly suspected, the workup should include a CBC with differential and urinalysis. However, leukocytosis may be found in a multitude of abdominal problems, including gastroenteritis. Abdominal radiographs sometimes reveal an appendicolith. Ultrasonography or CT may also be useful. However, clinical judgment and serial examinations over several hours are the most important diagnostic modalities.

6. If uncertainty exists, obtain a surgical consult, admit the patient to the hospital for observation, or arrange to have the child reexamined within roughly 6 to 18 hours or sooner if at all worse.

7. As with any abdominal disorder of unclear cause, it is important to inform the family that there is a possibility of appendicitis or other problem, and that the diagnosis may become clear only after several more hours.

O. Foreign bodies in the GI tract.

1. Most swallowed objects are small enough to pass through the GI tract without difficulty, but some remain in the esophagus or the stomach.

2. If a foreign body lodges in the esophagus, the child may hypersalivate and refuse to swallow. Metallic objects are seen on a plain roentgenogram, but others require radiocontrast material to outline them.

3. Endoscopic removal is indicated for foreign objects lodged in the esophagus.
4. Most foreign bodies that reach the stomach go through the remainder of the intestine uneventfully. Children who have ingested sharp objects, however, need close observation and repeated roentgenographic examinations. Button batteries with corrosive potential may need to be extracted if they are not excreted spontaneously within a day or two.

P. Pyloric stenosis.

1. Pyloric stenosis characteristically occurs at the age of 2 to 6 weeks in a firstborn male infant, with vomiting described as projectile. However, pyloric stenosis can present in an infant from 1 week to several months of age and may occur in girls and boys. The initial vomiting may not be projectile, and the infant who has been weakened with prolonged vomiting and malnutrition may be too weak to vomit forcefully.
2. Palpate the abdomen when the infant is completely relaxed, preferably immediately after a vomiting episode. The pyloric mass is elusive and may be located anywhere from the midepigastrium to the right upper quadrant under the liver.
3. If an experienced examiner cannot find the mass on repeated examination, abdominal radiographs or ultrasound may be diagnostic.
4. Surgical consultation should be obtained.

Q. Intussusception.

1. Intussusception occurs most commonly in infants approximately 5 to 10 months of age.
2. The child characteristically pulls the knees up to the abdomen, cries with pain, and then relaxes. These paroxysms occur 15 to 20 minutes apart, and the child may sleep during the interval. Vomiting is common, and a stool mixed with blood and mucus is often passed during the first 12 hours of illness.
3. A sausage-shaped mass may be palpated in the abdomen.
4. If upright or decubitus films of the abdomen reveal air-fluid levels diagnostic of intestinal obstruction, attention should be directed to the treatment of dehydration with replacement of fluids, and an early operation.
5. If the abdomen is not distended or tender, and if the child is seen during the first 24 hours, a barium enema may be not only diagnostic but effective in reducing the intussusception.

R. Incarcerated hernia. Inguinal hernias are common in children under 1 year of age. When a child has presenting symptoms of a swollen, tender scrotal mass in which the diagnosis could be an incarcerated hernia, sedation and Trendelenburg's position may be sufficient to achieve reduction. Surgical repair can then be undertaken electively. Precautions should be given to the parents, however, regarding incarceration. If the hernia cannot easily be reduced, surgical consultation should be obtained to consider immediate surgery.

S. Torsion of the testis (See also Chapter 19). Torsion of the testis is suspected when an infant cries out suddenly and is found to have a swollen, tender testis. Older boys complain of sudden onset of testicular pain, frequently after exercise. Doppler ultrasonography and nuclear scanning may be useful, but neither is fully sensitive, and scanning frequently requires an excessive amount of time.

Operative detorsion should be performed within 6 hours if the testis is to be salvaged. At the time of the operation, the testis is untwisted and orchiopexy performed. Contralateral orchiopexy is also necessary to prevent future torsion of the other testis.

T. GI tract bleeding.

1. In the newborn, small amounts of blood may be vomited or passed in the stool secondary to the ingestion of maternal blood. Vitamin K deficiency is another possibility, although this has become rare with the prophylactic administration of vitamin K.

2. In older infants, anal fissures can cause blood streaking of the stool. History indicates the passage of a hard stool with crying. Place the infant in the prone position and retract the buttocks to see the fissure. Treatment consists of stool softeners, local application of soothing ointments, and reassurance to the parents.

3. Bleeding from a peptic ulcer can occur in older children. See Chapter 18 for full discussion.

4. Meckel's diverticulum may be suspected when no other source of lower intestinal tract bleeding is identified. Bleeding from a Meckel's diverticulum usually will stop spontaneously, but transfusion may be needed. Resection on an elective basis may be required.

APPENDIX A

Symptom-Oriented
Clinical Pathways

ACEP CLINICAL POLICIES

In recent years, a number of organizations have formulated practice guidelines for a variety of clinical conditions. Many terms have been applied to these guidelines: clinical pathways, critical pathways, rules, standards, policies, protocols, algorithms, decision trees, and scoring systems. They have been formulated by insurance companies, governmental entities, medical staffs, and professional organizations.

The emergence of guidelines is not without controversy. Although they do offer the clinician an opportunity to enhance the quality of care, some feel that their use stifles creativity and fosters "cookbook medicine." Guidelines can be used to enhance cost-effectiveness, but the potential exists for them to be manipulated to limit expensive but necessary care. The protocols may not easily be applied to atypical cases. Also, there is the concern that anything less than perfect adherence to the guidelines may be a cause of potential medical-legal liability.

Despite these issues, guidelines are here to stay. If formulated correctly, they offer all of us the opportunity to enhance our clinical effectiveness in the service of our patients.

It is the opinion of the authors that guidelines are best written by the physicians who will use them. Thus, we believe that inclusion of the clinical guidelines formulated by the American College of Emergency Physicians (ACEP) represents a valuable addition to our book.

ACEP has issued a number of Clinical Policies. This chapter includes those that are available as of publication date. Each policy contains a preface explaining that policy, the actual policy itself, often an appendix, and a bibliography. Each policy is accompanied by a Quality Assurance Form that can be helpful to the physicians implementing the policy in their own practice, as well as a Quick Reference Form that summarizes the essential points of the particular policy. *It is these Quick Reference Forms that are reprinted in this chapter.*

*We urge the reader to obtain the entire current set of policies from ACEP, since the Quick Reference Forms reprinted in this book are only **outlines** of the full policies.**

It must be emphasized that no guideline, whether those written by ACEP or any other entity, constitutes the medical-legal "standard of care." There must always be room for variation in medical practice and adaptation of clinical evaluation and treatment to the individual patient. However, clinical pathways can offer an invaluable assistance to us in our efforts to provide the best possible care to our patients.

The next paragraph, as well as the Quick Reference Forms that follow, is reprinted from the official ACEP documents and is copyrighted by the American College of Emergency Physicians:

> The rules and guidelines for patient management emphasize those findings with the potential for high risk to the patient. No single finding should be considered independently in the process of making a clinical diagnosis. Some actions are separated by a slash mark (/), which means that either action may be appropriate in a given clinical situation at the discretion of the clinician. The order in which items appear in the rules and guidelines is arbitrary and not meant to imply the order in which they should be performed. In using this clinical policy, it may be helpful to think of *Rules* as broad categories that should be recorded as pertinent positives or negatives, whereas *Guidelines* are detailed or expanded lists that are meant to prompt the physician to consider many possibilities. Documentation should be sufficient to reflect the clinical decision-making process. It is unrealistic to expect a physician to perform or document every item in the guidelines for any individual patient.

---

*American College of Emergency Physicians, Sales & Service Dept., P.O. Box 619911, Dallas, Tex., 75261-9911. Phone: 800-798-1822.

American College of Emergency Physicians

Quick Reference Form and Quicklist

Product No. 04146A

for the

*Clinical Policy
for the Initial Approach
to
Patients Presenting With
Acute Blunt Trauma*

Acute Blunt Trauma Quick Reference Form

For age 12 and above with blunt trauma who are not obviously pregnant. The policy is NOT for initial evaluation of a severely traumatized patient but is to be used after initial resuscitation, stabilization and evaluation have taken place.

Circle line number if yes. **Underlined actions are rules.** Actions not underlined are guidelines.

Chief Complaint

Acute Blunt trauma

History of Injury

1. major mechanism or suspected major mechanism of injury .... LBIV, O₂, MON, OX, spinal immobilization, Hct, UAB

2. vehicular crash (especially involving single vehicle) .... evaluate for precipitating event (medical, alcohol, toxin, psychiatric)

3. prehospital hypotension or altered level of consciousness .... LBIV, O₂, spinal immobilization, Hct, UAB, DPL or Abd CT

4. significant prehospital blood loss .... <u>Hct</u>, LBIV, O₂, MON, T&S

Review of Symptoms—Other Current Symptoms and Complaints

5. chest pain .... LBIV, O₂, MON, OX/ABG, cardiac enzymes, CXR, ECG

6. shortness of breath .... **LBIV, O₂, MON, OX/ABG, <u>CXR</u>,** Hct, ECG

7. numbness/weakness .... **spinal immobilization, spinal x-rays,** neurosurgical consult, ORTHO

Vital Signs

8. significant tachycardia or hypotension .... **LBIV, O$_2$, MON, Hct**

.... airway evaluation and management, assess for cardiac tamponade and tension pneumothorax, serial Hcts, OX/ABG,

.... LYTES, BUN, CREAT, amylase, PT, PTT, T&S/C, UAB, C-spine X-ray, CXR, pelvic x-ray, ECG, OG/NG, CATH,

.... CVP, DPL or Abd CT (if stabilized) or laparotomy, isotonic fluid resuscitation, transfuse blood, SURGC

9. unexplained persistent tachycardia .... **SURGC,** IV, O$_2$, MON, serial Hcts, OX/ABG, TOX, CXR, pelvic x-ray, DPL or Abd CT, admit

10. temperature <35°C(95°F) .... **hypothermia evaluation and management**

Physical Examination

11. altered level of consciousness .... LBIV, O$_2$, MON, airway evaluation and management,

.... head trauma evaluation and management, C-spine evaluation and management,

.... rapid glucose determination or dextrose IV, Hct, OX/ABG, LYTES , BUN, CREAT, amylase,

.... ethanol screen, TOX, C-spine X-ray, CXR, pelvic x-ray, ECG, OG/NG, CATH,

.... DPL or Abd CT, head CT, opiate antagonist, SURGC, neurosurgical consult

12. Appearance:external bleeding/open wounds .... **attempt hemostasis,** wound evaluation and repair, assess tetanus prophylaxis

13. Appearance:pale and diaphoretic .... **LBIV, O$_2$, MON, Hct,** OX, spinal immobilization,T&S, UAB, ECG

14. Face:massive facial trauma or gross instability .... **LBIV, O$_2$, immobilize C spine, airway eval and management, C-Spine X-ray,**

.... MON, avoid NG tube placement, close observation

15. Neck:hoarseness .... **airway evaluation and management**

16. Neck:tracheal deviation .... LBIV, O$_2$, MON, OX/ABG, CXR, thoracostomy

17. Neck:tenderness .... spinal immobilization, C-spine x-ray

18. Neck:JVD .... assess for cardiac tamponade and tension pneumothorax

19. Chest:new or symptomatic dysrhythmia,excluding sinus tachycardia .... **IV, O$_2$, MON, OX, CXR, ECG,**

.... cardiac enzymes, manage dysrhythmias, surgical consult, admit

Continued

20. Chest:dyspnea .... **IV, O$_2$, MON, OX/ABG, CXR**, ECG

21. Chest:traumatic deformity or abnormal chest movement .... **IV, O$_2$, MON, OX, CXR,** airway eval & management, ABG, ECG

22. Chest:subcutaneous emphysema or crepitus .... **IV, O$_2$, MON, OX, CXR,** ECG, thoracostomy

23. Chest:tenderness .... IV, O$_2$, CXR, ECG

24. Chest:unequal or diminished breath sounds .... **O$_2$, CXR**, OX/ABG, thoracostomy

25. Abdomen-moderate to severe abdominal tenderness ..... **Hct, UAB,** LBIV, O$_2$, MON, spinal immobilization, serial Hcts, LYTES, BUN,
.... amylase, PT, PTT, T&S/C, CXR, pelvic x-ray, ECG, OG/NG, CATH, DPL or Abd CT, SURGC

26. Abdomen:pelvic tenderness or instability .... **pelvic x-ray,** UAB, DPL or Abd CT

27. Rectal:lax sphincter tone .... spinal evaluation and management

28. Rectal:gross rectal blood .... **IV, Hct, pelvic exam(female), SURGC, admit,** O$_2$, MON, T&S, pelvic x-ray, DPL or Abd CT

29. Male genitalia and rectal:meatal blood or high-riding prostate .... **urethral injury evaluation**

30. Male:perineal hematoma .... **pelvic x-ray**

31. Female:perineal hematoma or non-menstrual(by history) vaginal bleeding .... **pelvic exam, pelvic x-ray,** pregnancy test

32. Flank:ecchymosis or tenderness or mass .... serial Hcts, UAB, lumbar spine x-ray, IVP or Abd CT

33. Back:tenderness or deformity .... spinal immobilization, spinal x-ray based on location of finding

34. Extremities:open fracture .... **ORTHO/SURGC,** distal NV status, immobilize, WC, x-ray, antibiotic, tetanus?, dressings, admit

35. Extremities:deformity .... assess distal NV status, immobilization, x-ray

36. Extremities:point tenderness .... x-ray

37. Extremities:NV compromise distal to fracture/deformity .... **x-ray, ORTHO/SURGC, admit,** manipulate for pulses, immobilize

38. Neuro:motor or sensory abnormality(not secondary to extremity injury) .... **spinal immobilization, spinal imaging,**
.... CT of head, neurosurgical/ORTHO consult

Diagnostic Testing

39. C-spine x-ray:cervical fracture, malalignment, or prevertebral soft tissue swelling ....**spinal immobilization,** ....**neurosurgical/ORTHO consult,** thoracic/lumbar spine x-rays, admit

40. CXR:hemothorax ....**Hct, SURGC, admit,** ECG, thoracostomy

41. CXR:pneumothorax ....Hct, ECG, thoracostomy, SURGC, admit

42. CXR:pulmonary contusion ....**O₂, MON, OX/ABG, SURGC, admit,** airway evaluation and management

43. CXR:OG/NG tube deviation,apical capping,obfuscation of the aortic knob,wide mediastinum, or depressed left mainstem bronchus
....**evaluate possible aortic injury,** upright CXR–compare to old CXR, aortogram/thoracic CT

44. CXR–flail chest segment ....**O2, MON, OX/ABG, SURGC, admit,** airway evaluation and management

45. CXR–ruptured diaphragm ....**LBIV O₂, MON, Hct, T&C, thoracostomy, SURGC, admit**
.... airway evaluation and management, serial Hcts, OX/ABG, LYTES, BUN, creatinine, amylase, PT,PTT, UAB,
.... C-spine x-ray, pelvic x-ray, ECG, OG/NG, isotonic fluid resuscitation,transfuse blood

46. Pelvic x-ray–fracture of individual pelvic bone w/o break in pelvic ring(includes single ramus fracture) .... IV, serial Hcts,
.... T&S/C, UAB, DPL or Abd CT, ORTHO/SURGC, admit

47. Pelvic x-ray–break in pelvic ring,or acetabular fracture ....**LBIV, MON, Hct, T&C, UAB, ORTHO/SURGC, admit,**
.... O₂, serial Hcts, LYTES, BUN, creatinine, PT,PTT, CATH, DPL or Abd CT,
.... PASG suit application, isotonic fluid resuscitation, transfuse blood

48. Hct–low or falling Hct ....**LBIV, SURGC,** T&C, transfuse blood, admit

49. Urine for blood–gross hematuria ....**SURGC, admit,** BUN,creatinine, cystogram, IVP/Abd CT

50. Urine for blood–microscopic hematuria with hypotension or significant back, flank, pelvic, or abdominal trauma ....IVP/AbdCT

51. ECG:new ischemic changes ....**IV, O₂, MON, CXR, admit,** OX/ABG, cardiac enzymes, consult

52. ECG:new dysrhythmia,excluding sinus tachycardia ....**IV, O₂, MON, CXR, admit,**
.... manage dysrhythmia, OX/ABG, cardiac enzymes, consult

Continued

53. DPL or abdominal CT-positive lavage or evidence of intra-abdominal injury .... **LBIV, Hct, T&S/C, SURGC, admit,**
.... O_2, MON, airway evaluation and management, serial Hcts, OX/ABG, LYTES, BUN, creatinine, amylase, PT,PTT, UAB,
.... C-spine x-ray, CXR, pelvic x-ray, ECG, OG/NG, CATH, isotonic fluid resuscitation, transfuse blood

54. ABG/OX:hypoxia .... O_2, airway evaluation and management, CXR

55. amylase:elevated .... SURGC

56. NG/OG tube:gross blood(not from trauma of tube placement) .... **SURGC**, CBC, T&C

Assessment

Due to the great number of possible combinations and degrees of severity of injuries from blunt trauma, a complete exposition of rules and guidelines for all possible assessments of the victim of blunt trauma would make this document unusable for the practicing emergency physician. However, there are basic philosophies which apply:

1. **Patient instability mandates aggressive attempts at resuscitation and definitive(surgical) treatment.**
2. **Discovery of significant injury to one organ system necessitates an evaluation of the patient for other possible injuries(when patient condition allows).**
3. **Surgical consultants should be involved as early as possible in the care of the seriously traumatized patient.**
4. **Close observation, including serial examinations, is very important early on in the evaluation and management of the severely injured patient.**
5. **Blood component therapy, as opposed to the administration of whole blood, is to be encouraged, but the decision should be left to the individual practitioner.**

Abbreviations

Abd-abdominal
ABG-arterial blood gas
BUN-blood urea nitrogen
CATH-urinary catheter placement
CREAT-creatinine
CT-computerized axial tomography
CVP-central venous line access
CXR-chest x-ray
DPL-diagnostic peritoneal lavage
ECG-electrocardiogram

Hct-hematocrit
IV-IV access
LBIV-large bore IV access
LYTES-electrolytes
MON-cardiac monitor
NV-neurovascular
O_2-supplemental oxygen
OG/NG-oral gastric/nasal gastric tube placement
ORTHO-orthopedic consult

OX-pulse oximetry
PASG-pneumatic anti-shock garment
PT,PTT-protime,partial thromboplastin time
SURGC-surgical consult
TOX-toxicology screen
T&C-type and crossmatch
T&S- type and screen
UAB-urinalysis for blood
WC-wound culture

Notes:

Acute Blunt Trauma Quicklist

Significant findings which trigger actions:

Significant H&P	Bolded findings trigger rules (& possibly guidelines). Findings not bolded trigger only guidelines.	Reference number after findings refer to findings & actions on Quick Reference Form
Chief Complaint		**Lab and X-ray Findings:**
Blunt trauma		
History of Injury:	major mechanism or suspected major mechanism of injury 1	**C-spine x-ray**
	vehicular crash (especially involving single vehicle) 2	**cervical fracture, malalignment, or prevertebral soft tissue**
	prehospital hypotension or altered level of consciousness 3	**swelling** 39
	significant prehospital blood loss 4	
		Chest X-ray
Review of	chest pain 5	**hemothorax** 40
Symptoms:	**shortness of breath** 6	pneumothorax 41
	numbness/weakness 7	pulmonary contusion 42
		OG/NG tube deviation, apical capping, obfuscation of the aortic knob, wide mediastinum, or depressed left mainstem
Recent history:		
Past history:		
Allergies:		
Medications:		

Physical Exam		
		bronchus 43
		flail chest segment 44
Vital Signs: BP	significant tachycardia or hypotension 8	ruptured diaphragm 45
Pulse, Respirations	unexplained persistent tachycardia 9	**Pelvic X-ray**
Temperature:	temperature <35°C(95°F) 10	fracture of individual pelvic bone w/o break in pelvic ring 46
Level of		break in pelvic ring, or
Consciousness:	altered level of consciousness 11	acetabular fracture 47
Appearance:	external bleeding/open wounds 12	
	pale and diaphoretic 13	
		Hematocrit
Face:	massive facial trauma or gross instability 14	low or falling 48
Neck:	hoarseness 15	**Urine for blood**
	tracheal deviation 16	**gross hematuria** 49
	tenderness 17	microscopic hematuria with
	jugular venous distention 18	hypotension or significant back,
		flank, pelvic, or abdominal
Chest:	new or symptomatic dysrhythmia, exclude sinus tach 19	trauma 50

Continued

Abdomen:

dyspnea 20
traumatic deformity or abnormal chest movement 21
subcutaneous emphysema or crepitus 22
tenderness 23
unequal or diminished breath sounds 24
moderate to severe abdominal tenderness 25

Genitalia & Rectal:

pelvic tenderness or instability 26
rectal-lax sphincter tone 27
rectal-gross rectal blood 28
male genitalia and rectal-meatal blood or high-riding prostate 29
male-perineal hematoma 30
female genitalia and rectal-perineal hematoma or non-menstrual (by history) vag bleeding 31

Flank: ecchymosis or tenderness or mass 32
Back: tenderness or deformity 33
Extremities: open fracture 34
deformity 35
point tenderness 36
NV compromise distal to fracture/deformity 37
motor or sensory abnormality(not secondary to ext. inj) 38

ECG
new ischemic changes 51
new dysrhythmia, excluding sinus tachycardia 52

DPL or abdominal CT
positive lavage or evidence of intra-abdominal injury 53

ABG/OX
hypoxia 54

Amylase
elevated 55

NG/OG tube
gross blood(not from trauma of tube placement) 56

American College of Emergency Physicians

Quick Reference Form

Product No. 04157A

for the

*Clinical Policy
for the Initial Approach
to
Patients Presenting With
Penetrating Extremity Trauma*

Quick Reference Form: Penetrating Extremity Trauma

Solicit and record a history that includes: mechanism of injury, approximate age of wound, tetanus immunization status, and allergies. Conduct and record a physical examination that includes: inspection of the area of injury.

Circle line number if yes. **Highlighted actions are rules.** Actions not highlighted are guidelines.

History

Mechanism of injury:

1. Potential for foreign body in wound...**explore when anatomically feasible,** imaging
2. Potential for underlying injury..**explore when anatomically feasible,** imaging
3. High potential for infection due to contamination...**attempt decontamination,** antibiotic administration
4. Mammalian bite...rabies risk assessment, antibiotic administration appropriate for biting species
5. Human bite...assess for joint penetration when proximate to joint,
   ....possible delayed closure, antibiotic administration
   ....antibiotic administration to prevent infection
   ....with *Capnocytophagia canimorsus* (DF-2), **consult**
6. Dog bite to asplenic or immunosuppressed patient.................................
7. High-pressure injection injury...**consult**

Age of wound:

8. Delayed presentation...possible delayed closure, antibiotic administration

Comorbidity:

9. Valvular heart disease, immunosuppression, diabetes mellitus, internal prosthetic device ....antibiotic administration
10. Keloid formation ....consult/referral
11. Inadequate tetanus prophylaxis ....**provide tetanus prophylaxis**, refer to ACEP information paper on tetanus immunization

Physical Examination

Location of wound:

12. Over metacarpophalangeal joint or other joints..............**assess potential for joint penetration**, assess potential for human bite, immobilization, consult.
....imaging, antibiotic administration, immobilization, consult
13. Palmar puncture wound..imaging, consult, no weight bearing
14. Plantar puncture wound

Inspection, palpation, exploration, neurovascular examination, range of motion:

15. Nerve injury...immobilization, consult
16. Suspicion of significant vascular injury ....**control bleeding**, IV access, immobilization, consult
17. Tendon injury...immobilization, repair or consult
18. Deformity suggestive of underlying fracture...**image**, immobilization
19. Open fracture..**image**, antibiotic administration, immobilization, consult
....imaging, wound exploration, antibiotic administration, immobilization, consult
20. Suspicion of joint violation ....**joint irrigation or consult**, imaging, antibiotic administration, immobilization
21. Joint violation ....**attempt decontamination**, wound irrigation and cleansing,
22. Visible wound contamination ....debridement, antibiotic administration, consult

Continued

23. Foreign body in wound ....imaging, removal of foreign body
24. Significant avulsion injury ....grafting, consult

Disposition

Admission ....**transfer care to accepting physician**
Transfer ....**follow ACEP and other applicable transfer principles**
Discharge ....**provide referral for follow-up care, provide instructions regarding treatment and**
........................**circumstances that require return to ED,** advise patient about wound care,
........................signs and symptoms of infection, signs and symptoms of compartment
........................syndrome, the possibility of retained foreign body, methods for relieving
........................pain, signs and symptoms suggestive of occult bone or tendon injury, follow-up, suture removal, care of the immobilized
........................extremity/splint

Notes:

American College of Emergency Physicians

Quick Reference Form

Product No. 03086A

for the

*Clinical Policy
for the Initial Approach
to Adults
Presenting With a Chief
Complaint of Chest Pain,
With
No History of Trauma*

Quick Reference Form: Chest Pain Revision

For adults with chest pain with no history of trauma. This policy does *not* include history of proximate trauma; or visible lesions; or isolated breast disease; or pain of very brief duration (lasting for seconds only).

Circle line number if yes. **Bolded actions are rules.** Actions not bolded are guidelines.

Chief Complaint

Chest pain with no history of trauma

History

Pain

1. ongoing *and* severe *and* crushing *and* substernal *or* same as previous pain diagnosed as MI . . . . **IV access, supplemental oxygen, cardiac monitor, ECG, aspirin, nitrates, management of ongoing pain, admit,** serum cardiac markers (eg, CKMB), CXR, anticoagulation

2. severe *or* pressure *or* substantial *or* exertional *or* radiating to jaw, neck, shoulder, or arm .... **ECG,** IV access,
.... supplemental oxygen, cardiac monitor, serum cardiac markers (eg, CKMB), CXR, nitrates,
.... management of ongoing pain, admit
3. tearing, severe, and radiating to back .... **large–bore IV access, supplemental oxygen, cardiac monitor,**
.... **CXR, ECG,** differential upper extremity blood pressures, aortic
.... imaging, management of ongoing pain, admit
4. similar to that of previous pulmonary embolus .... **IV access, supplemental oxygen, cardiac monitor,**
.... **ABG/oximetry, anticoagulation/pulmonary vascular imaging, ECG,** CXR, admit
5. indigestion or burning epigastric .... ECG
6. pleuritic .... CXR, ECG
7. age (male>33 years, female>40 years) .... ECG

Associated Symptoms

8. syncope or near–syncope .... **ECG,** cardiac monitor, Hct
9. SOB, DOE, PND, or orthopnea .... **ECG,** ABG/oximetry, CXR
10. significant hemoptysis .... **CXR,** respiratory isolation, ABG/oximetry
11. nausea/vomiting .... ECG
12. productive or chronic cough .... respiratory isolation, CXR
13. palpitations .... cardiac monitor, ECG
14. significant weight change .... CXR
15. diaphoresis .... ECG

Continued

Past Medical History

16. previous MI .... **ECG**
17. coronary artery bypass graft/angioplasty .... **ECG**
18. cocaine use within last 96 hours .... **ECG**
19. previous positive cardiac diagnostic studies .... **ECG**
20. cardiac medications .... serum drug levels, ECG
21. diuretics .... potassium level, magnesium level
22. IV drug abuse .... ABG/oximetry, CXR, ECG
23. major risk factors for coronary artery disease (see Appendix A) .... ECG
24. major risk factors for pulmonary embolism (see Appendix A) .... ABG/oximetry, CXR,
.... pulmonary vascular imaging, venous imaging, ECG
25. major risk factors for thoracic aortic aneurysm/dissection (see Appendix A) .... CXR,
.... aortic imaging, ECG
26. major risk factors for pericarditis/myocarditis (see Appendix A) .... serum cardiac markers, CXR,
.... echocardiography, ECG
27. major risk factors for pneumothorax (see Appendix A) .... oximetry, CXR
28. major risk factors for pneumonia (see Appendix A) .... ABG/oximetry, CXR

Physical Examination

Vital Signs

29. irregular pulse .... **rhythm strip/cardiac monitor**, ECG

30. tachypnea (RR>24) . . . . ABG/oximetry, CXR, ECG
31. fever (>38°C/100.4°F) . . . . CXR
32. hypertension (>160/110) . . . . CXR, ECG
33. tachycardia (>100) . . . . ABG/oximetry, ECG
34. bradycardia (<60) . . . . IV access, ECG

Appearance

35. cyanosis with respiratory distress . . . . **IV access, supplemental oxygen, cardiac monitor, ABG, CXR,**
. . . . **ECG,** methemoglobin level, pulmonary vascular imaging, intubation, admit
36. diaphoresis . . . . **ECG,** IV access, ABG/oximetry, serum cardiac markers, CXR, admit

Cardiovascular

37. significant differential upper extremity blood pressures . . . . **large–bore IV access, CXR, ECG,**
. . . . supplemental oxygen, cardiac monitor, aortic imaging
38. new murmur . . . . **ECG,** CXR, echocardiography

Continued

39. pericardial rub . . . . **ECG,** serum cardiac markers, CXR, echocardiography

40. irregular rhythm . . . . **rhythm strip/cardiac monitor,** ECG

41. JVD . . . . CXR, ECG

42. S$_3$ gallop . . . . CXR, ECG

Pulmonary

43. unilateral diminished breath sounds . . . . **CXR,** ABG/oximetry

44. localized dullness to percussion . . . . CXR

45. pleural rub . . . . ABG/oximetry, CXR, ECG

46. unilateral rales . . . . supplemental oxygen, ABG/oximetry, CXR

47. bilateral rales . . . . IV access, supplemental oxygen, ABG/oximetry, CXR, ECG

48. wheezing . . . . supplemental oxygen, cardiac monitor, ABG/oximetry, FEV$_1$/PEF, CXR, ECG, ... bronchodilators

Extremities

49. signs of DVT: leg swelling, pain, tenderness, warmth, or erythema . . . . ABG/oximetry, CXR, ... pulmonary vascular imaging, venous imaging, ECG

50. bilateral edema . . . . CXR, ECG

Diagnostic Testing

51. cardiac monitor/ECG: new dysrhythmia . . . . **cardiac monitor,** IV access, supplemental oxygen, ... potassium level, magnesium level, serum cardiac markers, ECG, antidysrhythmic therapy

52. ECG: new injury . . . . **IV access, supplemental oxygen, cardiac monitor, assess for thrombolytic therapy** . . . . **(see Appendix B) or other reperfusion techniques, anticoagulation, aspirin, nitrates,** . . . . **management of ongoing pain, admit,** serial serum cardiac markers, CXR, cardiac imaging, serial ECGs, ... magnesium therapy if not given thrombolytics, β–blockers

53. ECG: new ischemic changes .... **IV access, supplemental oxygen, cardiac monitor, anticoagulation,**
.... **aspirin, nitrates, management of ongoing pain, admit,** comparison with previous ECG if available,
.... serial serum cardiac markers, CXR, serial ECGs, β–blockers

54. ECG: nondiagnostic ECG .... comparison with previous ECG if available, IV access, supplemental oxygen,
.... cardiac monitor, serial serum cardiac markers, CXR, serial ECGs, nitrates, management of ongoing pain

55. CXR: acute pulmonary edema .... **IV access, supplemental oxygen, cardiac monitor,**
.... **ABG/oximetry, ECG, preload/afterload reduction (eg, diuretics/nitrates),**
.... serum cardiac markers, management of ongoing pain, inotropic support, admit

56. CXR: wide mediastinum (new) .... **large–bore IV access, aortic imaging,** differential upper extremity blood pressure,
.... supplemental oxygen, cardiac monitor, blood type and crossmatch, surgical consult

57. CXR: large pneumothorax .... **reexpansion,** IV access, supplemental oxygen, ABG/oximetry, admit

58. CXR: small pneumothorax .... IV access, ABG/oximetry, serial CXRs, reexpansion, consult

59. CXR: new infiltrate .... respiratory isolation, supplemental oxygen, ABG/oximetry, appropriate cultures, sputum for Gram stain,
.... antibiotics, admit

60. CXR: new mass .... ABG/oximetry

61. CXR: new effusion .... ABG/oximetry, thoracentesis

62. ABG: new significant A–a gradient or new significant reduction in P_{O_2} .... **Supplemental oxygen, CXR,** IV access,
.... cardiac monitor, pulmonary vascular imaging, ECG, admit

63. VQ scan: high probability of pulmonary embolus .... **IV access, supplemental oxygen, cardiac monitor, ABG/oximetry, anticoagulation, admit,** assess for thrombolytic therapy (see Appendix B), ECG

64. VQ scan: intermediate, low, and normal in presence of high clinical suspicion .... IV access, supplemental oxygen, cardiac monitor,
.... venous imaging, pulmonary angiography, anticoagulation, admit

Assessment

65. unstable angina: new-onset exertional .... **ECG, aspirin,** IV access, supplemental oxygen, cardiac monitor, nitrates, consult/admit

66. unstable angina: ongoing or recurrent ischemia .... **IV access, supplemental oxygen, cardiac monitor, ECG, anticoagulation, aspirin, nitrates, management of ongoing pain, admit,** serial serum cardiac markers, CXR, cardiac imaging, serial ECGs, β–blockers

67. high clinical suspicion of MI with nondiagnostic ECG   **IV access, supplemental oxygen, cardiac monitor, anticoagulation, aspirin, nitrates, management of ongoing pain, admit,** serial serum cardiac markers, CXR, cardiac imaging, serial ECGs, magnesium therapy, β–blockers

68. high clinical suspicion of MI with bundle branch block .... **IV access, supplemental oxygen, cardiac monitor, assessment for thrombolytic therapy (see Appendix B) or other reperfusion techniques, anticoagulation, aspirin, nitrates, management of ongoing pain, admit,** serial serum cardiac markers, CXR, cardiac imaging, serial ECGs, magnesium therapy if not given thrombolytics, β–blockers

69. low clinical suspicion of MI with nondiagnostic ECG ..... IV access, supplemental oxygen, cardiac monitor, serial serum cardiac markers, CXR, cardiac imaging, serial ECGs, anticoagulation, β–blockers, aspirin, nitrates, management of ongoing pain, admit

70. acute MI with diagnostic ECG .... **IV access, supplemental oxygen, cardiac monitor, assessment for thrombolytic therapy (see Appendix B) or other reperfusion techniques, anticoagulation, aspirin, nitrates, management of ongoing pain, admit,** serial serum cardiac markers, CXR, cardiac imaging, serial ECGs, magnesium therapy if not given thrombolytics , β–blockers

71. aortic dissection .... **large–bore IV access, supplemental oxygen, cardiac monitor, blood type and crossmatch, ECG, management of blood pressure/cardiac contractility, management of ongoing pain, immediate surgical consultation, admit,** aortic imaging

72. pericarditis/myocarditis .... **ECG,** serum cardiac markers, CXR, echocardiography, consult/admit

73. pneumonia .... **CXR,** ABG/oximetry, appropriate cultures, sputum for Gram stain, antibiotics

74. pulmonary embolus .... **IV access, supplemental oxygen, cardiac monitor, ABG/oximetry, CXR, ECG, anticoagulation, admit,** assessment for thrombolytic therapy (see Appendix B), venous imaging, consultation for filter placement if history of recurrent pulmonary embolus

Continued

75. pneumothorax .... **CXR**, IV access, supplemental oxygen, ABG/oximetry, serial CXRs, reexpansion, consult/admit

76. acute pulmonary edema ...... **IV access, supplemental oxygen, cardiac monitor, ABG/oximetry, CXR, ECG, preload/afterload reduction (eg, diuretics/nitrates)**, serum .... cardiac markers, management of ongoing pain, inotropic support, admit

Disposition

77. admission .... **transfer care to accepting physician**

78. transfer .... **follow ACEP and other applicable transfer policies**

79. discharge .... **provide referral for follow–up care, provide instructions regarding treatment and circumstances that require return to emergency department**

Abbreviations		
A-a gradient=arterial to alveolar oxygen gradient	DVT=deep vein thrombosis	IV=intravenous
	DOE=dyspnea on exertion	JVD=jugular venous distension
ABG=arterial blood gas	ECG=electrocardiogram	MI=myocardial infarction
CXR=chest x-ray	FEV$_1$/PEF=forced expiratory volume	PND=paroxysmal nocturnal dyspnea
	1-second /peak expiratory flow	SOB=shortness of breath

Notes:

American College of Emergency Physicians

Quick Reference Form

Product No. 04156A

for the

*Clinical Policy
for the Initial Approach
to
Patients Presenting With
a Chief Complaint of
Nontraumatic Acute
Abdominal Pain*

Nontraumatic Acute Abdominal Pain Quick Reference Form

Solicit and record a history that includes: description of pain, associated symptoms, gynecologic history in women, past history.
Conduct and record a physical exam that includes: vital signs: blood pressure, pulse, respirations, temperature; cardiovascular, pulmonary, abdomen: palpation.

Circle line number if yes. **Underlined actions are rules.** Actions not underlined are guidelines.

Final ED Assessment

1. abdominal aortic aneurysm .... **large bore IV access x 2, supplemental oxygen, HCT, T&S/C, frequent assessment, consult, admit,**
...........................assess peripheral pulses, ELECT, BUN, creatinine, PT, PTT, diagnostic imaging, blood pressure management

2. abdominal pain of unknown etiology...observe or early follow-up

3. appendicitis...**consult, admit**, CBC, UA

4. bowel obstruction...**IV access, consult, admit**, rectal exam, ELECT, CBC, abdominal series, NG suction

5. cholecystitis (acute)/biliary obstruction.......................................**IV consult**, hepatic enzymes (liver function tests), amylase or lipase, CBC,
....diagnostic imaging, antibiotics, admit

6. cholelithiasis/biliary colic...diagnostic imaging, pain management

7. diverticulitis..**antibiotics**, consult/early follow-up

8. ectopic pregnancy...........................**consult**, IV, HCT, T&S, quantitative beta hCG, diagnostic imaging, culdocentesis, Rh immune globulin, admit

9. enteritis...advise occupational and public health precautions

10. hepatitis...assess hydration, PT, serologic testing, advise occupational and public health precautions

11. hernia..**evaluate for incarceration**

12. mesenteric ischemia ....**IV access, consult, admit**, ABG, ELECT, amylase, CBC, T&S, diagnostic imaging, ECG

13. ovarian torsion ....**consult, admit**, diagnostic imaging

14. testicular torsion ....**consult**, diagnostic imaging

15. pancreatitis ....oximetry/ABG, calcium, hepatic enzymes (liver function tests), amylase/lipase, glucose, CBC, hydration, pain management, consult

16. pelvic inflammatory disease or other sexually transmitted disease ....**disease specific therapeutic agent**, ...assess for pregnancy, CBC, ...serologic screening, evaluate need for HIV testing, UA, counsel regarding notification of partners/ public health precautions, ...pain management, consult

17. pyelonephritis ....**assess for pregnancy, antibiotics**, pain management

Disposition

18. admission ....**transfer care to accepting physician**

19. transfer ....**follow ACEP and other applicable transfer principles**

20. discharge ....**provide referral for follow-up care, provide instructions regarding treatment and circumstances** ....**that require return to ED**

Continued

Abbreviations

ABG	arterial blood gas	HCT	hematocrit
CBC	complete blood count	NG	naso-gastric
ECG	electrocardiogram	PT	protime
ELECT	electrolytes	PTT	partial thromboplastin time
		T&C	Blood type and crossmatch
		T&S	blood type and screen
		UA	urinalysis

Notes:

American College of Emergency Physicians

Quick Reference Form

Product No. 04197A

for the

*Clinical Policy
for the Initial Approach
to
Vaginal Bleeding*

Quick Reference Form: Vaginal Bleeding Clinical Policy

> For postmenarchal patients who present with a chief complaint of vaginal bleeding. This clinical policy does *not* include premenarchai females.

Circle line number if yes. **Bolded actions are rules.** Actions not bolded are guidelines.

Chief complaint

Vaginal bleeding in postmenarchal patients

History

Description of Bleeding

1. Heavy/significant bleeding · · · · · · · · · · · **inspection for tissue in cervical os/erosive lesions,** IV access, Hct, coagulation studies, β-hCG

2. Tissue/clot passage · inspection of tissue for fetal parts, tissue submission for pathologic analysis

Menstrual History

3. Premenopausal or perimenopausal · **β-hCG,** Hct

4. Postmenopausal · Hct, referral

Gynecologic History

5. IUD or hormonal contraceptive use—oral . . . . β-hCG, Hct, evaluate for STD and vulvovaginitis

6. IUD or hormonal contraceptive use—injected, implanted . . . . Hct, β-hCG, evaluate for STD and vulvovaginitis

7. Ectopic risk factors . . . . β-hCG, pelvic ultrasound, consult

8. PID risk factors . . . . β-hCG, evaluate for STD and vulvovaginitis

9. History of gynecologic malignancy, abnormal Pap smear, DES exposure . . . . **referral**, Hct

Obstetric History

10. 1st half of pregnancy or post elective termination . . . . β-hCG, Hct, Rh type, quantitative β-hCG, pelvic ultrasound

11. 2nd half of pregnancy . . . . **assess for fetal heart tones**, IV access, Hct, Rh type, blood type and screen, pelvic ultrasound for placental localization, consult

12. <6 weeks postpartum . . . . Hct, pelvic ultrasound

Associated Symptoms

13. Pain . . . . β-hCG, catheter urinalysis, evaluate for STD and vulvovaginitis, pelvic ultrasound, pain management

14. Weakness/syncope/near-syncope . . . . β-hCG, IV access, Hct

15. Bruising or bleeding tendencies . . . . Hct, platelet count, coagulation studies

16. Urinary symptoms . . . . catheter urinalysis, evaluation for STD and vulvovaginitis

17. Vaginal discharge . . . . evaluate for STD and vulvovaginitis or foreign body

Past Medical History

18. Coagulopathy/anticoagulation . . . . Hct, platelet count, PT, PTT

Physical Examination

Vital Signs

19. Significant tachycardia/hypotension . . . . **IV access, Hct, β-hCG, fluid resuscitation**, blood type and screen/crossmatch, consult

20. Fever . . . . evaluate for pelvic infection/STD/endometritis, CBC, catheter urinalysis, urine culture

Continued

Dermatologic

21. Ecchymoses, petechiae · Hct, platelet count, DIC panel, PT/PTT, D-Dimer

Abdominal Examination

22. Fetal heart tones · ultrasound for gestational age and placental localization

23. Tenderness · β-hCG, evaluate for pelvic infection/STD, pelvic ultrasound

24. Signs of peritoneal irritation · β-hCG, IV access, CBC, ultrasound, culdocentesis, consult

Pelvic Examination

25. Heavy/significant bleeding · · · · · · · · · · inspection for erosive lesions/tissue in cervical os, β-hCG, IV access, Hct, blood type and screen, consult

26. Adnexal/uterine mass or enlargement · β-hCG, evaluate for pelvic infection/STD, ultrasound

27. Cervical motion or uterine tenderness · β-hCG, evaluate for pelvic infection/STD

28. Bleeding vulvar/vaginal lesions · assess for traumatic etiology, referral for biopsy

29. Internal cervical os open · Hct, consult

30. Tissue/clot in cervical os in 1st half of pregnancy · tissue removal, consult

Diagnostic Testing

31. Positive β-hCG · Hct, Rh type, quantitative β-hCG, ultrasound

32. Rh typing in pregnancy–Rh negative · **evaluate for anti-D immune globulin (RhoGam) administration**

Diagnostic Testing

33. Pelvic ultrasound: intrauterine pregnancy .... Hct, Rh type, threatened abortion precautions

34. Pelvic ultrasound: no intrauterine pregnancy with positive β-hCG .... **consult,** Hct, Rh type, quantitative β-hCG, culdocentesis, ... ectopic precautions if discharged

35. Culdocentesis—nonclotting blood .... **IV access, Hct, blood type and screen/crossmatch, consult**

36. Hct—symptomatic anemia .... iron supplement, follow local transfusion guidelines, consult

37. Coagulation study—abnormal .... treat for specific deficiency, consult

38. STD evaluation—positive result or high clinical suspicion .... **β-hCG, follow CDC guidelines,** referral for HIV testing, test for syphilis, counseling

39. Fetal heart rate in 2nd half of pregnancy (<120 beats per minute or >160 beats per minute) .... **consult**

Continued

Assessment

Pregnancy-related (*1st half*) bleeding

40. Threatened abortion–intrauterine pregnancy confirmed .... Rh type, threatened abortion precautions
41. Threatened abortion–intrauterine pregnancy not confirmed ....**ectopic precautions if discharged,** Rh type, quantitative β-hCG, culdocentesis, ...pelvic ultrasound, consult
42. Inevitable abortion (internal os open) .... **consult,** Hct, Rh type, pelvic ultrasound
43. Incomplete abortion or post elective termination ....**send tissue, if any, to pathology. consult,** Rh type, pelvic ultrasound, ...removal of products of conception from cervix
44. Presumed completed abortion ....**referral to confirm completion, send tissue, if any, to pathology.** Rh type, quantitative β-hCG, pelvic ultrasound, ...ectopic precautions if discharged
45. Presumed fetal demise detected on ultrasound ....**consult,** Rh type, quantitative β-hCG
46. Ectopic pregnancy–presumed/probable ....**ultrasound/culdocentesis/consult,** IV access, Hct, blood type and screen/crossmatch, Rh type, ...quantitative β-hCG, admit/observation, ectopic precautions if discharged
47. Ectopic pregnancy–ultrasound consistent with ectopic ....**consult, ectopic precautions if discharged,** IV access, Hct, blood type and screen/crossmatch, ...Rh type, quantitative β-hCG, admit/observation
48. Molar pregnancy ....**consult,** ultrasound, quantitative β-hCG
49. Pregnancy related (*2nd half*) bleeding–abruptio placenta ....**fetal heart rate, IV access, Hct, blood type and screen/crossmatch, consult,** oxygen, ...continuous fetal monitoring, DIC screening, platelet count, PT, PTT
50. Pregnancy-related (*2nd half*) bleeding–placenta previa ...**fetal heart rate, Rh type, consult,** IV access, continuous fetal monitoring, Hct, blood type and screen
51. Pregnancy-related <6 weeks postpartum bleeding ....Hct, quantitative β-hCG, pelvic ultrasound, consult
52. Non-pregnancy related PID or other sexually transmitted disease ....**follow CDC guidelines,** syphilis testing, referral for HIV testing, ...counsel regarding notification of partners/public health precautions, pain management, consult
53. Suspected cancer ....consult

54. Bleeding disorders .... initiate treatment for specific bleeding disorder, consult
55. Anovulatory bleeding .... consult
56. Local perineal/vulvar/vaginal/cervical lesion .... culture lesion, consult
57. Uterine fibroids .... consult
58. Other medically related bleeding .... assess for liver, kidney, thyroid dysfunction, consult

Disposition

59. Admission .... **transfer care to accepting physician**
60. Transfer .... **follow ACEP and other applicable transfer policies**
61. Discharge .... **provide referral for follow-up care, provide instructions regarding treatment and circumstances that require return to**
.... **emergency department**

Abbreviations		**Notes:**
CBC=complete blood count	IUD=intrauterine device	
CDC=Centers for Disease Control and Prevention	PID=pelvic inflammatory disease	
DES=Diethylstilbestrol	PT=prothrombin time	
DIC=disseminated intravascular coagulation	PTT=partial thromboplastin time	
Hct=hematocrit	Rh=rhesus (blood factor)	
HIV=human immunodeficiency virus	STD=sexually transmitted disease	
IV=intravenous		

American College of Emergency Physicians

Quick Reference Form

Product No. 04176A

for the

*Clinical Policy
for the Initial Approach
to
Adolescents and Adults
Presenting to the Emergency
Department
With a Chief Complaint
of Headache*

Quick Reference Form: Headache Clinical Policy

For adolescent and adult patients who present with a chief complaint of headache. This clinical policy does *not* include patients with identified history of acute head trauma.

Circle line number if yes. **Bolded actions are rules.** Actions not bolded are guidelines.

Chief Complaint

Headache with no identified history of acute head trauma

History

Headache

1. Severe sudden (thunderclap) onset . . . . **CT if available, LP if CT negative or not available (CSF for cell count and xanthochromia)**,
. . . . consult

Continued

2. Potential carbon monoxide exposure .... **100% oxygen, carboxyhemoglobin level**, investigate source of exposure

3. Change from past headaches ....directed neurologic exam, neuroimaging

4. Change in functional level ....directed neurologic exam, electrolytes, glucose level, carboxyhemoglobin level,
....CSF syphilis test, neuroimaging, LP

5. Headache localized to the vertex ....CT, sinus imaging

6. History of benign primary headache disorder (migraine, tension, cluster) without change from previous episode ....See Assessment

7. History of HIV/immunocompromise ....MRI or CT (with and without contrast if HIV positive), LP (CSF analysis including
....a syphilis test, and fungal and mycobacterial studies), antimicrobials

8. History of non-CNS malignancy ....directed neurologic exam, neuroimaging

9. History of neurosurgery or CNS shunt ....CT, LP, shunt evaluation, consult

Associated Symptoms

10. New neurologic symptoms .... **directed neurologic exam**, neuroimaging

11. Diplopia or visual field defects .... **ophthalmologic exam**, neuroimaging

12. Visual acuity changes .... **ophthalmologic exam**, tonometry, erythrocyte sedimentation rate

13. New onset seizure/syncope .... **cardiac monitor**, IV access, electrolytes, glucose or rapid serum glucose
..................................determination, carboxyhemoglobin level, neuroimaging, ECG, LP

14. Protracted or recurrent vomiting ....assess degree of hydration, electrolytes, carboxyhemoglobin level, CT, LP, antiemetics

Current Medications/Substance Abuse

15. Alcohol abuse ....neuroimaging

16. Anticoagulant use ....PT/PTT, CT

17. Chronic analgesic use ....consult

18. Chronic ergotamine use ....consult/admit

19. Sympathomimetic ....blood pressure monitoring, neuroimaging, consult

Past Medical History

20. Current or recent pregnancy .... directed neurologic exam, blood pressure monitoring, UA, neuroimaging, consult
21. History of AVM/aneurysm .... funduscopic exam, assess for meningeal signs, CT, LP

Physical Examination

Vital Signs

22. Fever .... **assess for meningeal signs,** CT, LP, antipyretics, antibiotics
23. Significant hypertension .... assess for end-stage organ damage, CT, LP (CSF for cell count and xanthochromia),
  .... management of blood pressure, consult, admit

Head

24. Sensitivity to dental percussion .... transillumination, sinus imaging, dental referral
25. Sinus tenderness .... transillumination, sinus imaging
26. Temporal artery/scalp tenderness .... reassess history for myalgias, arthralgias, jaw claudication; visual acuity, erythrocyte
  .... sedimentation rate, consult

Neck

27. Nuchal rigidity or other meningeal signs–suspect subarachnoid hemorrhage .... **CT if available, LP if CT negative or not available,**
  .... other neuroimaging studies, consult
28. Nuchal rigidity or other meningeal signs–suspect meningitis .... **LP, antibiotics if bacterial etiology suspected,** CT
29. Nuchal rigidity and fever .... **LP, antibiotics,** blood cultures, CT, antipyretics, consult, admit

Physical Examination

Neurologic

30. New neurologic finding including change in mental status .... **neuroimaging**, directed toxic-metabolic evaluation, IV access,
.... supplemental oxygen, cardiac monitor, serum sodium determination,
.... rapid glucose determination, carboxyhemoglobin level, LP, consult

31. New ataxia (including nystagmus) or abnormal gait .... **neuroimaging with special attention to posterior fossa,**
.... surgical consult

Eye

32. New corneal clouding .... **visual acuity, tonometry/consult**
33. New visual field defects .... **neuroimaging**, other neurologic imaging studies, consult
34. Ophthalmoplegia .... **neuroimaging**, consult

35. Papilledema . . . . **neuroimaging,** consult

36. Change in visual acuity . . . . swinging flashlight test (Marcus Gunn pupil), pinhole test, tonometry, glucose
. . . . determination, erythrocyte sedimentation rate (if age >50 years), consult

37. Ipsilateral ptosis and miosis (Horner's syndrome) . . . . carotid imaging, consult

38. Pain with extraocular movement . . . . swinging flashlight test (Marcus Gunn pupil), visual acuity, orbital CT,
. . . . ophthalmologic consult

Diagnostic Testing

39. Carboxyhemoglobin level–clinically significant elevation . . . . **treat for carbon monoxide toxicity (see Assessment),** consult

40. Tonometry–elevated intraocular pressure . . . . **evaluate for acute glaucoma,** consult

41. LP–significant numbers of WBCs . . . . **assess for meningitis/encephalitis (bacterial, fungal,**
. . . . **viral) or vasculitis,** antimicrobials, consult, admit

42. LP–bacterial organisms on Gram stain of CSF . . . . **IV access, antibiotics, admit,** electrolytes, serum glucose determination,
. . . . CBC, respiratory isolation

43. LP–positive India ink test or fungal antigen . . . . **treat as fungal meningitis (see Assessment),** assess for HIV

44. LP–positive acid-fast bacillus stain . . . . **respiratory isolation, treat as acid-fast bacillus meningitis,**
. . . . assess for HIV

45. LP–RBCs in CSF with no difference in red cell numbers between tube 1 and tube 4 . . . . . . **treat as subarachnoid hemorrhage**
. . . . **(see Assessment)**

46. LP–xanthochromic CSF . . . . **treat as subarachnoid/intracranial hemorrhage (see Assessment)**

47. LP–CSF protein >100 mg/dL . . . . assess for meningitis (including TB, syphilis, Lyme disease and
. . . . fungal), neoplasms, or multiple sclerosis

48. LP–increased intracranial pressure with normal CSF analysis . . . . assess for idiopathic intracranial hypertension (pseudotumor
. . . . cerebri), mass lesions

Continued

49. LP—significant decrease in CSF/serum glucose ratio .... treat as bacterial meningitis (see Assessment)
50. Neuroimaging—CNS mass lesion/midline shift .... **directed neurologic exam, consult, admit**, IV access, supplemental
.... oxygen, cardiac monitor, assess for increased intracranial pressure,
.... airway management, steroids, admit
51. Neuroimaging—new dilated/slit-like ventricles .... **consult LP**
52. Neuroimaging—normal with meningeal signs .... visual acuity, steroids, consult
53. Erythrocyte sedimentation rate—elevated (age >50 years) .... treat as sinusitis (see Assessment)
54. Sinus imaging—sinus fluid or mucosal thickening .... treat as sinusitis (see Assessment)
55. UA—3 + or greater protein in the 2nd half of pregnancy or recent postpartum patient .... **assess for pregnancy–induced hypertension (preeclampsia)**, consult, admit

Assessment

56. Subarachnoid hemorrhage .... **IV access, serial reassessment, consult, admit**, supplemental oxygen,
.... cardiac monitor, airway management, electrolytes, CBC, platelet count,
.... PT/PTT, management of blood pressure, elevate head of bed 30°,
.... Nimodipine, anticonvulsants
57. Subdural hematoma, acute .... **IV access, serial reassessment, consult, admit**, supplemental oxygen,
.... cardiac monitor, airway management, electrolytes, BUN/creatinine, CBC, PT/PTT,
.... blood type and screen, elevate head of bed 30°
58. Subdural hematoma, chronic .... **consult**

Assessment

59. Epidural hematoma, acute .... **IV access, serial reassessment, urgent neurosurgical consult, admit,**
.... supplemental oxygen, cardiac monitor, airway management, electrolytes,
.... BUN/creatinine, CBC, PT/PTT, blood type and screen, management of blood
.... pressure, elevate head of bed 30°

60. Intracerebral hemorrhage, acute .... **IV access, serial reassessment, consult, admit,** supplemental oxygen,
.... cardiac monitor, airway management, electrolytes, BUN/creatinine, CBC,
.... PT/PTT, management of blood pressure

61. Cerebellar hemorrhage, acute .... **IV access, serial reassessment, urgent neurosurgical consult, admit,**
.... supplemental oxygen, cardiac monitor, airway management, electrolytes, BUN/
.... creatinine, CBC, PT/PTT, blood type and screen, management of blood pressure

Continued

62. Non-hemorrhagic cerebrovascular accident . . . . **serial reassessment, consult/admit**, IV access, supplemental oxygen,
. . . . cardiac monitor, airway management, electrolytes, duplex doppler sonography

63. Cerebral venous sinus thrombosis . . . . **consult, admit**, heparinization, antibiotics

64. Carotid artery dissection . . . . **consult, admit**, CBC, PT/PTT

65. Meningitis, bacterial . . . . **antibiotics, admit**, CBC, PT/PTT, analgesics, antipyretics

66. Meningitis, viral . . . . antiviral medication, analgesics, consult, admit

67. Meningitis, fungal . . . . **consult**, IV antifungal medication, admit

68. Retro-orbital infection . . . . **antibiotics, consult, admit**

69. CNS abscess . . . . **consult**, antibiotics, admit

70. Sinusitis . . . . decongestants/vasoconstrictors, saline nasal spray, steroids, analgesics,
. . . . antibiotics, consult, admit

71. CNS tumor . . . . **consult**, steroids

72. Acute hydrocephalus . . . . **consult**, admit

73. Idiopathic intracranial hypertension (pseudotumor cerebri) . . . . LP, pharmacologic therapy, consult

74. Acute glaucoma . . . . **ophthalmology consult**, pharmacologic therapy

75. Optic neuritis . . . . **consult**, steroids

76. Carbon monoxide toxicity . . . . **100% oxygen**, investigate source of exposure, hyperbaric oxygen, admit

77. Temporal arteritis . . . . **steroids, consult**, admit

78. Febrile headache . . . . evaluate and treat source as indicated, antipyretic

79. Vasculitis . . . . steroids, consult, admit

80. Pregnancy induced hypertension . . . . consult

81. Primary headache syndromes: migraine, tension-type, cluster . . . antiemetics, analgesics, serotonin receptor modulators, sedatives,
. . . . steroids, oxygen, consult

Disposition

82. Admission .... transfer care to accepting physician
83. Transfer .... follow ACEP and other applicable transfer principles
84. Discharge .... provide referral for follow-up care, provide instructions regarding treatment
.... and circumstances that require return to ED

Abbreviations

AVM=arteriovenous
   malformation
BUN=blood urea nitrogen
CBC=complete blood count

CNS=central nervous
   system
CSF=cerebrospinal fluid
CT=computed tomography
ECG=electrocardiogram

IV=intravenous
LP=lumbar puncture
PT/PTT=protime, partial
   thromboplastin time
RBCs=red blood cells

TB=tuberculosis
UA=urinalysis
WBCs=white blood cells

Notes:

American College of Emergency Physicians

Quick Reference Form

Product No. 04147A

for the

*Clinical Policy
for the Initial Approach
to
Patients Presenting With a
Chief Complaint of
Seizure,
Who Are Not in Status Epilepticus*

Quick Reference Form: Seizure Clinical Policy

For patients 6 years or older who have had a seizure, and are not in status epilepticus.

This clinical policy is *not* intended for use with patients in whom seizure is due to eclampsia or to acute head trauma.

Circle line number if yes. **Bolded actions are rules.** Actions not bolded are guidelines.

Chief complaint

Patient 6 years or older who has had a seizure, and is not in status epilepticus.

History

1. Seizure history—known epileptic . . . . .seek exacerbants, antiepileptic drug levels

2. Seizure history—epileptic with new seizure type or pattern, or no previous workup . . . .**seek etiology/exacerbants**, evaluate as first seizure, antiepileptic
. . . . .drug levels

3. Seizure history—no previous seizure . . . . **evaluate as first seizure**

Continued

4. Circumstances—potential deceleration injury secondary to seizure .... C-spine immobilization, C-spine x-ray
5. Exacerbants—drug/toxins/occupational exposures .... toxicologic screen/levels
6. Exacerbants—ethanol use .... glucose determination

Medications

7. Patient taking antiepileptic drugs .... antiepileptic drug levels
8. Patient taking oral hypoglycemics/insulin .... **glucose determination**, administer dextrose
9. Patient taking anticoagulants .... coagulation studies, noncontrast head CT

Medical History

10. Recent head trauma .... noncontrast head CT
11. Diabetes .... glucose determination
12. Heart disease .... cardiac monitor, ECG
13. Coagulopathy/platelet disorder .... CBC, coagulation studies, noncontrast head CT, treat coagulopathy
14. History of electrolyte abnormalities .... electrolytes
15. History of renal failure .... electrolytes, BUN/creatinine
16. No recent menses in patient with reproductive potential .... pregnancy test
17. 2nd half of pregnancy .... assess blood pressure, deep tendon reflexes, and urine protein, assess fetal status, consult obstetrician
18. HIV positive/immunosuppression .... CBC, MRI or CT (with and without contrast), LP if not contraindicated by neuroimaging studies
19. Alcoholism .... electrolytes/magnesium level, BUN/creatinine, glucose determination, toxicologic screen, alcohol level, CBC, platelets, prothrombin time, ... noncontrast head CT, thiamine administration, magnesium administration

Physical Examination

20. Vital signs—temperature elevation .... drug screen, LP, antibiotics, manage temperature
21. Vital signs—abnormal respirations .... supplemental oxygen, ABG/pulse oximetry

22. Vital signs—bradycardia/tachycardia/irregular pulse .... cardiac monitor, ECG

23. Head—signs of recent trauma .... noncontrast head CT

24. Neck—cervical spine tenderness .... C-spine immobilization, C-spine x-ray

25. Neck—stiff neck on flexion .... blood culture, noncontrast head CT, LP, antibiotics

26. Neurologic examination—mental status not at baseline but improving .... **observe, reexamine, IV access**

27. Neurologic examination—mental status not at baseline and not improving ... IV access, oxygen/pulse oximetry, **electrolytes, glucose level, rapid glucose determination/administer dextrose**, noncontrast head CT, **observe, reexamine**, rectal temperature, cardiac monitor, ABG/carboxyhemoglobin, calcium level, magnesium level, BUN/creatinine, toxicologic screen/levels, alcohol level, CBC, UA, EEG, ECG, LP, opiate antagonist, thiamine administration, magnesium administration, consult/admit

28. New focal abnormality .... **IV access, noncontrast head CT, observe, reexamine, consult/admit**, supplemental oxygen, oximetry, electrolytes, calcium, BUN/creatinine, toxicologic screen, CBC, LP

Assessment

29. First seizure without known etiology or previously diagnosed seizure with change in pattern without attributable cause—With mental status returning to baseline **evaluate for pregnancy, serum sodium level, glucose determination, noncontrast head CT or schedule neuroimaging, provide referral for follow-up care or admit**, oxygen/pulse oximetry, cardiac monitor, electrolytes, calcium level, BUN/creatinine, toxicologic screen, CBC, RPR, HIV testing, UA, EEG, LP, antiepileptic drug, glucose, consult

Assessment—*continued*

30. First seizure without known etiology or previously diagnosed seizure with change in pattern without attributable cause—With mental status not returning to
baseline . . . . **reexamine, IV access, oxygen/pulse oximetry/ABG, evaluate for pregnancy, electrolytes, glucose determination/administer dextrose,**
. . . . **noncontrast head CT, observe/admit,** rectal temperature, cardiac monitor, ABG/carboxyhemoglobin, calcium level, magnesium level, BUN/creatinine,
. . . . toxicologic screen/levels, alcohol level, CBC, UA, EEG, ECG, LP, opiate antagonist, thiamine administration, magnesium administration, consult/admit

31. Previously diagnosed epilepsy . . . **observe, manage antiepileptic drug levels, provide referral for follow-up care,** evaluate for drug compliance, evaluate for drug
. . . . interaction, discuss any change in dosing with primary care physician

32. Alcohol-related seizure (that is not a first seizure) . . . . . . **observe, provide referral for follow-up care for seizure, electrolytes, magnesium level, rapid blood**
. . . . glucose determination or administer dextrose, CBC, thiamine administration, magnesium administration, treat ethanol withdrawal, refer for drug abuse
. . . . rehabilitation

33. Drug/toxin related seizure (that is not a first seizure) . . . . **observe, provide referral for follow-up care,** decontamination, specific antidotes/management,
. . . . treat for drug toxicity/withdrawal, refer for drug abuse rehabilitation
. . . .

Disposition

34. Admission .... transfer care to accepting physician

35. Transfer .... follow ACEP and other applicable transfer policies

36. Discharge .... provide referral for follow-up care, provide instructions regarding treatment and circumstances that require return to .... emergency department

Notes:

Abbreviations

ABG=arterial blood gas	HIV=human immunodeficiency virus
BUN=blood urea nitrogen	IV=intravenous
CBC=complete blood count	LP=lumbar puncture
C-spine=cervical spine	MRI=magnetic resonance imaging
CT=computed tomography	RPR=rapid plasma reagin
ECG=electrocardiogram	UA=urinalysis
EEG=electroencephalogram	

American College of Emergency Physicians

Quick Reference Form

Product No. 04160A

for the

*Clinical Policy
for the Initial Approach
to Patients
Presenting With
Acute Toxic Ingestion
or Dermal or Inhalation
Exposure*

Quick Reference Form: Acute Toxic Ingestion or Dermal or Inhalation Exposure

Solicit and record a history that includes: history of exposure, and past medical history. Conduct and record a physical exam that includes: vital signs (blood pressure, pulse, respirations, temperature), general appearance, weight (if age <6 years), neurologic mental status, cardiovascular, and pulmonary.

Circle line number if yes. **Bolded actions are rules.** Actions not bolded are guidelines.

History

1. Dermal exposure . . . **skin decontamination (may be performed prehospital), protection of health care worker,** complete disrobing . . . . of patient (proper disposal), assess for systemic exposure/toxicity, perform copious eye irrigation with water, decontamination of skin . . . . folds/creases

2. Gastrointestinal exposure–caustics . . . . **avoid emesis and gastric lavage,** dilute, endoscopy

3. Gastrointestinal exposure—hydrocarbons . . . . evaluate neurologic and pulmonary status
4. Most other toxic substances . . . . . **charcoal**, protection of health care worker, GI decontamination, specific drug or toxic substance levels,
. . . . radiopaque substances: KUB, drug bezoars, body packers: contrast study
5. Intentional ingestion . . . . **evaluation for potential suicidal risk**, patient restraint, patient supervision, psychiatric consultation
6. Accidental ingestion . . . . **evaluation for abuse or neglect**, protective service referral
7. Unknown potentially toxic substances . . . . . **charcoal**, GI decontamination, acetaminophen level, salicylate level, toxicologic blood screen,
. . . . toxicologic urine screen
8. Inhalation exposure . . . . protection of patient and health care worker, supplemental oxygen, humidification, ABG/oximetry/co-
. . . . oximetry/methemoglobin level/carboxyhemoglobin level, CXR

Physical Examination

9. Pulse <60 . . . . **IV access, cardiac monitor**, supplemental oxygen/ABG/oximetry, ECG
10. Pulse >120 (≥6 years), >140 (peds <6 years) . . . . . . **IV access, cardiac monitor**, supplemental oxygen/oximetry, ABG/cooximetry/methe-
. . . . moglobin level/carboxyhemoglobin level, ECG
11. Pulse-irregular . . . . **cardiac monitor**, IV access, ECG
12. Respirations <10 (adult), <xx (peds) See Attachment A . . . . **IV access, supplemental oxygen, cardiac monitor**, intubate,
. . . ventilate, rapid glucose determination, ABG/cooximetry/methemoglobin level/carboxyhemoglobin level, pulse oximetry, opioid antagonist
13. Respirations >24 (adult), >xx (peds) See Attachment A . . . . **IV access,** supplemental oxygen, cardiac monitor, ABG/oximetry,
. . . . salicylate level, CXR
14. Temperature >40°C . . . . **IV access, active cooling**, supplemental oxygen, cardiac monitor, assess for neuroleptic malignant
. . . . syndrome, ECG
15. Temperature <35°C . . . . IV access, supplemental oxygen, cardiac monitor, rapid glucose determination, ECG, treat hypothermia
16. General appearance-Cyanosis . . . . **IV access, supplemental oxygen, cardiac monitor, ABG/oximetry**, intubate, methemoglobin
. . . . level, measured oxygen saturation/cooximetry, CXR, ECG

Continued

17. Neuro-Decreased level of consciousness with no gag reflex . . . . **IV access, cardiac monitor, airway management,** rapid glucose determination

18. Neuro-Unresponsive to painful stimuli . . . . **IV access, supplemental oxygen, cardiac monitor, glucose administration/rapid glucose determination, ABG/oximetry,** ABG/cooximetry/carboxyhemoglobin level, toxicologic screen, urinalysis, abd x-ray for radiopaque toxic substances, opioid antagonist, thiamine

19. Neuro-Altered level of consciousness . . . . **frequent assessment,** rapid glucose determination, carboxyhemoglobin level, opioid antagonist, thiamine

20. Female with reproductive potential . . . . assess for pregnancy

21. HEENT-Miotic pupils . . . . IV access, opioid antagonist

22. HEENT-Oral burns of mucous membranes . . . . endoscopy, avoid emesis and gastric lavage

23. Pulmonary-Rales/rhonchi . . . . supplemental oxygen, cardiac monitor, ABG/oximetry, CXR

24. Pulmonary-Wheezes . . . . supplemental oxygen, cardiac monitor, ABG/oximetry, peak exp flow, CXR, beta agonist

25. Abdomen-rectal/vaginal drug packets . . . . **remove,** abdominal series x-ray, cathartics

26. Abdomen-Distended abdomen . . . . rectal examination, abd series x-ray, orogastric tube

27. Abdomen-Distended bladder . . . . bladder decompression

28. Skin-Pressure sores (erythema/vesicles) bullae . . . . assess for rhabdomyolysis/compartment syndrome, carboxyhemoglobin level

Diagnostic Testing

29. ABG-hypercapnia . . . . **ventilate,** intubate, opioid antagonist

30. ABG-hypoxemia .... **supplemental oxygen,** intubate, CXR, ECG
31. Urinalysis-dipstick positive for blood with few or no RBCs on microscopic .... evaluate/treat for rhabdomyolysis/hemolysis

Disposition

32. Admission .... **transfer care to accepting physician**
33. Transfer .... **follow ACEP and other applicable transfer principles**
34. Discharge .... **provide referral for follow-up care, provide instructions regarding treatment and circumstances that require**
.... **return to ED,** social services/protective services consult

Abbreviations		
Abd-abdominal	ECG-electrocardiogram	KUB-kidney, ureter, and bladder
ABG-arterial blood gas	ED-Emergency Department	Peak exp flow-Peak expiratory flow
CXR-chest x-ray	GI-gastrointestinal	
	IV-intravenous	

Notes:

American College of Emergency Physicians

Quick Reference Form

Product No. 04145A

for the

*Clinical Policy
for the Initial Approach
to
Children Under the Age of 2 Years
Presenting With Fever*

Fever Under 2 Months Quick Reference Form

> Document the fever history, associated symptoms and behavior, current medications,
> vital signs: temperature (location taken), pulse, respirations, weight; observation of
> interaction of child with caregiver or environment, and exam of the head, neck, and chest.

Circle line number if yes. **Underlined actions are rules.** Actions not underlined are guidelines.

Chief Complaint

1. Fever: reported core temperature >38°C (100.4°F)..................**CBC, UA, BC, UC, CXR, LP, consult/admit**

Associated Symptoms

2. cough.. chlamydial culture or antigen testing of nasopharynx, RSV culture, CXR

3. vomiting............................... assess type (e.g. **projectile, regurgitative**) **and relationship to feeding** , **assess degree of dehydration**, **examine abdomen**, UA, ELECT, CBC

4. diarrhea.................................. **assess degree of dehydration**, CBC, fecal leukocytes, stool for culture, ova, parasites

5. first seizure......................... **examine for source of fever**, **serum sodium**, **glucose**, UA , **BC**, **UC**, **LP**, **consult**,
.... serum Ca, BUN, CREAT, CBC, CXR, CT scan, antibiotics, admit

6. reported abnormal behavior (irritability, lethargy, feeding prob, inconsole)................. **observe behavior**, **consult**
.... IV, ELECT, glucose determ, CBC, UA, BC, UC, CXR, LP, antibiotics, admit

Past Medical History

7. immune suppression .... **CBC, BC**, UA, UC, CXR, LP, antibiotics, admit

8. sickle cell disease .... **CBC, BC**, RETIC, UA, UC, CXR, antibiotics, consult/admit

9. congenital anomalies, chronic disease, or implants.. entity specific evaluation

Continued

Physical Examination

10. observed behavior when held by parent/caregiver: persistent irritability with inconsolability or paradoxical irritability, lethargy, weak or shrill cry, moaning, continual cry, opisthotonos.................................. **ELECT, serum glucose, UA, BC, CXR, LP,**
.... CBC, UC, antibiotics, admit

11. vital signs: age 0-4 weeks with temperature >38°C(100.4°F) or <36°C(96.8°F) & no source.......... **UA, BC, UC, CXR, LP, follow-up**
.... **within 24 hours if not admitted**, serum glucose, CBC, external cooling if >40.6°C(105°F), antipyretic, antibiotics, admit

12. vital signs: age 1-24 months with temperature >40°C(104°F) & no source............. **record exam of abdomen, skin, and extremities,**
.... serum glucose, CBC, UA, BC, UC, CXR, LP,
.... external cooling if temperature >40.6°C(105°F), antipyretic, antibiotics, follow-up within 24 hours if not admitted

13. skin-generalized rash & macular or maculopapular................ **obtain history of exposure, immunizations, prolonged fever, CBC**

14. generalized hemorrhagic rash (purpuric, petechial).................. **BUN/CREAT, UA, BC, antibiotics, admit,** tick exposure?,
.... serum glucose, CBC(+platelets), PT/PTT, UC, stool occult blood, LP

15. head & neck: bulging fontanelle or meningismus................... **BC, LP, IVantibiotics, admit**, CBC, UA, UC, CXR, CT scan

16. head & neck: facial cellulitis .... **IVantibiotics, admit**

17. extremities: limping, unable to use, or inflammed joint .... passive **ROM, tenderness?, xray,**
.... CBC, ESR, BC, ARTHRO, consult/admit

Lab and Xray

18. lumbar puncture: organisms on Gram stain of CSF or WBC >9 or WBC>29 (0-4weeks)................ **Rx as meningitis,** ELECT

Assessment

19. heat stroke .... **rapid cooling, manage heat stroke, admit**

20. facial cellulitis (no penetrating wound) .... **IV antibiotics for H. influenzae, S. aureus, & group A strep, admit,** CBC, BC

21. omphalitis (neonatal) .... **IV antibiotics for group A&B strep, S. aureus, & Gram-neg. enteric rods, consult, admit**

22. meningitis .... IV, ELECT, serum glucose, IVantibiotics for group B strep, *E. coli*, Listeria monocytogenes, & *N. meningitides*, admit, IV fluids at 3/4 maintenance after stabilize, CBC, PT/PTT platelets, BC, steroids, IV antibiotics for *H. influenzae* (age 4-8 weeks)

23. meningitis with diarrhea .... RX meningitis, antibiotics-salmonella, replace fluids

24. sepsis .... IV, acidosis?, hypoglycemia?, coagulopathy?, IV antibiotics for meningitis

25. septic arthritis .... IV antibiotics for Group B strep & *S. aureus*, admit

26. septic arthritis of hip .... IV antibiotics for *H. influenzae* & *S. aureus*, admit, surg/ortho consult

27. osteomyelitis .... consult prior to starting antibiotics (bone cultures?)

28. pneumonia (age <2 weeks) .... IV, IV antibiotics for group B strep, Gram-negative bacilli, admit, O₂, ABG/pulse oximetry

29. pneumonia (2-8 weeks) ... IVantibiotics for chlamydia, *S. pneumoniae*, *H. influenzae*, & *S. aureus*, admit, O₂, ABG/pulse oximetry

30. moderate to severe dehydration .... oral rehydration or IV fluids, ELECT, CBC, UA, BC, UC, CXR, admit

31. localized source of fever .... treat as indicated, consult

Notes:

Abbreviations
ABG	arterial blood gas
ARTHRO	arthrocentesis analysis
BC	blood culture
BP	blood pressure
CXR	chest xray
ELECT	electrolytes
ESR	erythrocyte sedimentation rate
IV	IV access
LP	lumbar puncture
LFT	liver function tests
O₂	supplemental oxygen
PT/PTT	protime,partial thromboplastin time
RETIC	reticulocyte count
UA	urinalysis
UC	urine culture

Fever 2 Months to 2 Years Quick Reference Form

> Document the fever history, associated symptoms and behavior, current medications, vital signs: temperature (location taken) pulse, respirations, weight; observation of interaction of child with caregiver or environment, and exam of the head, neck, and chest.

Circle line number if yes. **Underlined actions are rules.** Actions not underlined are guidelines.

Chief Complaint
Reported temperature >38°C (100.4°F) & the following

Associated Symptoms
1. vomiting .... **assess degree of dehydration, examine abdomen,** UA
2. vomiting <6 months .... **assess type (e.g., projectile, regurgitative) and relationship to feeding,** ELECT, CBC
3. diarrhea .... **assess degree of dehydration,** CBC, fecal leukocytes, stool for culture, ova, parasites
4. first seizure: & <6 months or 6-24 months not meeting criteria for febrile seizure
   .... **examine for source of fever, serum sodium, glucose, UA, BC, UC, LP, consult,**
   .... serum Ca, BUN, CREAT, CBC, CXR, CT scan, antibiotics, admit
5. first seizure: & age 6-24 months meeting definition of febrile seizure .... ELECT, serum glucose, CBC, UA, BC, UC, LP
6. reported abnormal behavior (irritability, lethargy, feeding prob, inconsole) .... **examine for source, observe behavior**
   .... glucose determ, CBC, BC, CXR, LP

Past Medical History
7. immune suppression .... CBC, BC, UA, UC, CXR, LP, antibiotics, admit
8. sickle cell disease .... CBC, BC, RETIC, UA, UC, CXR, antibiotics, consult/admit
9. congenital anomalies, chronic disease, or implants .... entity specific evaluation

Physical Examination

10. observed behavior when held by parent/caregiver: persistent irritability with inconsolability or paradoxical irritability, lethargy, weak or shrill cry, moaning, continual cry, opisthotonos .... **serum glucose, UA, BC, CXR, LP**

11. vital signs: temperature >40°C(104°F) no source .... ELECT, urine tox, CBC, UA, BC, UC, antibiotics, admit

.... **record exam of abdomen, skin, and extremities.**

.... if temperature >40.6°C(105°F), antipyretic, antibiotics, follow-up within 24 hours if not admitted

.... serum glucose, CBC, UA, BC, UC, CXR, LP, external cooling

12. skin–generalized rash & macular or maculopapular ... **obtain history of exposure, immunizations, prolonged fever,** CBC

13. generalized hemorrhagic rash(purpuric,petechial) .... **BUN/CREAT, UA, BC, antibiotics, admit** tick exposure?,

.... serum glucose, CBC(+platelets), PT/PTT, UC, stool occult blood, LP

14. head & neck: bulging fontanelle or meningismus .... **BC, LP, IV antibiotics, admit** , CBC, UA, UC, CXR, CT scan

15. head & neck: facial cellulitis .... **IV antibiotics, admit**

16. extremities: limping, unable to use, or inflamed joint .... **passive ROM, tenderness?, xray,**

.... CBC, ESR, BC, ARTHRO, consult/admit

Lab and Xray

17. lumbar puncture: organisms on Gram stain of CSF or WBC>9 .... **Rx as meningitis,** ELECT

Assessment

18. heat stroke .... **rapid cooling, manage heat stroke, admit**

19. facial cellulitis (no penetrating wound) .... **IV antibiotics for** *H. influenzae, S. aureus,* & group A strep, admit, CBC, BC

20. omphalitis (neonatal) .... **IV antibiotics for group A & B strep,** *S. aureus,* & Gram-neg. enteric rods, consult, admit

.... IV, ELECT, serum glucose, IV antibiotics for *E. coli, H. influenzae, S. pneumoniae,*

21. meningitis .... & *N. meningitidis* , admit, CBC, PT/PTT platelets, steroids

Continued

22. meningitis with diarrhea .... RX meningitis, antibiotics-salmonella, replace fluids
23. sepsis .... IV, acidosis?, hypoglycemia?, coagulopathy?, IV antibiotics for meningitis
24. septic arthritis .... IV antibiotics for *H. influenzae* & *S. aureus*, admit
25. septic arthritis of hip .... IV antibiotics for *H. influenzae* & *S. aureus*, admit, surg/ortho consult
26. osteomyelitis .... consult prior to starting antibiotics (bone cultures?)
27. pneumonia .... antibiotics for *S. pneumoniae*, *H. influenzae*, & *S. aureus*, O_2 ABG/ pulse oximetry, admit
28. moderate to severe dehydration .... oral rehydration or IV fluids, ELECT, CBC, UA, BC, UC, CXR, admit
29. localized source of fever .... treat as indicated

Notes:

Abbreviations

ABG ——— arterial blood gas	IV ——— IV access
ARTHRO - arthrocentesis analysis	LP ——— lumbar puncture
BC ——— blood culture	LFT ——— liver function tests
BP ——— blood pressure	O_2 ——— supplemental oxygen
CXR ——— chest xray	PT/PTT —— protime,partial thromboplastin time
ELECT —— electrolytes	RETIC —— reticulocyte count
ESR ——— erythrocyte sedimentation rate	UA ——— urinalysis
	UC ——— urine culture

APPENDIX B

Suggested Readings

General emergency medicine textbooks

Bosker G et al, editors: *The manual of emergency medicine therapeutics,* St Louis, 1995, Mosby.

May HL et al, editors: *Emergency medicine,* ed 2, Boston, 1992, Little, Brown.

Rosen P et al, editors: *Emergency medicine: concepts and clinical practice,* ed 4, St Louis, 1997, Mosby.

Rund DA et al, editors: *Essentials of emergency medicine,* ed 2, St Louis, 1996, Mosby.

Shock

Assalia A, Schein M: Resuscitation for haemorrhagic shock, *Br J Surg* 80:213, 1993.

Bickell WH et al: A comparison of immediate versus delayed fluid resuscitation for hypotensive patients with penetrating torso trauma, *N Engl J Med* 331:1105-1109, 1994.

Bochner BS, Lichtenstein LM: Anaphylaxis, *N Engl J Med* 324:1785-1790, 1991.

Califf RM, Bengtson JR: Cardiogenic shock, *N Engl J Med* 330:1724-1730, 1994.

Pollack CV: Prehospital fluid resuscitation of the trauma patient, an update on the controversies, *Emerg Med Clin North Am* 11:61-70, 1993.

Rackow EC, Astiz ME: Pathophysiology and treatment of septic shock, *JAMA* 266:548-554, 1991.

Overview of major trauma

American College of Surgeons, Committee on Trauma: *Advanced trauma life support program for physicians,* Chicago, American College of Surgeons, 1993.

Thoracic trauma

Foil MB et al: The asymptomatic patient with suspected myocardial contusion, *Am J Surg* 160:638, 1990.

Jackimczyk K: Blunt chest trauma, *Emerg Med Clin North Am* 11:81, 1993.

Jorden RC: Penetrating chest trauma, *Emerg Med Clin North Am* 11:97, 1993.

Mathiesen DJ, Grillo H: Laryngotracheal trauma, *Ann Thorac Surg* 43:254, 1987.

Peper WA, Obeid FN, Horst HM: Penetrating injuries of the mediastinum, *Am Surg* 52:359, 1986.

Orthopedic trauma

Ashkenaze DM, Ruby LK: Metacarpal fractures and dislocations, *Orthop Clin North Am* 23:19, 1992.

Jerrard DA: Pelvic fractures, *Emerg Med Clin North Am* 11:147, 1993.

Marshall JL, Baugher WH: Stability examination of the knee, *Clin Orthop* 146:78, 1980.

O'Brien ET: Acute fractures and dislocations of the carpus, *Orthop Clin North Am* 15:237, 1984.

Rogers LF, Hendrix RW: Radiographic imaging in orthopedics, *Orthop Clin North Am* 21:3, 1990.

Hand injuries

Blair WF, Steyers CM: Extensor tendon injuries, *Orthop Clin North Am* 23:141, 1992.

Clark DP, Scott RN, Anderson IWR: Hand problems in an accident and emergency department, *J Hand Surg* 10:297, 1985.

Margles SW: Principles of management of acute hand injuries, *Surg Clin North Am* 60:665, 1980.

Overton DT, Uehara DT: Evaluation of the injured hand, *Emerg Med Clin North Am* 11:585, 1993.

Steinberg DR: Acute flexor tendon injuries, *Orthop Clin North Am* 23:125, 1992.

Ophthalmologic emergencies

Bertolinin J, Pelucio M: The red eye, *Emerg Med Clin North Am* 13:561, 1995.

Gossman MD, Roberts DM, Barr CC: Ophthalmic aspects of orbital injury, *Clin Plast Surg* 19:71, 1992.

Griffin JR: Acute iritis, *Postgrad Med* 88:117, 1989.

Janda AM: Sudden nontraumatic visual loss, *Postgrad Med* 91:111, 1992.

Kearns P: Traumatic hyphema, *Br J Ophthalmol* 75:137, 1991.

Lavrich JB, Nelson LB: Disorders of the lacrimal system apparatus, *Pediatr Clin North Am* 40:767, 1993.

Linden JA, Renner GS: Trauma to the globe, *Emerg Med Clin North Am* 13:581, 1995.

O'Hare TH: Blow out fractures, *J Emerg Med* 9:253, 1991.

Stern AL, Pamel GJ, Benedetto LG: Physical and chemical injuries of the eyes and eyelids, *Dermatol Clin* 10:785, 1992.

Stern GA et al: Effect of topical antibiotic solutions on corneal epithelial wound healing, *Arch Ophthalmol* 101:644, 1983.

Anesthesia, analgesia, and sedation

Barkin RM: Analgesia for children: options and choices, *Ann Emerg Med* 18:592, 1989.

Feld LH, Negus JB, White PF: Oral midazolam preanesthetic medication in pediatric patients, *Anesthesiology* 73:831, 1990.

Meyer G, Henneman PL: Buffered lidocaine, *Ann Emerg Med* 20:218, 1991.

Murphy MF: Regional anesthesia in the emergency department, *Emerg Med Clin North Am* 6:783, 1988.

Wright SW et al: Midazolam use in the emergency department, *Am J Emerg Med* 8:97, 1990.

Soft tissue infections

Callaham ML: Prophylactic antibiotics in common dog bite wounds: a controlled study, *Ann Emerg Med* 9:410, 1980.

Dreyfuss UY, Orthop M, Singer M: Human bites of the hand, *J Hand Surg* 10:1985, 1985.

Edlich RF et al: Principles of emergency wound management, *Ann Emerg Med* 17:1284, 1988.

Hunt TC: The physiology of wound healing, *Ann Emerg Med* 17:1265, 1988.

Lindsay D: Soft tissue infections, *Emerg Med Clin North Am* 10:737, 1992.

Cardiac emergencies

American Heart Association: *Textbook of advanced cardiac life support,* Dallas, 1994, The Association.

Drugs for cardiac arrhythmias, *Med Lett Drugs Ther* 38:75-82, 1996.

Every NR et al: A comparison of thrombolytic therapy with primary coronary angioplasty for acute myocardial infarction, *N Engl J Med* 325:1253-1260, 1996.

Grines CL et al: A comparison of immediate angioplasty with thrombolytic therapy for acute myocardial infarction, *N Engl J Med* 328:673-679, 1993.

The GUSTO Investigators: A clinical trial comparing primary coronary angioplasty with tissue plasminogen activator for acute myocardial infarction (GUSTO 11b), *N Engl J Med* 336:1621-1628, 1997.

The GUSTO Investigators: An international randomized trial comparing four thrombolytic strategies for acute myocardial infarction, *N Engl J Med* 329:673-682, 1993.

Intravenous amiodarone, *Med Lett Drugs Ther* 37:114-115, 1996.

Lange RA, Hillis LD: Immediate angioplasty for acute myocardial infarction, *N Engl J Med* 328:726-727, 1993.

O'Keefe JR Jr. et al: Early and late results of coronary angioplasty without antecedent thrombolytic therapy for acute myocardial infarction, *Am J Cardiol* 64:1221-1230, 1989.

Reteplase (Retavase), *Med Lett Drugs Ther* 39:17-18, 1997.

Respiratory emergencies
Pneumonia

Arbo M, Keusch GT: Newer therapeutic uses of the quinolone antibiotics: part I. Primary-care indications, *Pharmacy & Therapeutics* 1099-1108, July 1992.

Choice of Antibacterial Drugs, *Med Lett Drugs Ther* 38:26-34, 1996.

Goshman L: Brief update on new macrolide antibiotics: clarithromycin and azithromycin, *Pharmacy & Therapeutics* 1265-1273, Aug 1992.

Niederman MS et al: Guidelines for the initial management of adults with community-acquired pneumonia: diagnosis, assessment of severity, and initial antimicrobial therapy, *Am Rev Resp Dis* 148:1418-1426, 1993.

Nolan PE, Bass JB: New drugs for treating lung infection, *Chest* 94:1076-1079, 1988.

Reed WW et al: Sputum Gram's stain in community-acquired pneumococcal pneumonia—a meta-analysis, *West J Med* 165:197-204, 1996.

Sue DY: Community-acquired pneumonia in adults, *West J Med* 161:383-389, 1994.

Pulmonary embolus

Hull RD et al: A noninvasive strategy for the treatment of patients with suspected pulmonary embolism, *Arch Intern Med* 154:289-297, 14, 1994.

Killewich LA et al: Value of lower extremity venous duplex examination in the diagnosis of pulmonary embolism, *J Vasc Surg* 17:934-938, 1993.

PIOPED Investigators: Value of the ventilation/perfusion scan in acute pulmonary embolism. Results of the prospective investigation of pulmonary embolism diagnosis (PIOPED), *JAMA* 263:2753-1759, 1990.

Stein PD et al: Clinical characteristics of patients with acute pulmonary embolism, *Am J Cardiol* 68:1723-1724, 1991 (analysis of data from the Prospective Investigation of Pulmonary Embolism Diagnosis [PIOPED] study).

Stein PD et al: Complications and validity of pulmonary angiography in acute pulmonary embolism, *Circulation* 85:462-468, 1992 (an analysis of PIOPED data).

Worsley DF et al: A detailed evaluation of patients with acute pulmonary embolism and low- or very-low-probability lung scan interpretations, *Arch Intern Med* 154:2737-1741, 1994 (an analysis of PIOPED data).

Genitourinary tract emergencies

Choice of antibacterial drugs, *Med Lett Drugs Ther* 38:26-34, 1996.

Sexually transmitted diseases, *Med Lett Drugs Ther* 37:117, 1995.

Stamm WE, Hooton TM: Management of urinary tract infections in adults, *N Engl J Med* 329:1328-1334, 1993.

Neurologic emergencies

Alteplase for thrombolysis in acute ischemic stroke, *Med Lett Drugs Ther* 38:99-100, 1996.

Hacke W et al: Intravenous thrombolysis with recombinant tissue plasminogen activator for acute hemispheric stroke. The European Cooperative Acute Stroke Study (ECASS), *JAMA* 274:1017-1025, 1995.

Kay R et al: Low-molecular weight heparin for the treatment of acute ischemic stroke, *J Engl J Med* 333:1588-1593, 1995.

The National Institute of Neurological Disorders and Stroke Study Group: Tissue plasminogen activator for acute ischemic stroke, *N Engl J Med* 333:1581-1587, 1995.

Transplantation emergencies

Carpenter CB, Lazarus JM: Dialysis and transplantation in the treatment of renal failure. In Isselbacher KJ et al, editors: *Harrison's principles of internal medicine,* ed 13, New York, 1994, McGraw-Hill.

Dienstag J: Liver transplantation. In Isselbacher KJ et al, editors: *Harrison's principles of internal medicine,* ed 13, New York, 1994, McGraw-Hill.

Finberg R: Infections in the immunocompromised host. In Isselbacher KJ et al, editors: *Harrison's principles of internal medicine,* ed 13, New York, 1994, McGraw-Hill.

Schroeder JS: Cardiac transplantation. In Isselbacher KJ et al, editors: *Harrison's principles of internal medicine,* ed 13, New York, 1994, McGraw-Hill.

Seaberg DC: The patient following organ transplantation taking immunosuppressive therapy. In Herr RD, Cydulka RK, editors: *Emergency care of the compromised patient,* Philadelphia, 1994, JB Lippincott.

Serody JS, Cohen MS: Infection in the immunocompromised host. In Brillman JC, Quenzer RW, editors: *Infectious disease in emergency medicine,* Boston, 1992, Little, Brown.

Thomas ED: Bone marrow transplantation. In Isselbacher KJ et al, editors: *Harrison's principles of internal medicine,* ed 13, New York, 1994, McGraw-Hill.

Trulock EP, Cooper JD: Lung transplantation. In Isselbacher KJ et al, editors: *Harrison's principles of internal medicine,* ed 13, New York, 1994, McGraw-Hill.

Dermatologic disorders

Bart BJ: Annular skin eruptions, *Postgrad Med* 96:37, 1994.

Barton LL, Friedman AD: Impetigo: a reassessment of etiology and therapy, *Pediatr Dermatol* 4:185, 1987.

Goldner R: Work-related irritant contact dermatitis, *Occup Med* 9:37, 1994.

Omerod AD: Urticaria—recognition, causes and treatment, *Drugs* 48:717, 1994.

Stevens DL et al: Severe group A streptococcal infections associated with a toxic shocklike syndrome and scarlet fever toxin, *N Engl J Med* 321:1, 1989.

Environmental emergencies

Auerbach PS, editor: *Wilderness medicine: management of wilderness and environmental emergencies,* St Louis, 1995, Mosby.

Curley G, Irwin RS: Disorders of temperature control: I, *Intensive Care Med* 1:5, 1986.

Demmler G et al: Brown recluse spider bites, *Am J Dis Child* 151:114, 1989.

Dexter WW: Hypothermia, *Postgrad Med J* 88:55, 1990.

Minton SA, Norris RL: Non-North American venomous reptile bites. In Auerbach PS, editor: *Wilderness medicine: management of wilderness and environmental emergencies,* St Louis, 1995, Mosby, pp 710-730.

Olshanker JS: Near drowning, *Emerg Med Clin North Am* 10:339, 1992.

Pennell T, Babu S, Meredith J: The management of snake and spider bites in the southeastern United States, *Am Surg* 53:201, 1987.

Sullivan JB, Wingert WA, Norris RL: North American venomous reptile bites. In Auerbach PS, editor: *Wilderness medicine: management of wilderness and environmental emergencies,* St Louis, 1995, Mosby, pp 680-709.

Poisoning, overdose, and envenomation

Anker AL, Smilkstein MJ: Acetaminophen: concepts and controversies, *Emerg Med Clin North Am* 12:335, 1994.

Curtis R, Barone J, Giacona N: Efficacy of ipecac and activated charcoal/cathartic, *Arch Intern Med* 144:48, 1984.

Kulig K: Initial management of ingestions of toxic substances, *N Engl J Med* 326:1677, 1992.

Temple AR: Acute and chronic effects of aspirin toxicity and their treatment, *Arch Intern Med* 141:364, 1981.

Wiley JF: Difficult diagnoses in toxicology: poisons not detected by the comprehensive drug screen, *Pediatr Clin North Am* 38:725, 1991.

Pediatric emergencies

APLS: the pediatric emergency medicine course, ed 2, Dallas, 1993, American College of Emergency Physicians and the American Academy of Pediatrics.

Barkin RM, Rosen P: *Emergency pediatrics: a guide to ambulatory care,* ed 4, St Louis, 1994, Mosby.

Miskowiak J, Burcharth F: The white cell count in acute appendicitis, a prospective blind study, *Dan Med Bull* 29:210-211, 1982.

Montgomery CJ et al: Plasma concentrations after high-dose (45 mg.kg^{-1}) rectal acetaminophen in children, *Can J Anaesth* 42:982-986, 1995.

Rappaport WD et al: Factors responsible for the high perforation rate seen in early childhood appendicitis, *Am Surg* 10:602-605, 1989.

Strange W et al: *Pediatric emergency medicine,* New York, 1996, American College of Emergency Physicians, McGraw-Hill.

Waisman Y: Prospective randomized double-blind study comparing L-epinephrine and racemic epinephrine aerosols in the treatment of laryngo-tracheitis (croup), *Pediatrics* 89:302-306, 1992.

INDEX

A

Abdominal aortic aneurysm, 159
Abdominal emergencies, 185-196
  concerns, 186-187
  diagnostic studies, 186
  disorders, 187-196
  general considerations, 185-187
  physical examination, 186
  symptoms, 185-186
  trauma, 46-48
    blunt *vs.* penetrating, 48
    diagnostic studies, 46-47
    general considerations, 46
    initial evaluation and
      stabilization, 46
    special considerations, 48
Abdominal pain
  AIDS and, 248
  gynecologic disorders with, 203
  Quick Reference Form, 390-392
Abdominal radiography
  with bowel obstruction, 186,
    190
  with constipation and fecal
    impaction, 194
  with diverticulitis, 191
  with GI gas, 194
  with ileus, 186
  with iron poisoning, 313
  with lead poisoning, 312
  with obstipation, 186
  with peptic disorders, 189
  with poisoning, overdose, 293
Abductor digiti V muscle, 73*f*
Abductor pollicis longus
  damage to, 76
  insertion of, 74*f*

Abortion
  inevitable, 205
  spontaneous, 205
  threatened, 205
Abrasions
  anesthesia of, 112
  corneal, 90
Abruptio placentae, 210
Abscesses, 113-116
  Bartholin's, 209
  cerebral, 252
  dental, 241
  perirectal, 195
  peritonsillar, 238
  treatment principles, 113-114
  tuboovarian, 206
Accidental tattoos, 112
ACEP; *see* American College of
    Emergency Physicians
Acetaminophen overdose, 303
  antidote, 295*t*
  Rumack-Matthew nomogram
    for, 303, 304*f*
Acetazolamide, 245
N-Acetylcysteine, 295*t*, 303
Acid-base disorders, 10-14
Acid diuresis, forced, 299, 299*b*
Acidosis
  adrenal crisis and, 219
  diabetic ketoacidosis, 216
  metabolic, 11-12
    poisoning and, 292
    respiratory compensation
      of, 165
  respiratory, 10-11
Aconitine, 327
Acquired immunodeficiency
    syndrome, 246-249
Acromioclavicular separation, 62
Activase; *see* Tissue plasminogen
    activator
Activated charcoal
  for acetaminophen overdose,
    303

Page numbers followed by *t* indicate
tables. Page numbers followed by *b*
indicate boxes. Page numbers followed
by *f* indicate figures.

Activated charcoal–cont'd
for poisonings, 297-298
Acute myocardial infarction,
125-130; *see also*
Myocardial infarction
Acute ventilatory failure, 166-167
Acyclovir
for genital herpes, 276
for herpes genitalis, 208
for herpes infections, 241
for herpes zoster infections, 277
Addisonian crisis, 219-220
Addison's disease, 222
Adenosine, 135*b*, 136
Adrenal crisis, 219-220
Adrenaline, 93
α-Adrenergics
for shock, 6, 7*t*
for tranquilizer overdose,
305-306
β-Adrenergics
for acute angle-closure
glaucoma, 245
for acute myocardial infarction,
129
for angina, 130
for atrial flutter, 138*b*, 139
in cardiogenic pulmonary
edema, 133
for croup, 355
for shock, 6, 7*t*
for supraventricular tachycardia,
136
Adult respiratory distress
syndrome, 178-179
Affective disorders; *see* Mood
disorders
Afterload reduction, 131
Airflow obstruction, 163
Airway management
in burns, 283
in cardiac arrest, 150
in head injuries, 53
in major trauma, 29
in shock, 6
in spinal injuries, 59
in thoracic trauma, 29
Airway obstruction
acute, 233

Airway obstruction–cont'd
fluid, 163
foreign body, 233, 234-235
laryngospasm, 233
upper, 166
Albuterol
for asthmatic bronchospasm,
133, 167, 170
for asthmatic bronchospasm in
children, 356
Alcohol, 214-215, 341-343; *see also*
Ethanol
ethyl, 317
intoxication
acute, 214
dialysis for, 299, 300*b*
forced diuresis for, 300*t*
simple, 341
treatment, 215
treatment, 215
withdrawal, 341-342
acute, 214
treatment, 215
Alkaline battery ingestion, 310
Alkaline diuresis, forced, 299,
299*b*
Alkaloids, plant, 327-328
Alkalosis
metabolic, 13-14
respiratory, 12-13
Allen's test, 73-74
Allergic reactions
to chemotherapy, 256
shock, 6
Alteplase, 128
Altered levels of consciousness,
211-221
Aluminum acetate, 208
Aluminum hydroxide, 189
Aluminum magnesium hydroxide,
328
Alveolar-arterial PO_2 gradient, 165
Amanita poisoning, 322
hemoperfusion for, 299, 301*b*
American College of Emergency
Physicians (ACEP)
Clinical Policies, 363-364
Quality Assurance Forms, 363
Quicklists, Acute Blunt Trauma,
365-374

American College of Emergency
    Physicians (ACEP)–cont'd
    Quick Reference Forms, 363,
        364
        Acute Blunt Trauma, 365-374
        Acute Toxic Ingestion or
            Dermal or Inhalation
            Exposure, 417-423
        Chest Pain Revision, 379-388
        children presenting with
            fever, 426-430
        Headache, 400-409
        Nontraumatic Acute
            Abdominal Pain, 389-392
        Penetrating Extremity
            Trauma, 375-378
        Seizure, 410-416
        Vaginal Bleeding, 393-399
AMI; *see* Acute myocardial
    infarction
Aminoglycosides
    for meningitis, 252
    for pyelonephritis, 198
Aminophylline, 168
Amiodarone, 147, 151
Amitriptyline overdose, 306
Ammonia, 235
Ammonium chloride, 309
Ammonium hydroxide ingestion,
    310
Amoxicillin
    for acute sinusitis, 240
    for bacterial otitis media, 239
    for lung infections, 174
    for orbital fractures, 82
    for otitis media in children, 358
    for pneumonia, 353
Amoxicillin-clavulinate
    for acute sinusitis, 240
    for bacterial otitis media, 239
    for lung infections, 176-177
Amphetamine overdose, 342
    dialysis for, 299, 300*b*
    forced diuresis for, 300*t*
    withdrawal, 342
Ampicillin
    for lung infections, 174, 176-
        177
    for meningitis, 232, 252, 352
    for pneumonia, 353

Amputations, hand, 79
Amylase
    pancreatitis and, 188
    septic shock and, 6
Amyl nitrate inhalation
    for cyanide intoxication, 315
    for hydrogen sulfide and
        carbon disulfide
        intoxication, 314
Analgesia, 92-105
Analgesics; *see also* Narcotics;
        specific analgesics
    for abdominal emergencies, 187
    for acute cystitis, 197
    for mushroom poisoning, 322
    for pancreatitis, 188
    parenteral
        for incision and drainage,
            114
        side effects, 103
    for tennis elbow, 64
Anaphylactic distributive shock, 6
Anaphylaxis, 170
Ancef; *see* Cefazolin
Anemia
    emergent, 258
    hemolytic, 259*b*
    red cell destruction, 258-261,
        259*b*
    syncope and, 222
Anesthesia, 92-105
    of abrasions, 112
    for incision and drainage, 114
    of palm or dorsal aspect of
        hand, 74
    of partial finger, 74
    for reduction of distal radius
        fractures, 64
    regional, 92-100
        complications of, 100-102
    topical, 93
    for wound care, 106
Angina, 130
    differential diagnosis, 126-127
    preinfarction, 130
    unstable, 130
Angiography
    with pulmonary embolism, 180
    with transient ischemic attack,
        230

Angiography—cont'd
  with vertigo, 225
Angioplasty, 129
Animal venoms, 317-328
Anistreplase, 129
Ankle injuries, 68
Antacids, 189
Anterior chamber paracentesis,
    244
Antibiotics; *see also specific*
    antibiotics
  for acute sinusitis, 240
  for Bartholin's abscess, 209
  for cholelithiasis or
    cholecystitis, 188
  for dermatologic problems, 279*t*
  for diarrhea, 192, 193
  for epididymitis, 199
  for herpes genitalis, 208
  for ingestion of caustics, 236
  for lung infections, 174-177
  for meningitis, 232
  for olecranon bursitis, 116
  for otitis externa, 240
  overdose, 299, 300*b*
  for pneumonia, 178
  prophylactic
    for bite wounds, 118
    for open fractures, 79
    for orbital fractures, 82
    for wound infection, 117
  for pyelonephritis, 198
  for shock, 6, 7*t*
  for soft-tissue infections, 113
  for wound infections, 117
Antibodies, antilymphocyte, 267
Anticholinergics
  for asthmatic bronchospasm,
    168
  overdose, 295*t*
  for suprapubic pain of bladder
    spasm, 197
Anticoagulation
  for acute myocardial infarction,
    129
  for pulmonary embolism, 181
Antidepressants overdose, 299,
    301*b*, 306

Antidotes, 294, 295*t*-296*t*
Antiemetics
  in chemotherapy, 255, 255*b*
  for headache, 228
Antifungal agents, 279*t*
Antihemophilic factor; *see* Factor
    VIII
Antihistamines
  for anaphylaxis, 170
  for peripheral vertigo, 225
  for shock, 6, 7*t*
Antiinflammatory drugs; *see also*
    Nonsteroidal
    antiinflammatory drugs
  for tennis elbow, 64
Antilymphocyte antibodies, 267
Antimotility agents, 192
Antirabies serum
  dosages for, 120*t*
  indications for, 119*t*
Antiseptics, 106
Antithymocyte globulin, 267
Antivenin
  for black widow bites, 321
  for snake bites, 320
Antivert; *see* Meclizine
Anusol, 195
Anxiety, 340-341
Aortic ballon pumps, 6, 7*t*
Aortic disease, 158-159
Aortic injuries, 42
Aortic valve disease, 221
Aortography
  with injuries to aorta and great
    vessels, 42
  with rib fracture, 34
  with thoracic aortic dissection,
    158
Aphonia, 86
Appendicitis, 187
  in children, 359
ARDS; *see* Adult respiratory
    distress syndrome
Aristocort; *see* Triamcinolone
    acetonide
Arm tourniquets, 78
ARS; *see* Antirabies serum
Arsenic poisoning, 315-316

Arsine gas poisoning, 315-316
Arterial blood gases
  age-correction formula, 165
  with altered levels of
      consciousness, 214
  assessment of, 164-165
  with cardiogenic pulmonary
      edema, 132
  formulas for interpreting, 165
Arterial contusions, 160, 160*f*
Arterial embolization, 155-156
Arterial ischemia, 155
Arterial trauma, 161-162
Arteriography, 161
Arteriosclerosis obliterans, 156
Arteriovenous malformations, 228
Arthrocentesis, 67
Arthropod bites, 321-322
Aspergillus, 267
Aspiration
  gastric, 184
  nasogastric, 188, 189
  needle
    of olecranon bursitis, 116
    of pericardial tamponade, 43,
        44*f*
    of perirectal abscess, 195
    of thrombosed external
        hemorrhoids, 195
Aspirin
  for myocardial infarction, 128
  for stroke, 231
Asthma, 168-170
  pediatric, 354-355
Atarax; *see* Hydroxyzine
Atenolol, 138*b*, 139
ATG; *see* Antithymocyte globulin
Athlete's foot, 274
Ativan; *see* Lorazepam
Atracurium, 105
Atrial fibrillation, 138*b*, 139*f*, 139-
    140
Atrial flutter, 137*f*, 137-139, 138*b*
Atrial tachycardia, multifocal,
    136-137, 137*f*
Atrioventricular block, 141-144
  first-degree, 141, 142*f*
  Mobitz I (Wenckebach, 142,
      143*f*

Atrioventricular block—cont'd
  Mobitz II, 142, 143*f*
  second-degree, 141-142, 142,
      143*f*
  third-degree, 142, 144*f*
  treatment, 141*b*, 142, 143-144
Atropine, 104
  for AV block, 143-144
  for bradydysrhythmias, 133
  for diarrhea, 192
  for mushroom poisoning, 323*t*
  for organophosphate
      poisoning, 311
  pediatric dosages, 349
  in plants, 327
  for premature ventricular
      contractions, 145
  for pulseless electrical activity
      and asystole, 151
  for sinus bradycardia, 141, 141*b*
Atropine sulfate, 295*t*, 296*t*
Auditory hallucinations, 332, 339
AV block; *see* Atrioventricular
    block
Avulsions
  hand, 79
  tooth, 87
Axis; *see* Nizatidine
Azactam, 176
Azathioprine, 266
Azithromycin
  for lung infections, 177
  for pneumonia, 178
  for streptococcal pharyngitis,
      238
  for urethritis in male, 198
Aztreonam, 176

B
Babinski's sign, 212
Bacitracin
  for bacterial conjunctivitis, 243
  for corneal abrasion, 90
  for perforated eardrum, 87
Bacterial infections
  conjunctivitis, 242-243
  meningitis, 231

Bacterial infections—cont'd
  otitis media, 239
  in transplant recipients, 267
  vaginosis, 208
Bactrim; *see* Trimethoprim-
    sulfamethoxazole
Bactroban; *see* Mupirocin
Bag-valve-mask ventilation,
    150-151
Ballet fracture, 68
Barbiturates
  overdose, 303-305, 342
    dialysis for, 299, 300*b*
    hemoperfusion for, 299, 301*b*
  withdrawal, 342
Barotrauma, 289-290
Bartholin's abscess, 209
Battered child, 358-359
Battery acid exposure, 88-89
Bell's palsy, 229
Benadryl; *see* Diphenhydramine
Bends, 289
Benign positional vertigo, 223
Benzathine penicillin
  for streptococcal pharyngitis,
    238
  for syphilis, 278
  for tonsillitis and pharyngitis,
    358
Benzocaine, 233
Benzodiazepines
  abscesses and, 114
  for eclamptic seizures, 210
  overdose, 295*t*
  sedation and, 104, 330
  for seizures, 226
Betamethasone
  for dermatologic problems, 279*t*
  relative potencies, 169*t*
Bethanechol overdose, 295*t*
Biaxin; *see* Clarithromycin
Bicarbonate, 217
Bier block, 64
Bilirubin, 186, 188
BiPAP; *see* Biphasic airway
    pressure
Biphasic airway pressure
  for ARDS, 179
  for cardiogenic pulmonary
    edema, 132

Bismuth suppositories, 195
Bite wounds, 118-121
Black elder, 325*t*
Black widow, 321
Bladder injuries, 50
Bladder rupture, 50
Bladder spasm, 197
Bleach ingestion, 310
Bleeding, 162; *see also*
    Hemorrhage
  from ear and nose, 54
  from external auditory canal, 83
  from limb wound, 161
  in mouth, 111
  sentinel bleed, 227
  vaginal, 203-204
    Quick Reference Form,
    394-399
Bleomycin sulfate, 255, 256*b*
Blood flow obstruction, 163
Blood gases; *see* Arterial blood
    gases
Blood pressure
  epistaxis and, 236
  equation for, 3
Blood urea nitrogen, 214
Blunt trauma
  abdominal, 48
  acute
    Quicklist, 372-374
    Quick Reference Form,
    366-371
  arterial contusions with, 160
  to eye, 91
Bone infarction, 260, 260*t*
Bone marrow transplantation, 270
Bowel obstruction, 190
Bowel sounds, 186
Boxer's fracture, 65
Brachial plexus injury, 61
Bradycardia
  refractory, 133
  sinus, 140*f*, 140-141
Bradydysrhythmias, 130, 133
Branhamella catarrhalis, 172
Breathing; *see also* Airway
    management
  diminished breath sounds, 163
  in major trauma, 29-30

Breathing—cont'd
  shortness of breath, 248
  in thoracic trauma, 33
Bretylium
  for premature ventricular
      contractions, 146
  for pulseless ventricular
      tachycardia, 151
  for ventricular fibrillation, 150*b*,
      151
  for ventricular tachycardia,
      146*b*, 147
Bromide overdose
  dialysis for, 299, 300*b*
  forced diuresis for, 300*t*
Bronchial rupture, 41-42
Bronchiolitis, in infants, 357
Bronchitis
  bacterial causes, 172-173
  chronic, 170
  definition of, 171
Bronchodilators, 167
Bronchoscopy, 41
Bronchospasm, 167-171
  pediatric, 356-357
  treatment, 133, 167-168, 170
Brown recluse spider bites,
    321-322
Buccal mucosa, lacerations of, 111
Bullous impetigo, 277
BUN; *see* Blood urea nitrogen
Bupivacaine, 34
Burns
  caustic, 235-236, 310
  chemical
    of conjunctiva and cornea,
        88-89
    pulmonary burn, 182-183
  electrical, 285
  pulmonary, 182-183, 283
  thermal, 281-285
Burow's Solution; *see* Aluminum
    acetate
Bursitis
  olecranon, 115-116
  trochanteric, 66
Busulfan, 255, 256*b*
Butoconazole, 207
Butyrophenones, 255, 255*b*

C

CABG; *see* Coronary artery bypass
    grafting
CaEDTA; *see* Calcium disodium
    edathamil
Calcaneal fractures, 68
Calcium
  altered levels of consciousness
      and, 214
  falsely elevated serum levels, 23
  hypercalcemia, 21-23
  hypocalcemia, 23-24
Calcium channel blockers
  for atrial flutter or fibrillation,
      138, 138*b*, 139
  for supraventricular tachycardia,
      135*b*, 136
Calcium chloride
  for aconitine, 328
  pediatric dosages, 349
  for verapamil-induced
      hypotension, 138
Calcium disodium edathamil, 312
Calcium gluconate, 321
Calf vein thrombosis, 157
Campylobacter
  antibiotics for, 193
  diarrhea and, 192
Cancer; *see* Oncologic
    emergencies
Candida
  AIDS and, 248
  in transplant recipients, 267
  vaginitis and, 207
CA overdose, 306-307
Carafate; *see* Sucralfate
Carbapenem-cilastatin
    combinations, 176
Carbenicillin, 252
Carbocaine; *see* Mepivacaine
Carbon disulfate overdose, 314
Carbon monoxide
  with altered levels of
      consciousness, 214
  poisoning, 183-184, 314
    headache and, 227
Carcinoma; *see* Oncologic
    emergencies

Cardiac arrest, 149-151
  evaluation and treatment, 150*b*,
    150-151, 151*b*
  management in children,
    348-349
Cardiac compression
  in child, 349
  closed-chest, 150
  in infant, 349
Cardiac disorders
  anaphylactic shock and, 6
  in cancer, 256-257
  chemotherapy and, 256
  presenting as psychiatric
    disorders, 336*b*
  regional anesthesia and,
    101-102
Cardiac dysrhythmias; *see*
    Dysrhythmias
Cardiac emergencies, 125-154
  in cancer, 256-257
  syncope and, 221-222
Cardiac enzymes, 126
Cardiac ischemia
  acute, 125
  initial treatment of, 127
  without acute infarction, 130
Cardiac monitoring, 43
Cardiac tamponade, 43-44
Cardiogenic pulmonary edema,
    131-133
Cardiogenic shock, 3-4, 4*t*,
    130-131
  treatment, 7*t*, 130-131
Cardiopulmonary arrest, 149-151;
    see also Cardiac arrest
  in children, 348-349
Cardiopulmonary resuscitation,
    149
Cardiovascular disorders; *see*
    Cardiac disorders
Cardioversion; *see also*
    Defibrillation
  of atrial flutter, 138
  for dysrhythmia, 133
  of supraventricular tachycardia,
    136
  for tachycardias, 132

Cardioversion—cont'd
  of torsades de pointes, 149,
    149*b*
  of ventricular tachycardia, 147
Cardioverters/defibrillators,
    151-154
Carmustine, 255, 256*b*
Carotid sinus syndrome, 222
Casts, 60
  for distal radius fractures, 64
  for navicular fractures, 65
Cat bites, 118
  indications for rabies
    prophylaxis, 119*t*
Cathartics
  for constipation and fecal
    impaction, 194
  for poisoning, 298-299
Cat scratches, 118
Caustic ingestion, 235-236, 310
Cefaclor, 175
Cefadroxil, 175
Cefazolin, 175
Cefixime
  for gonococcal dermatitis, 271
  for gonococcal pharyngitis, 238
  for lung infections, 175
Cefizox; *see* Ceftizoxime
Ceflor; *see* Cefaclor
Cefobid; *see* Cefoperazone
Cefoperazone, 176
Cefotaxime
  for lung infections, 175
  for meningitis, 232, 252, 352
  for pneumonia, 353
Cefoxitin
  for lung infections, 175
  for pelvic inflammatory disease,
    206
Ceftazidime, 176
Ceftin; *see* Cefuroxime
Ceftizoxime, 176
Ceftriaxone
  for epididymitis, 199
  for gonococcal dermatitis, 271
  for gonococcal pharyngitis, 238
  for lung infections, 176
  for meningitis, 232, 352

Ceftriaxone—cont'd
  for otitis media in children, 358
  for pelvic inflammatory disease,
      206
  for pneumonia, 353
  for pyelonephritis, 198
  for urethritis in male, 198
Cefuroxime, 175
Cellulitis, 113
  AIDS and, 248
Central nervous system
  infections with cancer, 251-252
  pathology, 218-219
Central nervous system
    stimulants, 342
Central retinal artery, occlusion
    of, 244
Central venous pressure
    monitoring, 31
Central vertigo, 222-223
  causes, 223-224
Centruroides scorpion
    envenomation, 319, 320*t*
Cephalexin
  for impetigo, 277
  for lung infections, 175
  for open fractures, 79
  for wound infections, 117
Cephalic vein, 74*f*
Cephalosporins
  for acute cystitis, 197
  for acute sinusitis, 240
  for bacterial otitis media, 239
  for cat and dog bites, 119
  for lung infections, 175-176
  for meningitis, 252
  for olecranon bursitis, 116
  for orbital fractures, 82
  for pneumonia, 178
  for pyelonephritis, 198
  for wound infections, 117
Cephazolin, 79
Cerebellar infarction, 224
Cerebral abscess, 252
Cerebral herniation, 249-250
Cerebrovascular accident, 228
  sickle cell disease and, 260*t*
Cerebyx; *see* Fosphenytoin

Cervical carcinoma, 209
Cervical spine radiography
  with altered levels of
      consciousness, 214
  with closed head injuries, 54
Cetacaine; *see* Benzocaine
Chalazion, 245
Cheek lacerations, 111
Chemical exposure
  of conjunctiva and cornea,
      88-89
  pulmonary burn, 182-183
Chemotherapy
  allergic reactions, 256
  cardiac toxicity, 256
  effects of, 255-256
  gastrointestinal toxicity, 255,
      255*b*
  neurotoxicity, 256
  pulmonary toxicity, 255, 256*b*
  SIADH and, 254
Chest escharotomy, 281, 282*f*
Chest pain
  ischemic, 125-130
  Quick Reference Form, 379-388
Chest radiography
  with bronchiolitis in infants,
      357
  with cardiogenic pulmonary
      edema, 132
  with diaphragmatic rupture, 42
  with GI gas, 194
  with hemothorax, 41
  with ingestion of caustics, 235
  with pneumothorax, 38-39
  with pulmonary embolism, 180
  with rib fracture, 35
  with thoracic aortic dissection,
      127, 158
Chest wound, sucking; *see*
    Pneumothorax, open
Cheyne-Stokes respiration, 214
Chickenpox; *see* Varicella
Child abuse, 358-359
Children; *see* Pediatric
    emergencies
CHIPES, 291
Chlamydia pneumoniae, 173

Chlamydia trachomatis
pelvic inflammatory disease
with, 205
urethritis in male and, 198
Chloral hydrate overdose, 299,
300*b*
Chlorambucil, 255, 256*b*
Chloramphenicol, 232, 352
Chlorpromazine
in chemotherapy, 255, 255*b*
for heat stroke, 286
for mushroom poisoning, 323*t*
overdose, 305
for psychotic agitation, 330,
339
Chokes, 289
Cholecystectomy, 188
Cholecystitis, 187-188
Cholelithiasis, 186, 187-188
sickle cell disease and, 260*t*
Cholinergic overdose, 292, 295*t*
Christmas disease, 263
Chronic obstructive pulmonary
disease, 170-171
Chvostek's sign, 24
Cimetidine
for anaphylaxis, 170
for peptic disorders, 189
for urticaria, 275
Cipro; *see* Ciprofloxacin
Ciprofloxacin
for acute cystitis, 197
for diarrhea, 193
for gonococcal dermatitis, 271
for gonococcal pharyngitis, 238
Ciprofloxazone, 177
Circulation management, 30
in thoracic trauma, 33
Claforan; *see* Cefotaxime
Clarithromycin
for lung infections, 177
for pneumonia, 178, 353
Clavicular fractures, 60-61
Clindamycin
for bacterial vaginosis, 208
for pelvic inflammatory disease,
206
Clinical pathways, symptom-
oriented, 363-430

Clinical Policies, 363-364
Clinitest tablets, 310
Clostridium difficile, 193
Clostridium tetani, 116
Clotrimazole
for dermatologic problems, 279*t*
for fungal infections, 276
for thrush, 241
for yeast vaginitis, 207, 208
Cloxacillin, 278
Coagulation disorders, 261-263
Coagulation pathway, 262*f*
disorders of, 261-263
Coagulation studies, 194
Cocaine
intoxication, 342
topical anesthesia with, 93
withdrawal, 342
"Coffee grounds" emesis, 193
Cognitive (organic disorders,
335-338
etiology, 334, 336*b*
Cognitive function
normal, psychoses with,
338-340
testing, 332-333, 337
Colchicine, 327
Colic, renal, 200
Colitis
diarrhea and, 193
pseudomembranous, 193
Colles' fractures, 64
Coma
causes, 212, 214-221
deep, 212
hyperthyroid crisis and, 220
metabolic, 211-232
myxedema, 220
overdose and, 292
pediatric hypoglycemic,
353-354
Common digital nerve block, 96*f*
Common extensor tendon, 76
Compazine; *see* Prochlorperazine
Compensation for shock, 4-5
Compensatory venoconstriction,
loss of, 222
Complete blood count
with altered levels of
consciousness, 214

Complete blood count–cont'd
　with gastrointestinal
　　hemorrhage, 194
Computed tomography
　with abdominal trauma, 46, 47
　with acute sinusitis, 240
　with altered levels of
　　consciousness, 214
　with appendicitis, 187
　with bladder injuries, 50
　with cholelithiasis or
　　pancreatitis, 186
　with closed head injuries, 54
　with encephalitis, 252
　with genitourinary tract
　　obstruction, 186
　with headache, 228
　with injuries to aorta and great
　　vessels, 42
　with laryngeal trauma, 86
　with meningitis, 232, 253
　with pancreatitis, 188
　with renal colic, 200
　with renal injuries, 49, 50
　spinal, 59
　with stroke, 230
　with thoracic aortic dissection,
　　159
　with ureteral injuries, 50
　with vertigo, 225
Confusion, 219
Congestive heart failure
　hyponatremia and, 16
　physical examination, 126
　sickle cell disease and, 260*t*
Conjunctiva, chemical exposure
　of, 88-89
Conjunctivitis
　bacterial, 242-243
　viral, 243
Consciousness
　altered levels of, 211-221
　　causes, 211-212
　　etiology, 212
　　general considerations,
　　　211-212
　　laboratory and radiologic
　　　investigations, 214
　　physical examination,
　　　212-214

Consciousness–cont'd
　altered levels of–cont'd
　　treatment, 214
　evaluation of, 53
Constipation, 194
Contact dermatitis, 280
Continuous positive airway
　　pressure
　for ARDS, 179
　for cardiogenic pulmonary
　　edema, 132
Contrast studies
　with foreign bodies in airway or
　　esophagus, 234
　with ingestion of caustics, 235
　with peptic disorders, 189
Contusions
　arterial, 160, 160*f*
　myocardial, 42-43
Convulsions, 55
　pediatric, 350-351
Cooling sprays, 114
COPD; *see* Chronic obstructive
　　pulmonary disease
Coral snakes, 317, 318*f*, 319
Cordarone; *see* Amiodarone
Cornea
　abrasion of, 90
　chemical exposure of, 88-89
Coronary artery bypass grafting
　for acute myocardial infarction,
　　129
　for angina, 130
　for cardiogenic shock, 131
Corpine, 323*t*
Corticosteroids; *see also* Steroids
　for croup, 355
　for dermatologic problems, 279*t*
　for herpes zoster infections, 277
　for meningitis, 352
　for mushroom poisoning, 323*t*
　relative potencies, 169*t*
　for spinal injuries, 59
　for tennis elbow, 64
　for toxic epidermal necrolysis,
　　278
　for urticaria, 275
Cortisporin, 240
Cough, in AIDS, 248

Coumadin, 181
Coxsackievirus infection, 271-272
  stomatitis and, 241
CPAP; *see* Continuous positive
    airway pressure
Creatine phosphokinase, in acute
    myocardial infarction, 126
Creatinine, altered levels of
    consciousness and, 214
Cricothyrotomy, 32
Crohn's disease, 193
Crotamiton, 277
Croup, 355
Cryptococcus
  AIDS and, 248
  in transplant recipients, 267
Cushingoid appearance, 219
Cyanide overdose, 295*t*, 314-315
Cyanosis, 292
Cyclopeptides, 323*t*
Cyclophosphamide, 255, 256*b*
Cycloplegics, 90
Cyclosporine, 267, 268
Cystitis, 197
Cystospaz; *see* Hyoscyamine
Cysts, ovarian, 207
Cytomegalovirus, in transplant
    recipients, 267
Cytotec; *see* Misoprostol
Cytoxan; *see* Cyclophosphamide

D

Dapsone, 322
Darvon; *see* Propoxyphene
D-dimer, 180
Decadron; *see* Dexamethasone
Decandron; *see* Dexamethasone
Decompression illness, 289-290
Deep vein thrombosis, 158
Deferoxamine, 296*t*, 313
Defibrillation; *see also*
    Cardioversion
  in cardiac arrest, 149, 150*b*, 151
Defibrillators, 154
Degenerative diseases presenting
    as psychiatric disorders,
    336*b*

Dehydration, 15
  in children, 349-350
  hyponatremia and, 16
  syncope and, 222
Delirium, 337-338; *see also*
    Encephalopathy
Delirium tremens, 214
Delusions, 331
Demeclocycline, 17
Dementia, 338
Demerol; *see* Meperidine
Dental abscess, 241
Dental caries, 241
Dental infections, 241
Dental trauma, 87
Depersonalization, 332
Depression, major, 338, 340
Derealization, 332
Dermal exposure, Quick
    Reference Form, 418-423
Dermatitis
  atopic, 279*t*, 279-280
  contact, 280
  gonococcal, 271
  mild, 280
  moderate-to-severe, 280
Dermatologic disorders, 271-280
  medications for, 279*t*, 279-280
Dermatophytoses, 276
Descending thoracic aorta, injury
    to, 160
Desipramine overdose, 306
Desonide, 279*t*
Desoximetasone, 279*t*
Detergent exposure, conjunctiva
    and cornea, 88-89
DEV; *see* Duck embryo vaccine
Dexamethasone
  for cerebral edema, 55
  in chemotherapy, 255, 255*b*
  for hyperthyroid crisis, 221
  lead poisoning and, 312
  for meningitis, 352
  for mushroom poisoning, 323*t*
  relative potencies, 169*t*
Dextrose, 215
DHE-45; *see* Dihydroergotamine
Diabetes
  acute cystitis with, 197

Diabetes–cont'd
  pediatric, 353-354
  prophylactic antibiotics with,
    117
Diabetic hyperglycemia, 216-217
Diabetic hypoglycemia, 215
Diabetic ketoacidosis, 216
  pediatric, 354
The Diagnostic and Statistical
    Manual of Mental Disorders,
    fourth edition, 333-334
Diagnostic peritoneal lavage, 46,
    47
Dialysis
  for poisonings, 299, 300*b*
  with severe hypermagnesemia,
    25
Diamox; *see* Acetazolamide
Diaphragmatic rupture, 42
Diarrhea, 191, 192-193
  AIDS and, 248
  infectious, 191-192
  travelers', 192
Diazepam
  for black widow bites, 321
  for CA overdose, 307
  for convulsions, 55
  for convulsions in children, 351
  for eclamptic seizures, 210
  for hyperventilation syndrome,
    182
  for mushroom poisoning, 323*t*
  for PCP intoxication, 308
  for peripheral vertigo, 225
  sedation with, 104, 330
  for seizures, 226
Dicloxacillin
  for cat and dog bites, 119
  for dermatologic problems, 279*t*
  for impetigo, 277
  for olecranon bursitis, 116
  for open fractures, 79
  for wound infections, 117
Dieffenbachia, 325*t*
Digital artery, 72*f*
Digitalis overdose, 295*t*, 309-310
Digital nerve, 72*f*
Digital nerve block, 95-96, 96*f*

Digoxin
  for atrial fibrillation, 140
  for atrial flutter, 138*b*, 139
  for supraventricular tachycardia,
    136
Digoxin-specific antibody FAB
    fragments, 295*t*, 310
Dihydroergotamine, 228
Dilantin; *see* Phenytoin
Dilaudid; *see* Hydromorphone
Diltiazem
  for atrial fibrillation, 140
  for atrial flutter, 138, 138*b*
  for supraventricular tachycardia,
    135*b*, 136
Dimercaprol
  for arsenic poisoning, 316
  for lead poisoning, 312
  for mercury poisoning, 314
Diphenhydramine
  for anaphylaxis, 170
  as antidote, 295*t*
  for peripheral vertigo, 225
  for poison oak and poison ivy,
    280
  for urticaria, 275
Diphenoxylate overdose, 296*t*
Diphenoxylate with atropine, 192
Diplopia, 81
Disequilibrium, 223
Dislocation
  of elbow, 63
  of hip, 66
  patellar, 66
  shoulder, 61-62
  temporomandibular joint, 241
Disopyramide, 149
Disposition, 345-346
Disseminated intravascular
    coagulation
  with abruptio placentae, 210
  cancer and, 253, 257
Distal radius (Colles' fractures, 64
Distributive shock, 4, 4*t*
  anaphylactic, 6
  septic, 6
  treatment, 6, 7*t*
Diuresis, forced, 299, 299*b*
  drugs helped by, 300*t*

Diuretics
   for cardiogenic pulmonary
      edema, 132
   hyponatremia and, 16
Diverticulitis, 190-191
Diving injuries, 87
Dizziness, 222-225
Dobutamine, 131
Dog bites, 118
   indications for rabies
      prophylaxis, 119*t*
Doll's eyes, 212
Domeboro; *see* Aluminum acetate
Dopamine
   for AV block, 144
   for cardiogenic shock, 131
   for hypotension, 170
   pediatric dosages, 349
   for sinus bradycardia, 141, 141*b*
Doppler ultrasonography
   with thrombophlebitis, 157
   with torsion of spermatic cord,
      201
   with transient ischemic attack,
      230
Doriden; *see* Glutethimide
Dorsal carpal ligament, 73*f*
Dorsal interosseous muscle, 74*f*
Doxycycline
   for Bartholin's abscess, 209
   for cat and dog bites, 118-119
   for epididymitis, 199
   for pelvic inflammatory disease,
      206
   for pneumonia, 178
   for urethritis in male, 198
DPL; *see* Diagnostic peritoneal
      lavage
Droperidol
   in chemotherapy, 255, 255*b*
   for nausea and vomiting, 192
Drowning, 290
Drug abuse; *see also* Overdose;
      Poisoning
   reactions presenting as
      psychiatric disorders, 336*b*
   toxicology studies, 214
Drug eruption, 271
Drug overdose; *see* Overdose

Drugs; *see also specific drugs*
   associated with hemolysis, 259*b*
   causing hemolytic anemias,
      259*b*
   for dermatologic problems, 279*t*
   for dysrhythmia, 133
   pediatric access, 348
   pediatric dosages, 349
   for psychiatric emergencies, 330
Drug syndromes, 341-343
DSM-IV; *see The Diagnostic and
      Statistical Manual of Mental
      Disorders*, fourth edition
Duck embryo vaccine
   dosages, 120*t*
   indications, 119*t*
Duricef; *see* Cefadroxil
Dysphagia, 248
Dysphonia, 86
Dysrhythmias, 133-149
   bradydysrhythmias, 130, 133
   in cancer, 256
   overdose and, 292
   syncope and, 221
   tachydysrhythmias, 130, 132
   ventricular, 307
Dysuria, 197

E
Ear
   bleeding from, 54, 83
   foreign body in, 235
   infections of, 238-240
Eardrum perforation, 86-87
Eastern Cottonmouth snake, 318*f*
Eclampsia, 210
Econazole, 279*t*
Ectopic pregnancy, 204-205
Edema, 15
   cardiogenic pulmonary,
      131-133
EDTA; *see* Ethylenediaminetetra-
      acetic acid
Effusion, 239
Ehlers-Danlos syndrome, 158
Elavil; *see* Amitriptyline
Elbow injuries, 63-64
Elderly, mental status
      examination, 345

Electrical burns, 285
Electric shock, 285
Electrocardiography
    with acute myocardial
        infarction, 126
    with angina, 126, 130
    with atrial fibrillation, 139
    with atrial flutter, 137
    with atrioventricular block,
        141-142, 142*f*, 143*f*, 144*f*
    with hypercalcemia, 22
    with hypocalcemia, 24
    with hypothermia, 287, 288*f*
    with multifocal atrial
        tachycardias, 136
    with myocardial contusion,
        42-43
    with paroxysmal
        supraventricular
        tachycardia, 135
    with premature ventricular
        contractions, 144
    with pulmonary embolism, 180
    with sinus bradycardia, 140
    with sinus tachycardia, 133
    with torsades de pointes, 147
    with transplanted heart, 268
    with ventricular tachycardia,
        146
Electrocution, 45
Electrolyte disorders, 10-25
Electrolytes
    with altered levels of
        consciousness, 214
    calculations, 316
    with gastrointestinal
        hemorrhage, 194
Embolectomy, 182
Embolism
    pulmonary, 179-182
    sickle cell disease and, 260*t*
Embolization, arterial, 155-156
Emesis, 189
    "coffee grounds," 193
    indications for, 294, 297*b*, 298*b*
Eminase; *see* Anistreplase
Emphysema, 170
    subcutaneous, 39
Encephalitis, 252

Encephalopathy
    hepatic, 219
    hypertensive, 218-219
    metabolic, 211-221
Endocarditis
    infective, 117
    marantic, 253
Endocrine conditions, 219-221
    presenting as psychiatric
        disorders, 336*b*
    syncope and, 222
Endoscopy
    with gastrointestinal
        hemorrhage, 194
    with ingestion of caustics, 235
    with peptic disorders, 189
Endotracheal intubation
    access in children, 348
    for cardiogenic pulmonary
        edema, 132, 133
    for elevated intracranial
        pressure, 55
    for flail chest, 35
    for hypoventilation, 166
    for PCP intoxication, 308
    with pulmonary burn, 183
    for pulmonary contusion, 41
    for thoracic trauma, 29
Enterobacter, 231
Envenomation, animal, 317-328
Environmental emergencies, 281-
    290
Enzymes
    cardiac, 126
    liver
        cholecystitis and, 186
        GI hemorrhage and, 194
        pancreatitis and, 188
Epidemic keratoconjunctivitis,
    243
Epididymitis, 199, 201
Epidural hematoma, 54
Epiglottitis, 355-356
Epinephrine; *see also* Adrenaline
    for anaphylaxis, 168, 170
    for asthma, 168
    for asthmatic bronchospasm,
        168, 170, 356, 357
    for AV block, 144

Epinephrine—cont'd
contraindications, 106
for COPD, 168
for digital nerve blocks, 95
for local infiltration block, 92
pediatric dosages, 349
for pulseless electrical activity
and asystole, 151
reaction to, 102
for sinus bradycardia, 141, 141*b*
for urticaria, 275
for ventricular fibrillation, 150*b*,
151
for wound care anesthesia, 106
Epistaxis, 236-237
Epstein-Barr virus, in transplant
recipients, 267
Eruptions
drug, 271
of febrile illness, 271, 272*t*
skin, 247-248
Erythema multiforme, 275
Erythrocytosis, 257
Erythromycin
for bacterial otitis media, 239
for cat and dog bites, 119
for dermatologic problems, 279*t*
for diarrhea, 193
for impetigo, 277
for lung infections, 177
for otitis media in children, 358
for pneumonia, 178, 353
for streptococcal pharyngitis,
238
for tonsillitis and pharyngitis,
358
for wound infection, 117
Escape beats, 145
Escharotomy
chest, 283, 284*f*
extremities, 283
Escherichia coli, 352
antibiotics for, 193
diarrhea and, 192
in transplant recipients, 267
Esmolol
for acute myocardial infarction,
129
for atrial flutter, 138*b*, 139

Esmolol—cont'd
for supraventricular tachycardia,
136
Esophageal reflux, 127
Esophageal spasm, 127
Esophagogastric perforation, 235
Esophagus, foreign body in,
234-235
Ethanol; *see also* Alcohol
as antidote, 295*t*, 296*t*
for methanol and ethylene
glycol overdose, 317
Ethchlorvynol overdose, 299,
301*b*
Ethyl alcohol; *see* Ethanol
Ethylenediaminetetraacetic acid,
22-23
Ethylene glycol overdose, 316-317
antidote, 295*t*
dialysis for, 299, 300*b*
Eurax; *see* Crotamiton
Expiratory wheezing, 163
Extensor tendons
of hand, 71, 73*f*, 74*f*
injury repair, 79
of wrist, 72, 73*f*, 74*f*
damage to, 76
External genitalia disorders,
201-202
External pacing
for AV block, 144
for refractory bradycardias, 133
for sinus bradycardia, 141, 141*b*
Extraocular muscle entrapment,
81
Extraperitoneal ruptures, 50
Extremities
escharotomy of, 283
lower
injuries to, 65-69
regional nerve blocks, 99-100
Penetrating Extremity Trauma
Quick Reference Form,
376-378
suture removal, 109
suture size, 107
upper
injuries, 60-65
regional nerve blocks, 95-98

Eyelid injuries, 91
  lacerations, 91, 112
  suture removal, 109
Eyes
  blunt trauma to, 91
  examination of, 88, 252
    with head injuries, 53
  foreign bodies of, 89-90
  movement of, with head
    injuries, 53-54

F

Facial injuries, 81-87
  fractures, 81-85
  suture material for, 107
Factor VIII deficiency, 261-263
Faintness, 223
Famotidine, 189
Fear reaction, 102
Febrile illness; *see also* Fever
  eruptions of, 271, 272*t*
  with rash, 271-275, 272*t*
Fecal impaction, 194
Feelings of influence, 332
Felon, 114, 115*f*
Femoral nerve block, 99, 100*f*
Femoral shaft fractures, 66
Fentanyl
  for perirectal abscess, 195
  sedation with, 103
Ferrous gluconate overdose, 296*t*
Ferrous sulfate overdose, 296*t*
Fever
  with AIDS, 247, 247*t*
  in child
    evaluation, 347
    Quick Reference Forms,
      425-427, 426-430
  eruptions, 271, 272*t*
  with rash, 271-275, 272*t*
Fingers
  flexor tendons of, 71, 71*f*, 72*f*
    function test, 76, 76*f*, 77*f*
  partial anesthesia of, 74
  tourniquets, 78, 78*f*
Flagyl; *see* Metronidazole
Flail chest, 33, 34-36, 35*f*

Flexor tendons
  of fingers, 71, 71*f*, 72*f*
    function test, 76, 76*f*, 77*f*
  injury repair, 79
  of wrist, 70, 71*f*
Floxacin, 199
Floxin; *see* Ofloxacin
Fluconazole, 207
Fludrocortisone, 169*t*
Fluids; *see also* Hydration
  in airways, 163
  cardiogenic shock and, 130-131
  for dehydration in children, 350
  for diabetic hyperglycemia, 216
  for diabetic ketoacidosis in
    children, 354
  hypovolemic shock and, 8, 9
  with injuries to aorta and great
    vessels, 42
  for shock, 6, 7*t*
  for thermal burns, 282, 284
Flumazenil, 104, 295*t*
Fluocinolone acetonide, 279*t*
Fluocinonide, 279*t*
Fluoroquinolones
  for acute cystitis, 197
  for epididymitis, 199
  for lung infections, 177
Fluphenazine overdose, 305
Foley catheterization, 30-31
Folliculitis, 248
Food poisoning, 191
Foot injuries, 68-69
Forearm injuries, 64
Foreign bodies
  airway or esophageal, 233,
    234-235
  in eye, 89-90
  inground, 112
  in nose or ear canal, 235
  in pediatric GI tract, 359-360
  in wounds, 118
Fortaz; *see* Ceftazidime
Fosphenytoin, 226
Fractures
  ankle, 68
  arterial contusions with, 160,
    160*f*
  ballet, 68

Fractures—cont'd
  boxer's, 65
  calcaneal, 68
  clavicular, 60-61
  distal radius (Colles'), 64
  elbow, 63
  facial, 81
  facial bone, 81-85
  femoral shaft, 66
  of fifth metatarsal base, 68
  hand, 79
  hip, 65
  of humerus, 62-63
  mandibular, 83
  maxillary, 83-84
  metacarpal, 65
  midface, 84
  nasal, 84-85
  navicular, 65
  olecranon, 63-64
  open hand, 79
  orbital, 81-82, 82*f*
  patellar, 66
  pelvic, 69
  of penis, 51
  phalangeal, 69
  pubic, 69
  radius-ulna shaft, 64
  rib, 33-34
  scapular, 61
  of symphysis, 83
  tibial shaft, 68
  tooth, 87
Free water calculation, 350
Frenulum, 111
Frostbite, 287
Functional disorders, 333
Functional psychoses, 338
Fungal infections
  dermatologic, 276
  in transplant recipients, 267
Furosemide
  for cardiogenic pulmonary
    edema, 132
  for PCP intoxication, 309

G

Gall bladder disorders
  cholecystitis, 187-188

Gall bladder disorders—cont'd
  cholelithiasis, 186, 187-188,
    260*t*
  diagnostic studies, 186
Gamma benzene hexachloride, 277
Garamycin; *see* Gentamicin
Gas, gastrointestinal, 194
Gastric aspiration, 184
Gastroenteritis, 191-193
Gastrointestinal gas, 194
Gastrointestinal hemorrhage,
    193-194
  pediatric, 201
Gastrointestinal irritants, 323*t*
Gastrointestinal tract
  chemotherapy and, 255
  foreign bodies in, in children,
    359-360
  hypercalcemia and, 22
  hyperkalemia and, 19
Genital herpes, 208-209, 276
Genitourinary tract emergencies,
    197-210
  disorders of external genitalia,
    201-202
  infections, 197-199
  obstruction, 186
  trauma, 49-52
Gentamicin
  for bacterial conjunctivitis, 243
  for meningitis, 352
  for pyelonephritis, 198
German measles; *see* Rubella
Giardia, in transplant recipients,
    267
Glasgow Coma Scale, 212, 213*f*
Glaucoma, acute angle-closure,
    244-245
Glucagon, 215
Glucocorticoids, 22
Glucose
  altered levels of consciousness
    and, 214
  diabetic hyperglycemia,
    216-217
  diabetic hypoglycemia, 215
Glutethimide overdose, 305
Glycosides, 328
Gonococcal infections, 198-199
  dermatitis, 271

Gonococcal infections—cont'd
  pharyngitis, 237-238
Graft-versus-host-disease, 270
Grave mental disability, 343-344
Grease and paint gun injuries, 80
Great auricular nerve block, 95
Great vessels, injuries to, 42
Guidelines, 364
Gustatory hallucinations, 332
Gynecologic disorders, 204-210
  symptoms, 203-204
Gyromitrin, 323*t*

H

Haemophilus
  antibiotic prophylaxis, 232
  in transplant recipients, 267
Haemophilus influenzae, 171, 172,
    231, 352
Haldol; *see* Haloperidol
Hallucinations, 332, 339
Hallucinogens, 342-343
Haloperidol
  in chemotherapy, 255, 255*b*
  overdose, 295*t*, 305
  for psychotic agitation, 330,
    339
Haloprogin, 276
Hand
  deep infections of, 115
  dorsum of, 71-72, 73*f*
    anesthesia of, 74
  functional anatomy of, 70-72
  motor function evaluation,
    75-77
  palm of, 71, 72*f*
  sensation evaluation, 74-75, 75*f*
  vascular status evaluation, 73-74
Hand-foot-and-mouth disease,
    271-272
Hand injuries, 65, 70-80
  avulsions and amputations, 79
  diagnosis, 72-77
  general principles, 70
  lacerations, 76, 77
  nerve injuries, 79
  open fractures, 79
  suture material for, 107

Hand injuries—cont'd
  tendon injuries, 79
  treatment, 77-80
  vascular, 79
HDCV; *see* Human diploid cell
    vaccine
Headache, 227-228
  AIDS and, 248
  cluster, 227
  Quick Reference Form, 401-409
  tension, 227
  vascular, 227
Head and neck
  emergencies, 233-241
  infection, 237-240
  regional nerve blocks, 93-95
Head injuries, 53-55
Health care workers, precautions
    for, 249
Heart failure; *see also* Cardiac
    arrest
  in cancer, 256
  congestive
    hyponatremia and, 16
    physical examination, 126
    sickle cell disease and, 260*t*
  hyperthyroid crisis and, 220
Heart transplantation, 268-269
Heat cramps, 286
Heat exhaustion, 286
Heat stroke, 286
Heat syncope, 286
Heavy metals poisoning, 311-314
Heimlich maneuver, 166, 233
Hematocele, 51
Hematologic emergencies,
    258-261
  oncologic, 257
Hematoma
  epidural, 54
  septal, 84-85
  subdural, 54-55
Hematuria, 49, 186
  sickle cell disease and, 260*t*
Hemodialysis, 317
Hemolysis
  chronic, 260*t*
  drugs associated with, 259*b*
Hemolytic anemias, 259*b*

Hemoperfusion, 299, 301*b*
Hemopericardium, 43
Hemophilia A, 261-263
Hemophilia B, 263
Hemorrhage
  in cancer, 257
  central vertigo and, 224
  gastrointestinal, 193-194
    pediatric, 201
  intracerebral, 228
  retinal, 260*t*
  subarachnoid, 227
Hemorrhagic hypovolemic shock,
    8-9
Hemorrhagic stroke, 228-229
Hemorrhoids, 195
Hemostasis, 236-237
Hemothorax, 40-41
  treatment, 35-36, 41
Heparin
  for acute myocardial infarction,
    129
  for angina, 130
  for deep vein thrombosis, 158
  low-molecular-weight, 181
  for pulmonary embolism, 181
  for stroke, 231
Hepatic encephalopathy, 219
Hepatic failure, 219
Hepatic infarction, 260*t*
Hepatitis, 260*t*
Hepatitis B, 267
Hepatitis C, 267
Hernias
  incarcerated, 360-361
  inguinal, 360-361
Herniation
  cerebral, 249-250
  diaphragmatic, 42
Herpes genitalis, 208-209
Herpes simplex
  AIDS and, 247
  cutaneous infection, 276
  in transplant recipients, 267
Herpes simplex keratitis, 243
Herpes simplex stomatitis, 241
Herpesvirus infection,
    dermatologic, 276-277

Herpes zoster
  cutaneous infections, 276-277
  in transplant recipients, 267
Hip injuries, 65-66
Hippocrates, reduction method
    of, 61
Histamine$_1$ blockers, 275
Histamine$_2$ blockers
  for anaphylaxis, 170
  for gastrointestinal hemorrhage,
    194
  for peptic disorders, 189
  for urticaria, 275
Histoplasma
  AIDS and, 248
  in transplant recipients, 267
Hoarseness, 86
Holly, 324*t*
Homatropine drops
  for acute anterior uveitis, 245
  for foreign bodies in eye, 90
Homicidal risk, 343
Hordeolum, 245
HRIG; *see* Human rabies immune
    globulin
Human bites, 118
Human chorionic gonadotropin,
    in ectopic pregnancy, 204
Human diploid cell vaccine
  dosages for, 120*t*
  indications for, 119*t*
Human immunodeficiency virus;
    see also Acquired
      immunodeficiency
      syndrome
  clinical staging, 246
  diarrhea and, 193
Human rabies immune globulin
  dosages for, 120*t*
  indications for, 119*t*
Humerus fractures, 62-63
Humidity
  bronchiolitis and, 357
  croup and, 355
Hydration; *see also* Fluids
  for asthma, 356
  for erythema multiforme, 275
  for hypernatremia, 15
  hyponatremia and, 15-16

Hydrocarbon overdose, 310-311
  indications for emesis, 294,
    297*b*, 298*b*
Hydrocele, 51
Hydrocortisone
  for anaphylaxis, 170
  for asthmatic bronchospasm,
    168
  for hypercalcemia, 22
  for hypothyroid crisis, 220
  relative potencies, 169*t*
Hydrocyanic acid overdose, 295*t*
Hydrogen sulfide overdose, 314
Hydromorphone
  for incision and drainage, 114
  for perirectal abscess, 195
Hydroxyurea, 255, 256*b*
Hydroxyzine
  for nausea and vomiting, 192
  for poison oak and poison ivy,
    280
  for sedation with meperidine,
    103
  for urticaria, 275
Hyoscyamine, 197
Hypercalcemia, 21-23
Hyperglycemia, diabetic, 216-217
Hyperkalemia, 18-20
  adrenal crisis and, 219
Hypermagnesemia, 24-25
Hypernatremia, 14*t*, 14-15
Hypernephroma, 257
Hypersensitivity to regional
    anesthesia, 102
Hypertension
  eclamptic seizures and, 210
  headache and, 227
Hypertensive encephalopathy,
    218-219
Hyperthermic states, 286-287
Hyperthyroid crisis, 220-221
Hypertonia not resulting from
    sodium, 16
Hypertonic saline, 18
Hyperventilation, 164
  for elevated intracranial
    pressure, 55
Hyperventilation syndrome, 164,
    182

Hypesthesia, of hand, 75
Hyphema, 91
Hypnotics, 342
Hypocalcemia, 23-24
Hypoglycemia
  altered levels of consciousness
    with, 214
  cancer and, 253
  diabetic, 215
  syncope and, 222
Hypoglycemic coma, pediatric,
    353-354
Hypokalemia, 20-21
Hypomagnesemia, 25
Hyponatremia, 15-18
  adrenal crisis and, 219
  etiology, 16, 17*t*
  mild, 254
  severe, 254
  sodium deficit calculation, 350
  treatment, 17-18, 254
Hyposthenuria, 260*t*
Hypotension
  adrenal crisis and, 219
  drug-induced, 127
  poisoning and, 292
  treatment, 170
  verapamil-induced, 138
Hypothermia, 287-289
  cardiac arrest and, 149
  open thoracotomy in, 45
Hypothyroid crisis, 220
Hypothyroidism, 222
Hypoventilation, 163, 164, 166
Hypovolemic shock, 3, 4*t*
  hemorrhagic, 8-9
  hemothorax and, 40
  with pelvic fractures, 69
  treatment, 6, 7*t*
Hypoxia, 218
  with drowning, 290
  hemothorax and, 40

I

Ibotenic acid, 323*t*
I&D; *see* Incision and drainage
Ideas of references, 332

Idiopathic thrombocytopenic purpura, 261
Iliac vein thrombosis, 157
Ilium, fractures of, 69
Illusions, 332
Imipenem, 176
Imipramine overdose, 306
Imitrex; *see* Sumatriptan
Immersion injury, 290
Immunization
  against rabies, 119*t*, 120*t*, 121
  against tetanus, 116
Immunodeficiency; *see also* Acquired immunodeficiency syndrome
  sickle cell disease and, 260*t*
Immunosuppression, 266
Immunosuppressive agents, 266-267
Imodium; *see* Loperamide
Impedance plethysmography, 157
Impetigo, 277
  AIDS and, 248
Inapsine; *see* Droperidol
Incarcerated hernia, 360-361
Incision and drainage, 113
  anesthesia for, 114
  for perirectal abscess, 195
  for peritonsillar abscess, 238
  for thrombosed external hemorrhoids, 195
Inderal; *see* Propranolol
Indoles, 323*t*
Indomethacin, 116
Infants; *see also* Pediatric emergencies
  bronchiolitis in, 357
  external cardiac compression in, 349
  febrile
    evaluation of, 347
    Quick Reference Forms, 425-427, 428-430
  ventilation in, 349
Infarction
  acute myocardial, 125-130
  bone, 260*t*
  cerebellar, 224
  hepatic, 260*t*

Infarction—cont'd
  pulmonary, 260*t*
  right ventricular, 131
  transplanted heart, 269
Infections; *see also specific infections*
  in bone marrow transplantation, 270
  in cancer, 258
  deep, of hand, 115
  dental, 241
  distal fat pad, 114, 115*f*
  genitourinary tract, 197-199
  gonococcal, 198-199
  head and neck, 237-240
  herpesvirus, 276-277
  nongonococcal, 198-199
  oral, 241
  in organ transplants, 268
  presenting as psychiatric disorders, 336*b*
  pulmonary, 171-178
    sickle cell disease and, 260*t*
  skin lesions, AIDS and, 247-248
  soft-tissue, 113-121
  in transplanted lung, 269
  in transplant recipients, 267
  traumatic wound, 116-121
  urinary tract, 186
  wound, 117-118
Infectious diarrhea, 191-192
Infective endocarditis, 117
Infestations, 277
Infraorbital nerve block, 93-95, 94*f*
Inguinal hernia, 360-361
Inhalation disorders, 182-184
Inhalation injury, 283
  acute toxic exposure, Quick Reference Form, 418-423
Inorganic phosphate, 23
Inotropic agents, 131
Inspiratory stridor, 163
Insulin
  for diabetic hyperglycemia, 216-217
  for diabetic ketoacidosis in children, 354
Intercostal nerve block
  complications of, 100

Intercostal nerve block—cont'd
  for flail chest, 36
  for rib fracture, 34
Interrupted vertical mattress
    technique, 77
Intoxications; *see also* Overdose;
    Poisoning; *specific intox-
    icants*
  water, 16
Intracerebral hemorrhage, 228
Intracranial pressure, 55, 218
  cancer and, 249-250
Intraocular pressure, 242
Intraosseous medication, access in
    children, 348
Intraperitoneal ruptures, 50
Intravenous pyelography
  with bladder injuries, 50
  with genitourinary tract
    obstruction, 186
  with renal colic, 200
  with renal injuries, 49-50
Intravenous urography, 50
Intussusception, 360
Ipratropium bromide
  for asthmatic bronchospasm,
    168
  for COPD with bronchospasm,
    171
Iridocyclitis, 245
Iritis, 245
Iron poisoning, 313
Iron salt overdose, 296*t*
Ischemia
  arterial, 155
  cardiac, 125, 127
    without acute infarction, 130
  transient ischemic attack, 228-
    231
Ischemic chest pain, 125-130
Ischemic optical neuropathy, 244
Ischemic stroke
  definition, 228
  headache and, 227
  treatment, 230-231
Isoniazid overdose
  dialysis for, 299, 300*b*
  forced diuresis for, 300*t*

Isoproterenol
  for AV block, 144
  for bradydysrhythmias, 133
  pediatric dosages, 349
  for sinus bradycardia, 141, 141*b*
  for torsades de pointes, 149,
    149*b*
Isoxazoles, 323*t*
IVP; *see* Intravenous pyelography

J

Jerusalem cherry, 325*t*
Jimsonweed, 325*t*
Joint trauma, 60-69; *see also specific
    joints*
Junctura tendinum, 73*f*

K

Kabikinase; *see* Streptokinase
Kaposi's sarcoma, 248
Keflex; *see* Cephalexin
Kefurox; *see* Cefuroxime
Kefzol; *see* Cefazolin
Kenalog; *see* Triamcinolone
    acetonide
Keratitis, herpes simplex, 243
Keratoconjunctivitis, epidemic,
    243
Kerosene ingestion, 310-311
Ketoacidosis, diabetic, 216
  pediatric, 354
Ketorolac, 200
Kidney; *see also under* Renal
  transplantation, 268
Klebsiella pneumoniae, 173
Knee injuries, 66-68
Kwell; *see* Gamma benzene hexa-
    chloride

L

Labetalol, 218
Labyrinthitis, 223
Laceration repair, 106-112
  buccal mucosa, 111
  cheek, 111
  eyelids, 91, 112

Laceration repair—cont'd
  facial, 107
  hand, 76, 77, 107
  lip, 111, 112*f*
  oral mucosa, 111
  scrotum, 52
  skin, 107, 109, 110*f*
  stellate or V-shaped, 110, 110*f*
  suture material, 107
  suture removal, 109
  suture technique, 107, 108*f*-109*f*
  tongue, 111
  vascular, 159
Lacrimal canaliculus injuries, 91
β-Lactam/β-lactamase inhibitors,
      176-177, 178
β-Lactams, 174-177
Laetrile overdose, 295*t*
Large bowel obstruction, 190
Laryngeal trauma, 86
Laryngoscopy
  with foreign body in airway or
      esophagus, 234
  with laryngeal trauma, 86
Laryngospasm, 170
  airway obstruction caused by,
      233
Lateral femoral cutaneous nerve
      block, 99-100, 100*f*
Laxatives, 194
Lead lines, 312
Lead poisoning, 311-312
Legionella pneumophila, 174
Leukeran; *see* Chlorambucil
Leukocytes, fecal, 192
Leukocytosis
  with appendicitis, 187
  in cancer, 257
  with cholelithiasis or
      cholecystitis, 188
  with pelvic inflammatory
      disease, 206
Levophed; *see* Norepinephrine
Lidex; *see* Fluocinonide
Lidocaine
  for abrasions, 112
  for digital nerve block, 95
  for incision and drainage, 114
  for laryngospasm, 170, 233

Lidocaine—cont'd
  for local infiltration block, 92,
      93
  for median nerve block, 97
  pediatric dosages, 349
  for premature ventricular
      contractions, 145, 146
  for pulseless ventricular
      tachycardia, 151
  for reduction of fracture
      hematoma, 65
  for septal hematoma, 84
  for stomatitis, 241
  for ventricular dysrhythmia,
      307
  for ventricular fibrillation, 150*b*,
      151
  for ventricular tachycardia,
      146*b*, 147
  for wound care anesthesia, 106
Life-threatening psychiatric
      conditions, 343-344
Lightning, 285
Lip lacerations, 111
  through-and-through, 111, 112*f*
Listeria, 267
Listeria monocytogenes, 352
  meningitis and, 252
Lithium carbonate overdose, 306
Liver disorders; *see also under*
      Hepatic
  diagnostic studies, 186
Liver enzymes
  cholecystitis and, 186
  GI hemorrhage and, 194
  pancreatitis and, 188
Liver transplantation, 269
Local infiltration block, 92-93
Lomotil; *see* Diphenoxylate;
      Diphenoxylate with
      atropine
Lomustine, 255, 256*b*
Loperamide, 192
Lorazepam
  for CA overdose, 307
  for convulsions in children, 351
  for eclamptic seizures, 210
  sedation with, 330
  for seizures, 226

Lotrimin; *see* Clotrimazole
Lower extremities
  injuries to, 65-69
  regional nerve blocks, 99-100
Loxapine succinate overdose, 295*t*
Loxitane; *see* Loxapine succinate
Loxosceles, 321-322
LSD; *see* Lysergic acid diethyl-
  amide
Ludiomil; *see* Maprotiline
Lumbar puncture
  with headache, 228
  with meningitis, 253
Lung; *see also under* Pulmonary
  transplantation, 269
Lye exposure
  conjunctiva and cornea, 88-89
  ingestion, 235, 310
Lyme disease, 272
Lymphadenopathy, acute, 113
Lymphangitis, 113
Lyovac *Latrodectus*, 321
Lysergic acid diethylamide,
  342-343

M

Maalox, 189
Macrobid; *see* Nitrofurantoin
Macrolides
  for lung infections, 177
  for pneumonia, 178
Magnesium
  hypermagnesemia, 24-25
  hypomagnesemia, 25
  for peptic disorders, 189
Magnesium sulfate
  for asthmatic bronchospasm,
    168
  for constipation and fecal
    impaction, 194
  for eclamptic seizures, 210
  for mercury poisoning, 314
  for pulseless ventricular
    tachycardia, 151
  for torsades de pointes, 149,
    149*b*
  for ventricular fibrillation, 150*b*,
    151

Magnetic resonance angiography
  with transient ischemic attack,
    230
  with vertigo, 225
Magnetic resonance imaging
  with thoracic aortic dissection,
    159
  with vertigo, 225
Magnet rate, 153
Malathion poisoning, 296*t*, 311
Mandible, 83, 84*f*
Mandibular fractures, 81, 83
Mandibular nerve block, 93, 94*f*
Manic episodes, 339
Mannitol
  for acute angle-closure glau-
    coma, 245
  for elevated intracranial
    pressure, 55
  lead poisoning and, 312
  for myoglobinuria, 308
Maprotiline overdose, 306
Marantic endocarditis, 253
Marcaine; *see* Bupivacaine
Marfan's syndrome, 158
Marijuana, 342-343
MAST; *see* Military antishock
    trousers
MAT; *see* Multifocal atrial
    tachycardia
Maxillary fractures, 83-84
  clinical signs, 81
  Le Fort I, 83, 85*f*
  Le Fort II, 83, 85*f*
  Le Fort III, 84, 85*f*
Maximal force, 330
Measles, 272-273
Meckel's diverticulum, 361
Meclizine, 225
Median nerve
  anatomy of, 71, 71*f*, 72*f*
  motor branch, 71, 72*f*
  motor branch damage, 76
  sensation and, 74, 75*f*
Median nerve block, 96*f*, 96-97,
    97*f*
Medications; *see also* Drugs; *specific*
    medications
  for dermatologic problems, 279*t*

Mediflow lens, 89
Mefoxin; *see* Cefoxitin
Mellaril; *see* Thioridazine
Ménière's disease, 223
Meningismus, 352
Meningitis, 228, 231-232
    cancer and, 252, 252*t*, 252-253
    headache and, 227
    pediatric, 352
Meningococcemia, 231, 273
Meningococcus, antibiotic pro-
        phylaxis, 232
Meniscus tears, 67
Mental disability, grave, 343-344
Mental nerve block, 93, 94*f*
Mental status, altered, 248
Mental status examination, 329,
        331, 344
Meperidine
    for incision and drainage, 114
    sedation with, 103
Mepivacaine, 92, 93
Meprobamate overdose, 299,
        300*b*, 300*t*
Mercury poisoning, 314
Mesoridazine overdose, 305
Metabolic acidosis, 11-12
    poisoning and, 292
    respiratory compensation of,
        165
Metabolic alkalosis, 13-14
Metabolic coma, 211-232
Metabolic disorders
    in cancer, 253-254
    presenting as psychiatric
        disorders, 336*b*
Metabolic encephalopathies, 211-
        221
Metacarpal fractures, 65
Metatarsal fracture, 68
Methacholine overdose, 295*t*
Methanol overdose, 316-317
    antidote, 296*t*
    dialysis for, 299, 300*b*
Methemoglobin overdose, 296*t*
Methocarbamol, 321
Methotrexate, 267
    pulmonary toxicity, 255, 256*b*

Methsuximide overdose, 299,
        301*b*
Methyl alcohol; *see* Methanol
Methylene blue, 296*t*
Methylprednisolone
    for anaphylaxis, 170
    for asthmatic bronchospasm,
        168
    for ischemic optical
        neuropathy, 244
    relative potencies, 169*t*
Methylxanthine, 168
Metoclopramide
    in chemotherapy, 255, 255*b*
    for headache, 228
Metoprolol
    for acute myocardial infarction,
        129
    for atrial flutter, 138*b*, 139
Metronidazole
    for bacterial vaginosis, 208
    for colitis, 193
    for pelvic inflammatory disease,
        206
    for yeast vaginitis, 208
Miconazole
    for fungal infections, 276
    for yeast vaginitis, 207
Micturition syncope, 222
Midazolam
    for incision and drainage, 114
    sedation with, 104
Midface fractures, 84
Migraine, 227, 228
Military antishock trousers
    for hemorrhagic hypovolemic
        shock, 8
    for hypotension, 170
Milk of Magnesia, 194
Mineral enemas or suppositories,
        194
Misoprostol, 189
Mistletoe, 325*t*, 328
Mithramycin, 22
Mitomycin C, 255, 256*b*
Mitral valve disease, 221
MMH; *see* Monomethylhydrazine
Moban; *see* Molindone
Molindone overdose, 295*t*

Monobactams, 176
Monomethylhydrazine, 323*t*
Mood disorders, 339-340
Moraxella catarrhalis, 172-173
Morgan lens, 89
Morphine
  for cardiac ischemia, 127
  for incision and drainage, 114
  for perirectal abscess, 195
  for renal colic, 200
  sedation with, 103
Morphine sulfate
  for cardiac ischemia, 127
  for cardiogenic pulmonary
    edema, 132
Motor function evaluation, 54
Mouth; *see also under* Oral
  bleeding in, 111
Multifocal atrial tachycardia,
    136-137, 137*f*
Mupirocin, 277
Muscarine, 323*t*
Muscimol, 323*t*
Muscular paralysis, 104-105
Mushroom poisoning, 322, 323*t*
Mycobacteria, in transplant
    recipients, 267
Mycobacterium avium, 174
Mycobacterium avium complex,
    174
Mycobacterium intracellulare, 174
Mycobacterium tuberculosis, 174
Mycoplasma pneumonia, 172, 173
Mycostatin; *see* Nystatin
Mylanta, 189
Myleran; *see* Busulfan
Mylicon; *see* Simethicone
Myocardial contusion, 42-43
Myocardial infarction
  acute, 125-130
  thrombolytic therapy for, 128
  treatment of, 128-129
Myoglobinuria, 308
Myxedema coma, 220

N

Nafcillin, 278
Nalmefene, 309

Naloxone, 296*t*
Naphazoline, 243
Narcotics; *see also specific narcotics*
  for headache, 228
  for incision and drainage, 114
  overdose
    antidote, 296*t*
    cancer and, 253
  for perirectal abscess, 195
  for renal colic, 200
  sedation with, 103
Nasal fractures, 84-85
Nasogastric aspiration, 188, 189
Nasogastric intubation, 31, 194
Nasopharyngeal pack, 237
Nausea and vomiting, 192
Navicular fractures, 65
Near drowning, 290
Neck; *see* Head and neck
Needle aspiration
  of olecranon bursitis, 116
  of pericardial tamponade, 43,
    44*f*
  of perirectal abscess, 195
  of thrombosed external
    hemorrhoids, 195
Neisseria catarrhalis, 172
Neisseria gonorrhoeae
  pelvic inflammatory disease
    with, 205
  urethritis in male and, 198
Neisseria meningitidis, 231, 352
Neomycin
  for bacterial conjunctivitis, 243
  for corneal abrasion, 90
  for perforated eardrum, 87
Neoplastic diseases; *see also*
    Oncologic emergencies
  meningitis in, 252, 252*t*
  presenting as psychiatric dis-
    orders, 336*b*
Neosporin; *see* Neomycin
Neostigmine, 104
  overdose, 295*t*
Nerve blocks, 93-100
Nerve injuries, of hand, 79
Neurologic emergencies, 211-232
  oncologic, 249-252
  trauma, 53-59

Neurologic examination, 53-54, 55-56
  with altered levels of consciousness, 212-214
Neurologic monitoring in trauma, 30
Neuronitis, vestibular, 223
Neurotoxicity, chemotherapy, 256
Neurovascular disease, 222
Newborn infants; *see also* Infants; Pediatric emergencies
  febrile, 347
Nightshade, 324*t*
Nipride; *see* Nitroprusside
Nitrate/nitrite overdose, 296*t*
Nitrofurantoin, 197
Nitroglycerine
  for cardiogenic pulmonary edema, 132
  for myocardial infarction, 127
Nitroprusside
  for hypertensive encephalopathy, 218
  overdose, 295*t*
Nitrosoureas, 255, 256*b*
Nitrous oxide, inhaled, 114
Nizatidine, 189
Nocardia, 267
Noncardiogenic pulmonary edema, 178-179
Nondepolarizing agents, 104
Nongonococcal infections, 198-199
Nonpsychotic disorders, 334, 340-341
  differential diagnosis, 344, 345
Nonsteroidal antiinflammatory drugs
  for acute superficial thrombophlebitis, 157
  for olecranon bursitis, 116
  for temporomandibular joint disorders, 241
Nontraumatic Acute Abdominal Pain Quick Reference Forms, 389-392
Nontraumatic emergencies, 123-361

Norepinephrine
  for hypotension, 170
  pediatric dosages, 349
Norfloxacin, 197
Normodyne; *see* Labetalol
Noroxin; *see* Norfloxacin
Norpramin; *see* Desipramine
Nortriptyline overdose, 306
Nose
  bleeding from, 54
  foreign body in, 235
  fractures of, 84-85
Noxious gas poisoning, 314-316
Nuclear scanning, with torsion of spermatic cord, 201
Nursemaids' elbow, 63
Nylen-Barany test, 224
Nystagmus, 54
  overdose and, 292
Nystatin, 279*t*

O

Obstetrics and gynecology, 203-210
Obstipation, 186
Obstruction
  acute airway, 233
  of airflow, 163
  of blood flow, 163
  of central retinal artery, 244
  superior vena cava, 256
  upper airway, 166
  urinary tract, 200
Obstructive pulmonary disease, chronic, 170-171
Obstructive shock, 4, 4*t*
  treatment, 6, 7*t*
Octamethyl pyrophosphoramide poisoning, 311
Odynophagia, 238
  AIDS and, 248
Ofloxacin
  for acute cystitis, 197
  for gonococcal pharyngitis, 238
  for lung infections, 177
  for pelvic inflammatory disease, 206
  for urethritis in male, 199

OKT3, 267
Oleander, 325*t*
Olecranon bursitis, 115-116
Olfactory hallucinations, 332
Omeprazole, 189
OMPA; *see* Octamethyl
    pyrophosphoramide
Oncologic emergencies, 249-258
    adrenal crisis and, 219
    cardiopulmonary, 256-257
    general considerations, 249
    hematologic, 257
    infections, 258
    neurologic, 249-252
    psychiatric, 336*b*
    toxic and metabolic, 253-254
    vascular, 253
Ondansetron, 255, 255*b*
Open thoracotomy, 44-45
Ophthalmologic emergencies,
        242-245
    injuries, 88-91
Opiates
    for mushroom poisoning, 322
    overdose, 309, 342
    withdrawal, 342
Optical neuropathy, ischemic, 244
Oral infections, 241
Oral lesions, 248
Oral mucosa, lacerations of, 111
Orbital fractures, 81-82, 82*f*
Orchitis, traumatic, 51
Organic disorders; *see* Cognitive
        disorders
Organic mental disorders, 333
    classification of, 329
Organophosphate poisoning, 311
    antidote, 296*t*, 311
Organ transplant recipients,
        266-270
Organ transplants, 268-270
Orotracheal intubation, 32
Orthopedic trauma, 60-69
Osmolality, serum
    with altered levels of
        consciousness, 214
    calculations, 316
    formula for, 216
Osteomyelitis, 260*t*

Otitis, 238-240
Otitis externa, 240
Otitis media, 238
    childhood, 358
    with effusion, 239
Ovarian cysts, 207
Overdose, 291-328; *see also* Poi-
        soning
    drugs helped by forced diuresis,
        299, 300*t*
Overdrive pacing, 146
Oxalates, 328
Oxygenation assessment, 164-166
Oxygen saturation monitoring,
        transcutaneous, 164
Oxygen treatment, 165-166
    for asthmatic bronchospasm,
        167
    for cardiogenic pulmonary
        edema, 132
    for hydrogen sulfide and
        carbon disulfide
        intoxication, 314
    for shock, 6

P

Pacemakers
    implanted, 151-154
    for refractory bradycardias, 133
Pacing
    external
        for refractory bradycardias,
            133
        for sinus bradycardia, 141,
            141*b*
    overdrive, 146
    for torsades de pointes, 149,
        149*b*
Paint gun injuries, 80
Palm, 71, 72*f*
    anesthesia of, 74
Palmaris longus tendon, 70, 71*f*
Pamelor; *see* Nortriptyline
Pancreatic inflammation or
        obstruction, 186
Pancreatitis, 186, 188
Pancuronium, 104
Paraldehyde overdose, 299, 300*b*

Paralysis, 104-105
Paramethasone, 169*t*
Paraphimosis, 201*f*, 201-202
Parathion poisoning, 296*t*, 311
Paronychia, 114-115
Paroxysmal supraventricular
 tachycardia, 134*f*, 134-136
Partial thromboplastin time, 263,
 265
PASG; *see* Pneumatic antishock
 garments
Pasteurella multocida, 118-119
Patellar dislocations, 66
Patellar fractures, 66
PCP; *see* Phencyclidine
PEA; *see* Pulseless electrical
 activity
Pediatric emergencies, 347-361
 asthmatic bronchospasm,
  356-357
 convulsions, 350-351
 diabetes, 353-354
 diabetic ketoacidosis, 354
 drug delivery access, 348
 drug dosages, 349
 external cardiac compression,
  349
 fever
  evaluation of, 347
  Quick Reference Form,
   426-430
 GI tract bleeding, 201
 hypoglycemic coma, 353-354
 meningitis, 352
 pharyngitis, 357-358
 pneumonia, 352-353
 seizures, 350-351
Pediculosis, 277
PEEP; *see* Positive end-expiratory
 pressure
Pelvic fractures, 69
Pelvic inflammatory disease,
 205-206
Pelvic injuries, 69
Pelvic trauma, 48
Pemphigus vulgaris, 277-278
Penetrating trauma
 abdominal, 48

Penetrating trauma–cont'd
 arterial occlusions with, 160,
  161*f*
 head injuries, 55
 Quick Reference Form, 376-378
Penicillin
 for cat and dog bites, 118-119
 for ingestion of caustics, 236
 for lung infections, 174-175
 for meningitis, 232, 252
 for scarlet fever, 274
 for streptococcal pharyngitis,
  238
Penicillin V, for dermatologic
 problems, 279*t*
Penicillin VK
 for lung infections, 174
 for tonsillitis and pharyngitis,
  357
Penile trauma, 51
Pentazocine overdose, 296*t*
Pepcid; *see* Famotidine
Peptic disorders, 188-190
Perception, abnormal, 332
Perforations
 arterial, 159
 esophagogastric, 235
Pericardial tamponade, 33
 cardiac arrest and, 149
Peripheral vertigo, 222, 223, 225
Perirectal abscesses, 195
Peritoneal lavage, diagnostic, 46,
 47
Peritonsillar abscess, 238
Permanganate ingestion, 310
Perphenazine overdose, 305
Phalangeal fractures, 69
Pharmacologic therapy; *see also*
 Drugs; *specific pharmaceu-*
 ticals
 of dysrhythmia, 133
 in psychiatric emergencies, 330
Pharyngitis, 237-238
 pediatric, 357-358
Phenacetin overdose, 296*t*
Phenazopyridine
 for dysuria, 197
 intoxication, 296*t*

Phencyclidine, 342-343
    overdose, 307-308, 308-309
        forced diuresis for, 300*t*
        severe, 342
Phenergan; *see* Promethazine
Phenobarbital
    for convulsions in children, 351
    overdose, 300*t*
    for seizures, 226
Phenothiazines
    in chemotherapy, 255, 255*b*
    overdose, 305
    for peripheral vertigo, 225
Phenoxymethyl
    for streptococcal pharyngitis,
        238
    for tonsillitis and pharyngitis,
        357
Phenytoin
    for convulsions, 55
    overdose, 299, 301*b*
    for seizures, 226, 227
    for ventricular dysrhythmia,
        307
Pheochromocytoma, 222
Philodendron, 325*t*
Phlebotomy, 133
Physical protection, 329-330
Physostigmine
    for atropine, 328
    for mushroom poisoning, 323*t*
    overdose, 295*t*
Phytotoxins, 328
PID; *see* Pelvic inflammatory
        disease
Pilocarpine
    for acute angle-closure
        glaucoma, 245
    overdose, 295*t*
Pit vipers, 318-319
Placenta previa, 209
Plant toxins, 322-328
    commonly ingested, 326*b*-327*b*
    most ingested, 324*t*-325*t*
Platelet disorders, 261
Pleural space, violation of, 164
Pneumatic antishock garments
    for hemorrhagic hypovolemic
        shock, 8

Pneumatic antishock
        garments—cont'd
    for hypotension, 170
    for pelvic fractures, 69
Pneumococcus, 172
Pneumocystis, 267
Pneumocystis carinii, 174
    AIDS and, 248
Pneumomediastinum
    with pneumothorax, 39
    with tracheal or bronchial
        rupture, 39
Pneumonia
    AIDS and, 248
    antibiotic therapy for, 178
    atypical, 172, 173-174
    bacterial causes, 172-173,
        173-174
    classification of, 171-172
    definition of, 171
    diagnosis, 172
    mycobacterial, 174
    parasitic, 174
    pediatric, 352-353
    in transplanted lung, 269
    typical, 171, 172-173
Pneumopericardium, 39
Pneumothorax, 33, 36-40, 182
    with intercostal nerve block,
        100
    open, 33, 37
        diagnosis, 38-39
        treatment, 40
    with scapular injuries, 61
    simple, 36, 36*f*
    tension, 33, 37, 37*f*
        diagnosis, 38-39
        treatment, 40
    with tracheal or bronchial
        rupture, 39
    treatment, 35-36, 39-40
Poinsettia, 324*t*
Poisoning, 291-328
    activated charcoal for, 297-298
    antidotes for, 294, 295*t*-296*t*
    carbon monoxide, 183-184
    catharsis for, 298-299
    cholinergic, 292

Poisoning—cont'd
diuresis and dialysis for, 299,
299*b*
food, 191
general considerations, 291
identification, 292-293
management principles,
293-299
mushroom, 322
signs and symptoms of, 291-292
toxicology studies, 214
Poison ivy, 280
Poison oak, 280
Polyamines, 328
Polymyxin B sulfate, 87
Polypeptides, 328
Polystyrene sulfonate, 20
Positive end-expiratory pressure
for ARDS, 179
for pulmonary contusion, 41
Positive-pressure ventilation, 35
Posterior fossa tumors, 224
Posterior tibial nerve block, 100,
100*f*
Potassium
for diabetic hyperglycemia, 217
distribution alteration, 20
falsely elevated serum
measurements, 20
hyperkalemia, 18-20
hypokalemia, 20-21
inadequate intake, 20
increased excretion, 20
overdose, 295*t*
dialysis for, 299, 300*b*
Potassium iodide, 221
Potassium permanganate, 235
Pralidoxime, 296*t*, 311
Prednisolone
for acute asthmatic
bronchospasm, 356
relative potencies, 169*t*
Prednisone
for asthmatic bronchospasm,
168
for herpes zoster infections, 277
for ischemic optical
neuropathy, 244
relative potencies, 169*t*

Prednisone—cont'd
for toxic epidermal necrolysis,
278
Preeclampsia, 210
Preload enhancement, 130-131
Premature ventricular
contractions, 144-146, 145*f*
treatment, 145-146, 146*b*
Prepuce, manual reduction of,
201*f*, 202
Priapism
sickle cell disease and, 260*t*
spinal cord injury and, 56
Prilosec; *see* Omeprazole
Probenecid, 206
Procainamide
for atrial flutter, 138*b*
for premature ventricular
contractions, 146
for pulseless ventricular
tachycardia, 151
torsades de pointes and, 149
for ventricular fibrillation, 150*b*,
151
for ventricular tachycardia,
146*b*, 147
Procaine penicillin, 358
Procarbazine hydrochloride, 255,
256*b*
Prochlorperazine
in chemotherapy, 255, 255*b*
for headache, 228
for nausea and vomiting, 192
for peripheral vertigo, 225
Prolixin; *see* Fluphenazine
Promethazine
for nausea and vomiting, 192
for peripheral vertigo, 225
for sedation with meperidine,
103
Proparacaine, 89
Propoxyphene overdose, 296*t*
Propranolol
for atrial flutter, 138*b*, 139
for hyperthyroid crisis, 220
for mushroom poisoning, 323*t*
for refractory ventricular
dysrhythmia, 307
for supraventricular tachycardia,
136

Propranolol–cont'd
  for thoracic aortic dissection, 159
Propylthiouracil, 220
Prostaglandin inhibitors, 200
Prostatitis, acute, 199
Protein loss, 16
Prothrombin time, 261, 263
Proton pump inhibitors, 189
Protopam Chloride; *see* Pralidoxime
Protozoa, 267
Pseudodementia, 343
Pseudohyponatremia, 18
Pseudomembranous colitis, 193
Pseudomonas, 267
Psilocin, 323*t*
Psilocybin, 323*t*
Psoriasis, 248
PSVT; *see* Paroxysmal supraventricular tachycardia
Psychiatric emergencies, 329-346
  diagnostic categories, 333-334, 335*f*
  differential diagnosis, 344-345
  indications for medical hospitalization, 345
  indications for psychiatric hospitalization, 345-346
  life-threatening conditions, 343-344
  medical illnesses presenting as, 336*b*
  nonpsychotic disorders, 334, 340-341
    differential diagnosis, 344, 345
  principles of management, 330
Psychotic disorders, 334
  differential diagnosis, 344
  with normal cognition, 338-340
Psychotropic drug poisoning, 303-309
Pubic fractures, 69
Pubic rami fractures, 69
Pulmonary angiography, 180
Pulmonary burn, 182-183
Pulmonary contusion, 41

Pulmonary disorders
  in cancer, 257
  chemotherapy and, 255, 256*b*
  chronic obstructive pulmonary disease, 170-171
  radiation therapy and, 255
Pulmonary edema
  cardiogenic, 131-133
  definition, 131
  inflammatory causes, 179
  noncardiogenic, 178-179
  noninflammatory causes, 178
  opiate intoxication and, 309
Pulmonary embolism, 179-182
  cardiac arrest and, 149
  differential diagnosis, 127
Pulmonary infarction, 260*t*
Pulmonary infection, 171-178
  sickle cell disease and, 260*t*
Pulseless electrical activity, 151, 151*b*, 153*f*
Pulseless ventricular tachycardia, 150*b*, 151, 152*f*
Pulsus paradoxus, 43
Pupils
  dilatation of, 245
  with metabolic encephalopathies, 212
PVCs; *see* Premature ventricular contractions
Pyelonephritis, 197-198
Pyloric stenosis, 360
Pyrethrum/piperonyl butoxide, 277
Pyridium; *see* Phenazopyridine
Pyridostigmine overdose, 295*t*
Pyridoxine, 323*t*
Pyuria, 186
  renal colic with, 200

Q
Quality Assurance Forms, 363
Quick Reference Forms, 363, 364
  Acute Blunt Trauma, 365-374
  Acute Toxic Ingestion or Dermal or Inhalation Exposure, 417-423
  Chest Pain Revision, 379-388

Quick Reference Forms–cont'd
children presenting with fever, 426-430
Headache, 400-409
Nontraumatic Acute Abdominal Pain, 389-392
Penetrating Extremity Trauma, 375-378
Seizure, 410-416
Vaginal Bleeding, 393-399
Quinidine, torsades de pointes and, 149
Quinine/quinidine overdose
dialysis for, 299, 300*b*
forced diuresis for, 300*t*

R
Rabies, 121
immunization against, 119*t*, 120*t*, 121
postexposure prophylaxis
dosages for, 120*t*
indications for, 119*t*
Radial artery, 71, 71*f*
in "snuffbox," 73*f*, 74*f*
Radial nerve
sensory (superficial branch, 72, 75*f*
superficial ramus of, 72, 74*f*
Radial nerve block, 74, 98, 99*f*
Radiation effects, 254-256
Radioactive fibrinogen scanning, 157
Radiography; *see also* Abdominal radiography; Chest radiography
with abdominal trauma, 46
with altered levels of consciousness, 214
with elbow dislocation, 63
with foreign bodies in airway or esophagus, 234
with knee injuries, 67
with laryngeal trauma, 86
with mandibular fractures, 83
with nasal fractures, 84
with navicular fractures, 65
with orbital fractures, 82

Radiography–cont'd
with orthopedic trauma, 60
spinal, 59
with zygomatic arch fractures, 82
Radius fractures
distal radius (Colles' fractures, 64
radius-ulna shaft fractures, 64
Rales, 163
Ranitidine
for anaphylaxis, 170
for gastrointestinal hemorrhage, 194
for peptic disorders, 189
for urticaria, 275
Rash, 271-275, 272*t*
Rectal medication, access in children, 348
Rectal suppositories, for nausea and vomiting, 192
Red cell destruction anemias, 258-261, 259*b*
Reduction
for elbow dislocation, 63
method of Hippocrates, 61
for shoulder dislocation, 61-62
Reflexes, evaluation of, 54
Regional anesthesia, 92-100
complications of, 100-102
toxic reactions to, 101
Regional nerve blocks, 93-100
Reglan; *see* Metoclopramide
Rejection
heart transplant, 268
kidney transplant, 268
liver transplant, 269
lung transplant, 269
Renal colic, 200
Renal failure, 219
Renal function tests, 194
Renal injuries, 49-50
Resins, plant, 328
Respiratory acidosis, 10-11
Respiratory alkalosis, 12-13
Respiratory drive disorders, 163
Respiratory emergencies, 163-184
categorization of disorders, 163-165

Respiratory failure
  in cancer, 257
  with regional anesthesia,
    101-102
Respiratory system; *see also* Airway
    management
  compensation of acute meta-
    bolic acidosis, 165
  infections, 171-178
Retavase; *see* Reteplase
Reteplase, 129
Retinal detachment, 244
Retinal hemorrhage, 260*t*
Retroperitoneal trauma, 48
Revex; *see* Nalmefene
Rhonchi, 163
Rib fractures, 33-34
  with scapular injuries, 61
RID shampoo; *see* Pyrethrum/
    piperonyl butoxide
Rifampin, 232
Right ventricular infarction, 131
Ringer's solution, 170
Ringworm, 276
Riopan, 189
Road burns, 112
Robaxin; *see* Methocarbamol
Rocephin; *see* Ceftriaxone
Rodenticides, 328
Roentgenography; *see* Radiog-
    raphy
Romazicon; *see* Flumazenil
Roseola infantum, 273
Rubber banding thrombosed
    external hemorrhoids, 195
Rubella, 273
Rules, 364

S

Sacral fractures, 69
Sacroiliac joint dislocation, 69
Sagittal sinus thrombosis, 253
SAH; *see* Subarachnoid
    hemorrhage
Salicylate poisoning, 299-303,
    300*t*, 300*b*, 301*b*, 302*f*
Salmonella, 192

Scabies, 277
Scalp wounds
  soft-tissue, 55
  suture removal, 109
  suture size, 107
Scapular fractures, 61
Scapular rotation, 61-62
Scarlet fever, 273-274
Schiotz tonometer, 252
Schizophrenia, 338-339
Sciatic nerve block, 99, 100*f*
Scorpion envenomation, 319,
    320*t*
Scrotum
  incarcerated hernia and,
    360-361
  injury to, 51-52
Seborrhea, 248
Secondary survey, 30
Sedation, 102-104
  for hyperventilation syndrome,
    182
  for wound care, 106
Sedative hypnotics, 342
Sedatives, 104
Seizures, 225-227
  AIDS and, 248
  in cancer, 250
  with eclampsia and
    preeclampsia, 210
  pediatric, 350-351
  Quick Reference Form, 411-416
  syncope and, 221
Semustine, 255, 256*b*
Sensory dermatome, 57*f*
Sentinel bleed, 227
Sepsis, 218
Septa; *see* Trimethoprim-
    sulfamethoxazole
Septal hematoma, 84-85
Septic distributive shock, 6
Septra; *see* Trimethoprim-
    sulfamethoxazole
Serentil; *see* Mesoridazine
Serous otitis, 238, 239
Serum osmolality
  with altered levels of
    consciousness, 214

Serum osmolality–cont'd
  calculations, 316
  formula for, 216
Shigella
  antibiotics for, 193
  diarrhea and, 192
Shock, 3-9
  anaphylactic distributive, 6
  cardiogenic, 3-4, 4*t*, 7*t*, 130-131
  categories of, 3, 4*t*
  clinical pearls, 5-6
  definition of, 3
  distributive, 4, 4*t*
    anaphylactic, 6
    septic, 6
    treatment, 6, 7*t*
  hemorrhagic hypovolemic, 8-9
  hypovolemic, 3, 4*t*
    hemorrhagic, 8-9
  obstructive, 4, 4*t*, 6, 7*t*
  with renal injuries, 49
  septic distributive, 6
  in tension pneumothorax, 38
  treatment, 6-9, 7*t*
Shock wave trauma, 160, 161*f*
Shortness of breath, 248
Shoulder dislocation, 61-62
SIADH; *see* Syndrome of inappro-
      priate secretion of antidiu-
      retic hormone
Sickle cell disease, 260*t*, 260-261
Simethicone, 194
Sinus bradycardia, 140*f*, 140-141,
      141*b*
  PVCs with, 145
Sinusitis, 240
Sinus tachycardia, 133-134, 134*f*
Sitz baths
  for perirectal abscess, 195
  for thrombosed external
      hemorrhoids, 195
Skin eruptions, 247-248
Skin laceration
  suture removal, 109
  suture size, 107
  wound care, 109, 110*f*
Small bowel obstruction, 190
Snakebite, 317-320
Snellen eye chart, 88, 242

Sodium
  falsely low serum
      measurements, 18
  hypernatremia, 14-15
  hypertonic states not resulting
      from, 16
  hyponatremia, 15-18
  pseudohyponatremia, 18
Sodium bicarbonate
  for diabetic ketoacidosis, 354
  pediatric dosages, 349
  for salicylate poisoning, 302
Sodium iodide, 221
Sodium nitrite
  as antidote, 295*t*
  for cyanide poisoning, 315
  for hydrogen sulfide and
      carbon disulfide poi-
      soning, 314
Sodium thiosulfate
  as antidote, 295*t*
  for cyanide poisoning, 315
Soft-tissue infections, 113-121
Soft-tissue scalp wounds, 55
Solu-Cortef; *see* Hydrocortisone
Solu-Medrol; *see*
      Methylprednisolone
Somatic preoccupations, 332
Sorbitol, 298
Southern Copperhead snake, 318*f*
Spectazole; *see* Econazole
Spectinomycin, 271
Spermatic cord, torsion of, 201
Spider bites, 321-322
Spinal cord compression, 250-251
Spinal cord injuries, 55-59
  motor levels, 56*t*
  sensory dermatome, 57*f*
  sensory levels, 56*t*
Spinal injuries, 55-59
  classification of, 58*t*, 58-59
Spine, examination of, 55-59
Splinting; *see also* Casts
  shock and, 6, 7*t*
  sugar-tong, 64
Sprain, ankle, 68
SSSS; *see* Staphylococcal scalded
      skin syndrome
Staphylococcal scalded skin
      syndrome, 278

Staphylococcus aureus, 173
  infection, 117
  toxic epidermal necrolysis and, 278
  toxic shock syndrome and, 274
Stelazine; *see* Trifluoperazine
Stellate lacerations, 110, 110*f*
Steroids, 266-267
  for acute asthmatic broncho-spasm, 356
  adrenal crisis and, 219
  for anaphylaxis, 170
  for asthma, 168
  for asthmatic bronchospasm, 167-168
  for cerebral edema, 55
  for hypercalcemia, 22
Stevens-Johnson syndrome, 275
Stitches, interrupted, 77
Stomach, emptying, 294-297
Stomatitis, 241
Stones
  cholelithiasis, 186, 187-188
  urinary tract, 186
Stool guaiac
  with gastrointestinal hemorrhage, 194
  with peptic disorders, 189
Streptase; *see* Streptokinase
Streptococcal pharyngitis, 237-238
Streptococcus pneumoniae, 171, 172, 231
Streptococcus pyogenes, 173
Streptokinase
  for myocardial infarction, 128
  for pulmonary embolism, 182
Stroke, 228-231
  hemorrhagic, 228-229
  ischemic
    definition, 228
    headache and, 227
    treatment, 230-231
  syncope and, 221
Strongyloides, 267
Strychnine overdose, 299, 300*b*
Stupor, 214-221
Sty, 245
Subarachnoid hemorrhage, 227
Subclavian artery injury, 160

Subcutaneous emphysema
  with pneumothorax, 39
  with simple pneumothorax, 38
  with tracheal or bronchial rupture, 41
Sublimaze; *see* Fentanyl
Substance-related disorders, 341-343
Succinylcholine, 104
Sucking chest wound; *see* Pneumo-thorax, open
Sucralfate, 189
Sugar-tong splints, 64
Suicide
  attempted, 293
  risk, 343
  thoughts of, 332
Sulfacetamide
  for bacterial conjunctivitis, 243
  for corneal abrasion, 90
Sulfuric acid, 235
Sumatriptan, 228
Superficial cervical plexus block, 95
Superficial thrombophlebitis, 156-157
Superficial volar arch, 72*f*
Superior vena cava obstruction, 256
Supraorbital nerve block, 94*f*, 95
Supratrochlear nerve, 94*f*
Supraventricular tachycardia, 135*b*, 135-136
  paroxysmal, 134*f*, 134-136
Suprax; *see* Cefixime
Surgery; *see specific procedures*
Sutures
  corner, 110, 110*f*
  material, 107
  removal of, 109
  size, 107
  technique, 107, 108*f*-109*f*
  type, 107
Symphysis fractures, 83
Symphysis pubis, separation of, 69
Syncope, 221-222
  heat, 286
  micturition, 222
  vasovagal, 222

Syndrome of inappropriate
      secretion of antidiuretic
      hormone
   cancer and, 253-254
   hyponatremia and, 16
   treatment, 17, 254
Syphilis, 278

T

Tachycardias
   bronchospasm and, 167
   multifocal atrial, 136-137, 137*f*
   paroxysmal supraventricular,
      134*f*, 134-136
   shock and, 5
   sinus, 133-134, 134*f*
   treatment, 132
   ventricular, 146*f*, 146-147
   wide-complex, 133
Tachydysrhythmias, 130, 132
Tactile hallucinations, 332
Tagamet; *see* Cimetidine
Talwin; *see* Pentazocine
Tattoos, accidental, 112
Tazicef; *see* Ceftazidime
Tazidime; *see* Ceftazidime
Temporal arteritis
   headache and, 227
   ischemic optical neuropathy
      and, 244
Temporomandibular joint
      disorders, 241
TEN; *see* Toxic epidermal
      necrolysis
Tendon injuries, of hand, 79
Tennis elbow, 64
Tenosynovitis, 115
Tension headache, 227
Tension pneumomediastinum, 39
Tension pneumothorax, 33, 37, 37*f*
   cardiac arrest and, 149
   with tracheal or bronchial
      rupture, 39
   treatment, 40
TEPP; *see* Tetraethylpyrophos-
      phate
Terconazole, 207
Testis, torsion of, 201
   in children, 361

Tetanus
   immunization, 116
   prophylaxis, 116-117, 121
Tetracaine, 89, 93
Tetracyclic antidepressants over-
      dose, 306
Tetracycline
   for dermatologic problems, 279*t*
   for pneumonia, 178
   for syphilis, 278
Tetraethylpyrophosphate poison-
      ing, 311
Theophylline overdose, 299, 300*b*,
      301*b*
Thermal burns, 281-285
   criteria for admission, 282-283
   extent of injury, 281-282
   first-degree, 282
   how to estimate, 281, 282*t*
   minor, 283
   second-degree, 282
   severe, 283-285
Thiethylperazine, 255, 255*b*
Thioctic acid, 323*t*
Thioridazine overdose, 305
Thioxanthene overdose, 305
Thoracic aortic dissection, 158-
      159
   differential diagnosis, 126-127
Thoracic aortic injury, 160
Thoracic trauma, 32-45, 48
Thoracotomy
   for cardiac arrest, 150
   for cardiac tamponade, 43, 44
   for hemothorax, 41
   open, 44-45
Thorazine; *see* Chlorpromazine
Thought broadcasting, 332
Thought content, abnormal,
      331-332
Thought process, abnormal, 331
Thrombocytopenia, 261
   in cancer, 257
Thrombocytosis, 257
Thrombolytic therapy
   for ischemic stroke, 230-231
   for myocardial infarction, 128
   for pulmonary embolism,
      181-182

Thrombophlebitis, 156-158
  acute superficial, 156-157
  deep, 157-158
Thrombosed external
        hemorrhoids, 195
Thrombosis, 257
Thrush, 241
Thumb nerves, 96, 96*f*
Thyroid storm, 220-221
L-Thyroxine, 220
Tibial shaft fracture, 68
Ticarcillin-clavulanate, 176-177
Tigan; *see* Trimethobenzamide
Timber Rattlesnake, 318*f*
Timentin; *see* Ticarcillin-
        clavulanate
Timolol, 245
Tinnitus, 86
Tioconazole, 207
Tissue plasminogen activator
  for ischemic stroke, 230, 231
  for pulmonary embolism, 182
TMP/SMX; *see* Trimethoprim-
        sulfamethoxazole
Tofranil; *see* Imipramine
Tolnaftate, 276
Tongue lacerations, 111
Tonometry, 252
TonoPen, 242
Tonsillitis, 357-358
Tooth avulsion, 87
Tooth displacement, 87
Tooth fracture, 87
Topical anesthesia, 93
Topicort; *see* Desoximetasone
Torecan; *see* Thiethylperazine
Torsades de pointes, 147-149, 148*f*,
        149*b*
Torsion of spermatic cord, 201
Torsion of testis, 201
  in children, 361
Tourniquets, 161
  arm, 78
  finger, 78, 78*f*
Toxalbumins in plants, 328
Toxic epidermal necrolysis, 278
Toxic ingestion; *see also* Intoxica-
        tion; Overdose; Poisoning
  Quick Reference Form, 418-423
Toxicology studies, 214

Toxic plants, 324*t*-325*t*
Toxic reactions
  abnormalities in cancer,
        253-254
  to regional anesthesia, 101
Toxic shock syndrome, 274
Toxins, plant, 322-328, 326*b*
Toxoplasma, in transplant
        recipients, 267
t-PA; *see* Tissue plasminogen
        activator
Tracheal rupture, 41-42
Tracheostomy
  with burns, 283
  with tracheal or bronchial
        rupture, 41
Traction, passive, 61
Tranquilizer overdose, 305-306
Transcutaneous oxygen saturation
        monitoring, 164
Transesophageal
        echocardiography, 159
Transient ischemic attack, 228-231
Transplant recipients, 266-270
Transverse carpal ligament, 71, 72*f*
Trauma, 27-121
  abdominal, 46-48
  airway evaluation, 29
  blunt
    to eye, 91
    vs. penetrating, 48
  breathing and ventilation
        evaluation, 29-30
  circulation evaluation, 30
  dental, 87
  genitourinary tract, 49-52
  laryngeal, 86
  major, 29-31
  monitoring, 30-31
  neurologic, 53-59
  neurologic assessment, 30
  orthopedic, 60-69
  pelvic, 48
  penetrating, 48
    abdominal, 48
    arterial occlusions with, 160,
        161*f*
    head injuries, 55
    Quick Reference Form,
        376-378

Trauma—cont'd
penile, 51
presenting as psychiatric
disorders, 336*b*
retroperitoneal, 48
secondary survey, 30
thoracic, 32-45, 48
vascular, 159-162
wound infections, 116-121
Travelers' diarrhea, 192
Trendelenburg's position
with incarcerated hernia, 360
with verapamil-induced
hypotension, 138
Triamcinolone acetonide, 279*t*
Trichomonas infection, 208
Tricyclic antidepressants overdose,
306
hemoperfusion for, 299, 301*b*
Tridesilon; *see* Desonide
Trifluoperazine overdose, 305
Trifluridine, 243
Trigeminal nerve block, 93-95, 94*f*
Trilafon; *see* Perphenazine
Trimethobenzamide
in chemotherapy, 255, 255*b*
for nausea and vomiting, 192
Trimethoprim-sulfamethoxazole
for acute cystitis, 197
for acute sinusitis, 240
for bacterial otitis media, 239
for diarrhea, 193
for otitis media in children, 358
for pneumonia, 178
Trismus, 82
Trochanteric bursitis, 66
Troponin I and T, 126
Trousseau's sign, 24
Trunk sutures
removal, 109
size, 107
Tuberculosis
adrenal crisis and, 219
in transplant recipients, 267
Tube thoracostomy, 39-40
for hemothorax, 35-36
for pneumothorax, 35-36, 39
Tubocurarine, 104
Tuboovarian abscesses, 206

Tumors
headache and, 227
posterior fossa, 224
Tylenol; *see* Acetaminophen
Tympanic membrane perforation,
86, 87

U
Ulcers, 188-190
sickle cell disease and, 260*t*
Ulnar artery, 71, 71*f*, 72*f*
Ulnar nerve
anatomy of, 71, 71*f*, 72*f*
motor branch damage, 76-77
sensation and, 74, 75*f*
Ulnar nerve block, 96*f*, 97, 98*f*
Ulna shaft fractures, 64
Ultracef; *see* Cefadroxil
Ultrasonography
with abdominal trauma, 47
with appendicitis, 187
with cholelithiasis or
cholecystitis, 188
with cholelithiasis or
pancreatitis, 186
Doppler
with thrombophlebitis, 157
with torsion of spermatic
cord, 201
with transient ischemic
attack, 230
with ectopic pregnancy, 204
with genitourinary tract
obstruction, 186
with ovarian cysts, 207
with pancreatitis, 188
with pulmonary embolism, 180
with renal colic, 200
with spontaneous abortion, 205
Upper airway obstruction, 166
Upper extremities
injuries, 60-65
regional nerve blocks, 95-98
Ureaplasma urealyticum, 198
Ureteral injuries, 50
Urethral catheters, 69
Urethral injuries, 51
in male patients, 69

Urethritis, 198-199
Urethrography, 51
Urinalysis
    with altered levels of consciousness, 214
    with appendicitis, 187
    with diabetic ketoacidosis, 216
    with renal colic, 200
    with renal injuries, 49
Urinary retention, 200
    herpes genitalis and, 209
Urinary tract
    hypercalcemia and, 22
    infections of, 186, 197
    injury to, 69
    obstruction of, 200
    stones, 186
Urokinase, 182
Urticaria, 275
Uveitis, acute anterior, 245

V

Vagal stimulation, 135, 135*b*
Vaginal bleeding
    gynecologic disorders with, 203-204
    Quick Reference Form, 394-399
Vaginal discharge, 203-204
Vaginitis, 207-208
Vaginosis, bacterial, 208
Valium; *see* Diazepam
Valvular disease, 221
Vancomycin
    for colitis, 193
    for meningitis, 232
Varicella, 274-275
Varicella zoster infection, 247, 248
Varicosities, ruptured, 156
Vascular disorders, 261
    in cancer, 253
    emergencies, 155-162
    syncope and, 222
Vascular headache, 227
Vascular trauma, 159-162
    hand injuries, 79
    tibial shaft fracture and, 68
Vasocon; *see* Naphazoline

Vasodepressor syndrome, 222
Vasovagal syncope, 222
Vecuronium, 105
Vehicular accidents, 160
Vena caval interruption, 182
Venoconstriction, compensatory, loss of, 222
Venomous snakes, 317, 318*f*
Venoms, animal, 317-328
Venous disease, 156-158
Venous trauma, 162
Ventilation
    bag-valve-mask, 150-151
    in child, 349
    evaluation of, 29-30
    hyperventilation, 164
        controlled, 55
    hyperventilation syndrome, 164, 182
    hypoventilation, 163, 164, 166
    in infant, 349
    positive-pressure, 35
Ventilation-perfusion scanning, 180
Ventilatory failure, 166-167
Ventricular asystole
    cardiac arrest and, 151, 151*b*, 153*f*
    coarse, 151, 153*f*
    hyperkalemia and, 19
Ventricular dysrhythmias, 307
Ventricular ectopy, 146*b*
Ventricular fibrillation
    cardiac arrest and, 150*b*, 151, 152*f*
    coarse, 151, 152*f*
    fine, 151, 153*f*
    hyperkalemia and, 19
    open thoracotomy with, 45
    premature ventricular contractions and, 144
Ventricular tachycardia, 146*f*, 146-147
    premature ventricular contractions and, 144
    pulseless, 150*b*, 151, 152*f*
    treatment, 146*b*, 146-147
Verapamil
    for atrial flutter, 138, 138*b*

Verapamil—cont'd
for supraventricular tachycardia, 135*b*, 136
Vertebrobasilar artery insufficiency, 223
Vertigo, 86, 222-225
central, 222-223, 223-224
peripheral, 222, 223, 225
Vestibular neuronitis, 223
Viroptic; *see* Trifluridine
Viruses; *see also specific viruses*
conjunctivitis and, 243
meningitis and, 231
pneumonia and, 172
in transplant recipients, 267
viestibular neuronitis and, 223
Vision loss, 243*b*, 243-244
Vistaril; *see* Hydroxyzine
Visual hallucinations, 332
Vitamin K
for mushroom poisoning, 323*t*
for rodenticides, 328
Volar carpal ligament, 71, 72*f*
Volume expansion, 6, 7*t*
Vomiting, 191-193
AIDS and, 248
induced; *see* Emesis
Von Willebrand's disease, 263
V/Q scanning; *see* Ventilation-perfusion scanning
V-shaped lacerations, 110, 110*f*

W
Warfarin ingestion, 328
Water intoxication, 16
Wernicke-Korsakoff syndrome, 341
Wernicke's encephalopathy, 214, 215
Westermark's sign, 180
Wheezing, expiratory, 163
White blood cell counts, 186
Wolff-Parkinson-White syndrome, 139
supraventricular tachycardia with, 135
Wolff-Parkinson-White syndrome—cont'd
treatment, 140
Wood alcohol; *see* Methanol
Worms, 267
Wound care
bite wounds, 118-121
general principles of, 106-107
infections, 117-118
local infiltration blocks for, 92-93
penis, 51
scything, 111, 111*f*
special wounds, 109-112
suture material, 107
suture removal, 109
suture technique, 107, 108*f*-109*f*
trapdoor wounds, 111
untidy wounds, 109, 110*f*

WPW syndrome; *see* Wolff-
    Parkinson-White syndrome
Wrist
    dorsum of, 71-72, 73*f*
    extensor tendons of, 72, 73*f*, 74*f*
        damage to, 76
    flexor tendons of, 70, 71*f*
    injuries to, 65
    palmar surface of, 70-71, 71*f*
    radial aspect of, 72, 74*f*

X
Xeroform, 112

Y
Yeast vaginitis, 207
Yew, 324*t*

Z
Zantac; *see* Ranitidine
Zinacef; *see* Cefuroxime
Zithromax; *see* Azithromycin
Zofran; *see* Ondansetron
Zovirax; *see* Acyclovir
Zygomatic arch fractures, 82, 83*f*